BRITISH MEDICAL BULLETIN

VOLUME 54   NUMBER 4   1998

Screening

Scientific Editors

Catherine Peckham

Carol Dezateux

Series Editors
L K Borysiewicz PhD FRCP
M J Walport PhD FRCP

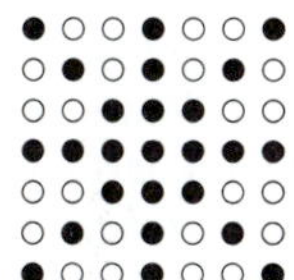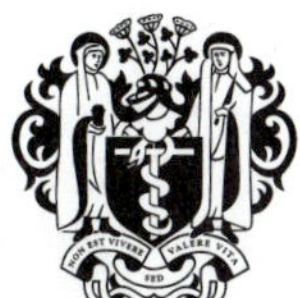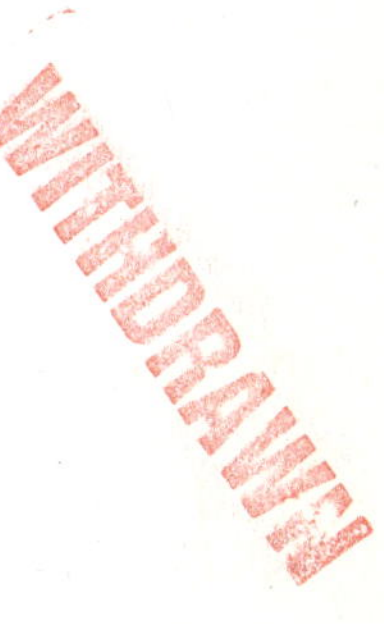

PUBLISHED FOR THE BRITISH COUNCIL BY
THE ROYAL SOCIETY OF MEDICINE PRESS LIMITED

ROYAL SOCIETY OF MEDICINE PRESS LIMITED
1 Wimpole Street, London W1M 8AE, UK
16 East 69th Street, New York, NY 10021, USA

British Library Cataloguing in Publication Data
A catalogue record for this book is available from the British Library
ISBN 1-85315-345–1
ISSN 0007-1420

Subscription information *British Medical Bulletin* is published quarterly in January, April, July and October on behalf of the British Council by the Royal Society of Medicine Press Limited. Subscription rates for Volume 54 (1998) are £142 Europe (including UK), US$240 USA, £146 elsewhere, £73 developing countries. Prices include postage by surface mail within Europe, by air freight and second class post within the USA*, and by various methods of air-speeded delivery to all other countries. Subscription orders and enquiries should be sent to: Publications Subscription Department, Royal Society of Medicine Press Limited, 1 Wimpole Street, London W1M 8AE, UK (Tel +44 (0)171 290 2928; Fax +44(0)171 290 2929).
*Periodicals postage paid at Rahway, NJ. US Postmaster: Send address changes to *British Medical Bulletin*, c/o Mercury Airfreight International Ltd, 365 Blair Road, Avenel, NJ 07001, USA.

Single copies (cased) and back numbers of issues published from 1996 are available at £45/US$73 and may be ordered from the Domus Medica, Royal Society of Medicine, 1 Wimpole Street, London W1M 8AE, UK (Tel +44(0)171 290 2960; Fax +44 (0)171 290 2969); from booksellers; or directly from the ditributors: Hoddle Doyle Meadows Limited, Station Road, Linton, Cambs CB1 6UX, UK (Tel +44 (0)1223 893855; Fax +44 (0)1223 893852).

Pre-1996 back numbers: Orders for any title published prior to 1996 should be sent to Jill Kettley, Subscriptions Manager, Harcourt Brace, Foots Cray, Sidcup, Kent DA14 5HP (Tel +44 (0)181 308 5700; Fax +44 (0)181 309 0807).

This journal is indexed, abstracted and/or published online in the following media: Adonis, Biosis, BRS Colleague (full text), Chemical Abstracts, Colleague (Online), Current Contents/ Clinical Medicine, Current Contents/Life Sciences, Elsevier BIOBASE/Current Awareness in Biological Sciences, EMBASE/Excerpta Medica, Index Medicus/Medline, Medical Documentation Service, Reference Update, Research Alert, Science Citation Index, Scisearch, SIIC-Database Argentina, UMI (Microfilms)

Editorial services and typesetting by BA & GM Haddock, Ford, Midlothian, Scotland
Printed in Great Britain by Bell & Bain Ltd, Glasgow, Scotland.

Screening

Scientific Editors
Catherine Peckham and Carol Dezateux

Acknowledgements

The planning committee for this issue of the *British Medical Bulletin* was chaired by Catherine Peckham and also included John Burn, Carol Dezateux and Kay-Tee Khaw.

The British Council and the Royal Society of Medicine Press are most grateful to them for their help and advice, and particularly to Professor Peckham and Dr Dezateux for their work as Scientific Editors.

Issues underlying the evaluation of screening programmes

Catherine S Peckham and **Carol Dezateux**

Department of Epidemiology and Public Health, Institute of Child Health, London, UK

Screening programmes have the potential to prevent premature death and disability and to improve quality of life, but they also have the potential for harm. Identifying worthwhile screening programmes, developing the correct strategies, and implementing them effectively is no easy task. A much more critical approach to screening is now being adopted and efforts are being made to ensure that new programmes of proven benefit and which are acceptable to the public, are effectively and equitably implemented in the community. We hope that this issue will stimulate further discussion and debate.

Screening has been defined as the systematic application of a test or enquiry, to identify individuals at sufficient risk of a specific disorder to benefit from further investigation or direct preventive action, amongst persons who have not sought medical attention on account of symptoms of that disorder[1]. The aim is to detect disease or pre-disease states but also, increasingly, genetic susceptibility to disease in either the individual being tested or their offspring. Screening differs from traditional medicine in that it aims to identify a disease or condition at an early stage, before medical advice is sought. This raises important ethical issues since individuals who considered themselves to be healthy may, after screening, be identified as potentially ill. Screening can only be justified, therefore, for disorders or conditions that are serious, a significant public health problem and for which treatment or intervention at this stage is more effective than when given to those seeking medical attention with symptoms or signs.

There has been an exponential rise in proposed new screening programmes, reflecting technological developments and the increasing assumption that early detection of disease is beneficial. However, decisions to start, continue or stop screening programmes must be informed by systematic review of the evidence. The screening process is complex and spans disease, detection, management and delivery, as well as long-term outcome. Evidence is also complex and frequently falls short of ideal. Each screening programme requires a policy, with continual review to allow for new research findings as well as technological

Correspondence to:
Professor C.S. Peckham,
Dept of Epidemiology
and Public Health,
Institute of Child Health,
30 Guilford Street,
London WC1N 1EH, UK

developments. At the same time, policy makers need to be in a position to respond in a timely, but informed, fashion to pressures to introduce screening, be they technology, consumer, media or clinician-led.

This issue of the *British Medical Bulletin* is devoted to screening and attempts to highlight some of the contemporary challenges arising from proposed and established screening programmes. Contributions have been sought to reflect screening at different stages of life and to illustrate the range and diversity of issues that arise in the conception and delivery of screening programmes, as well as some common themes that underpin them all.

The purpose of any screening programme needs to be made explicit and its introduction should not be driven by technological availability, clinical enthusiasm or misplaced public demand. It must be based on sound evidence that screening is effective and that the benefits derived outweigh any harm. New screening programmes should, where possible, be introduced within the context of a randomised controlled trial as observational studies may lead to biased assessment of outcome. Trials allow the potential risks to the population posed by screening programmes to be minimised[2] and this issue is explored in relation to neonatal screening for inborn errors of metabolism (*see* Carol Dezateux, p877). All too often screening is judged by the number of individuals detected with a particular disease or pre-disease state, rather than by measures of its impact in preventing or modifying disease. Early detection must not be an end in itself and the potential value of a screening programme should be fully established before its introduction. The successful implementation of a screening programme depends on public understanding of the benefits that accrue from screening as well as its limitations. There is a need for greater public participation in the research and development process to improve the way screening services are prioritised, commissioned and implemented[3].

The introduction of a new screening programme has major implications for the population being screened, as well as for health service resources. The benefits and disbenefits, including economic implications, of all screening programmes require careful appraisal. A National Screening Committee has been established in the UK, to develop screening policies based on all the available evidence[4]. This is supported through the work of the Population Screening Panel, an advisory committee of the National Health Service Research and Development Health Technology Assessment programme, which commissions reviews of new, as well as of existing, programmes[5]. These reviews help to set and prioritise the research agenda by presenting relevant information in an accessible and comprehensive format for policy makers. Table 1 summarises reviews, published or in progress, commissioned through this programme. Similar initiatives are ongoing in other European countries, the US and Canada[6,7].

Table 1 Systematic reviews of screening commissioned through the National Health Service Health Technology Assessment Programme[1]

Condition	Population to be screened	Publication date
Published reviews of specific screening programmes[33]		
Prostate cancer	Adult men	1997[8,9]
Fragile X	Pregnant women, newborn infants, young adults before conception	1997[34]
Inborn errors of metabolism	Newborn infants	1997[35,36]
Squint and amblyopia	Pre-school aged children	1997[37]
Congenital hearing impairment	Newborn infants	1997[38]
Down's syndrome	Pregnant women	1998[39]
Ovarian cancer	Adult women	1998[40]
Language delay	Children aged ≤ 7 years	1998[41]
*Commissioned reviews of specific screening programmes**		
Structural and other fetal abnormalities detected by ultrasound	Pregnant women	
Cystic fibrosis	Pregnant women, newborn infants, young adults before conception	
Haemoglobinopathies, including sickle cell disease and thalassaemia	Pregnant women, newborn infants, young adults before conception	
Hypercholesterolaemia	Children and adults	
Helicobacter pylori infection (to prevent gastric cancer or peptic ulcer)	Adults	

*Updated information can be obtained from the NHS R&D HTA website: http://www.soton.ac.uk/~hta/

The National Screening Committee recommended that routine screening for prostate cancer should be discouraged and that purchasers should not fund screening services for prostate cancer[4]. This decision was based on evidence from two commissioned systematic reviews[8,9]. However, the need for further evidence of the effectiveness of treatment in screen detected prostate cancer was emphasised, since interventions following a positive screening test exposed treated men to significant risks of incontinence and impotence. At the time the reviews were published, evidence that screening decreased mortality rates from prostate cancer was lacking. Subsequently, a significant reduction in mortality among those screened was reported at a conference from an as yet unpublished controlled trial of screening for prostate cancer carried out in the US[10]. While there has been debate about the validity of this conclusion, this does highlight the need to update systematic reviews when new information becomes available (*see* Sue Moss & Jane Melia, p791).

Introducing a screening programme

Before introducing a screening programme, the criteria summarised in Table 2 need to be considered. First formulated in 1968 by Wilson and Jungner for the World Health Organization[11], they have been expanded and modified subsequently to reflect and respond to contemporary screening issues[12].

Table 2 Criteria to be met by a screening programme

The condition should pose an important health problem and its natural history should be well understood. It should be recognisable at a latent or early symptomatic stage.

The test should be simple to administer, safe and reliable, inexpensive and acceptable to those screened. The distribution of test values should be known with cut-off levels agreed. There should be an agreed policy for the diagnostic investigation of those with positive screening results. The chance of physical or psychological harm to those screened should be less than the chance of benefit.

The treatment or intervention should be effective with evidence that earlier treatment results in better outcome.

The screening programme should be clinically, socially and ethically acceptable, with equity of access. The programme should be optimally cost-effective and managed and monitored within a quality assurance framework.

Adapted from National Screening Committee report[4].

The rationale for screening reflects both the incidence and prevalence of a condition, its projected trends in the population, as well as its consequences for affected individuals. The importance of information regarding the natural history of a condition for which screening is being proposed cannot be sufficiently emphasised: once screening has been introduced the opportunity to establish this has been lost. For example, screening for carcinoma of the cervix was introduced before the natural history of carcinoma *in situ* was established and it is still unclear how many women with this finding would develop carcinoma of the cervix[13]. Similarly, there has been much debate on the benefits or otherwise of screening for prostate cancer, given that many men with prostatic carcinomas identified through screening will die **with** their carcinoma rather than **from** it[14].

Which strategy for prevention?

A screening test is not a diagnostic test but serves to identify those who are at high risk of disease. Further tests will be required to confirm or refute the diagnosis. However, diagnostic confirmation is not always possible, particularly when the proposed screening test identifies individuals with increased risk of developing a condition at some future stage, rather than the early presence of the target condition. Examples of this include screening to prevent stroke by identifying individuals with raised blood pressure, screening to prevent hip fractures by identifying individuals with osteoporosis, and screening for developmental dysplasia of the hip by identifying newborns with hip instability. In these situations, the implication of a positive screen result is that all those identified above a certain threshold value or within certain defined categories will be treated, for example with statins, alendronate or abduction splinting appliances. Inevitably, even in screening programmes employing tests of high specificity, a substantial number of those treated would never have developed the outcome of interest. Thus, treatment effectiveness, safety and economic costs may be key drivers in determining screening policy. This raises the issue of whether interventions which aim to achieve primary prevention at a population level may be more cost-effective and appropriate[15]. Examples include the fortification of flour and cereals with folate to prevent neural tube defects[16], the promotion of weight-bearing exercise, such as walking, to prevent osteoporosis, or population-based dietary advice to prevent obesity.

The implications of test performance

Measures of test performance need to be estimated for any screening programme. Central to the rationale for screening is the detection rate (sensitivity) which measures the proportion of affected individuals identified through screening (those affected individuals not identified being referred to as false negatives). However, in policy terms, the false positive rate, that is the proportion of unaffected individuals wrongly identified as positive through screening, may be more important as these individuals will need further investigation and are potentially at risk of anxiety, misdiagnosis and unnecessary treatment. While failure to detect cases through screening may have medico-legal implications, the proportion of false positives may have important human and economic disbenefits. This proportion will depend on the frequency of the disease in the population being screened: the rarer the condition, the smaller the chance that those with a positive screening test are truly affected. However, a reduction in the false positive rate is usually only achieved at the expense of a rise in the false negative rate. Thus the screening test thresholds chosen for recall and follow up in any screening programme will depend on the goal of that programme, as well as on the implications of missing a true case or of a positive screening test result. For example, in antenatal screening for Down's syndrome using biochemical markers, diagnostic confirmation of a positive screening result requires an amniocentesis, which carries a small but, nonetheless, increased risk of fetal loss. In this programme, the maximum detection rate achievable for any given combination of serum markers is determined by a false positive rate, conventionally set at 5% to limit the number of women undergoing unnecessary amniocentesis (*see* Lyn Chitty, p839).

Even when perfectly implemented, there will always be false positives in any screening programme. For screening programmes that require repeat rather than one-off testing, the risk of a false positive screening result will increase with each successive test. For example, over the course of her lifetime, a woman is more likely to have a cervical smear result that incorrectly identifies her as having a condition that might develop into cervical cancer than she is of developing cervical cancer[17]. The full consequences of a false positive screening result are frequently not considered in the first waves of enthusiasm for screening, and are often limited to the medical and diagnostic implications. The potential anxiety caused by a positive screening test result should be assessed and consideration given to the ability or otherwise of the subsequent diagnostic process to fully reassure an unaffected individual that they are, after all, healthy.

The concept of a false positive and false negative result is a difficult one for the public to understand. A screening test, even one of high sensitivity, will give some false negative results when applied to a large number of individuals. As screening is limited to serious conditions, a false negative result will inevitably have important consequences for the individual, as false reassurance that all is well could delay referral for treatment when symptoms subsequently arise. Individuals need to be informed about the limitations of a screening test and advised that a negative test does not always exclude the condition. It comes as a great shock when a woman who has been screened for Down's syndrome and found to be at low risk subsequently gives birth to an affected child.

A related issue is that of unwanted information obtained in the course of screening. For example, minor sonographic features, such as echogenic cysts in the fetal bowel, may be discovered incidentally during antenatal ultrasound screening for major structural fetal anomalies. These are of uncertain significance, are managed differently in different centres and informed consent to screening for this has not usually been obtained. Wald has proposed that more focussed objectives are required in relation to the conditions being sought antenatally[18], thereby avoiding the ensuing anxiety for both parents and professionals.

The outcome of early treatment

An important criterion to be considered before screening is introduced is that treatment at this stage is more effective than that given after the condition has been clinically diagnosed. For example, with regard to screening for cystic fibrosis, uncertainty remains as to whether early detection and treatment improves the natural history of the condition[19,20]. This knowledge is critical when assessing the benefits or otherwise of introducing a neonatal screening programme[21].

The importance of avoiding biased assessment of outcome of early detection and treatment is well recognised in cancer screening programmes but has only recently been raised in the context of screening for genetic conditions, such as cystic fibrosis[20]. Bias may arise where comparisons are made between cases in screened and unscreened populations: those presenting clinically are likely to have a more severe form of the condition than those identified through screening, some of whom may have a milder disease with a better outcome. In this situation, screening will always appear to have a favourable outcome unless comparisons allow for differences in these prognostic characteristics, or there is uniform probability of ascertainment between screened and unscreened populations at the point when comparisons are made.

Information on the adverse effects of treatment is essential when assessing the risks inherent in screening and the balance of benefits and harms. This is because a large number of individuals may be treated as a result of a screening programme. For example, 8% of the target adult population have an absolute risk of heart attack greater than 3% per annum, the currently recommended treatment threshold for statins (*see* John Robson, p961). In Germany, the treatment thresholds defined for specific ultrasound appearances of the hip joint among newborn and young infants have led to 5–7% of the whole population being treated with abduction splinting appliances to prevent a condition which may at most affect 0.1–0.2%[22]. The public health implications of treatment on this scale are such that treatment thresholds need to be based on evidence from randomised trials unless there are compelling reasons why an exception should be made. It cannot be assumed that the same degree of risk is acceptable at a population level as is deemed acceptable in a clinical setting.

The cost effectiveness of screening

With increasing competition for scarce resources, more attention is being given to the cost-effectiveness of potential, as well as existing, screening programmes (*see* Jackie Brown & Martin Buxton, p993).

Screening programmes are expensive, resources for medical care and prevention limited, and screening policy decisions need to be made in the context of competing priorities. Resources spent on screening may compete with resources for acute clinical care and, where the latter are limited, this may influence screening policies (*see* Mike Robinson & Jack Hardcastle, p807; and Malcolm Law, p903). Economic evaluations provide information on the relative benefits and costs of screening strategies that may differ according to target population, screening test or service delivery. For example, a number of screening strategies for cystic fibrosis have been proposed, including preconceptional, antenatal and neonatal. Each screening strategy will have different effects on reproductive choice, birth prevalence, and outcome achieved through early diagnosis and treatment. It is, therefore, important that the objectives of a screening programme are made explicit (*see* Mark Wildhagen, Leo ten Kate & Dik Habbema, p857). Cost-effectiveness analyses may help identify the best configuration of screening services to adopt, but will need to be sensitive to advances in the management of previously lethal conditions. Decision analyses and economic modelling of screening strategies can help focus the policy research agenda and establish the rationale for and objectives of randomised controlled trials[23,24].

Evaluating anticipated risks as well as benefits

A full assessment of the potential benefits and harm associated with each stage in the screening pathway (screening, diagnosis and treatment) is required before screening for any condition is introduced, and this information should be made available to individuals before they are screened. However, the best way to communicate these risks in any given screening programme is not always clear. This important issue of communicating and interpreting risk is discussed by Richard Eiser (p779).

The inherent risks of screening include misdiagnosis, over-treatment, and the provocation of anxiety and fear. For example, there is increasing recognition that some individuals with false positive screening results experience considerable anxiety which does not necessarily diminish when the presumptive screening result is not confirmed. This anxiety may have long-lasting effects that vary between different screening programmes. For example, false positive screening results during pregnancy and the first months of life may be particularly difficult for parents, leading them to feel persistently anxious about the underlying health status of their child. However, anxiety is not only confined to those with false positive results. Individuals found to be hypertensive in a workplace screening programme had increased sickness absence, increased anxiety and reduced self perceived health status regardless of whether or not their hypertension required treatment[25,26].

From research to policy

Where there is good evidence that the benefits of screening outweigh the harms and that the condition is an important health priority, detailed specifications for a screening programme are required. Equity and uniformity in screening programmes are important and clear policies and guidelines need to be in place for the management of those individuals testing positive. It is not appropriate for individual clinicians or health authorities to formulate these policies. Access to good quality screening and diagnostic services is important and a system for quality assurance needs to be in place. Local variations in screening policies and screening and diagnostic services are well described which do not reflect local variation in disease prevalence or severity. Where disease prevalence varies with demographic factors in the population, such as sickle cell disorders, local variation may be justified. In the UK, four newborn screening laboratories responsible for testing 16% of births routinely test for cystic fibrosis[27]: the remainder do not. The provision of screening for Down's syndrome is another example of inequity: some districts provide serum screening free of charge, others charge and others only offer nuchal fold testing. This is inconsistent and confusing for pregnant women who often then seek further tests privately.

All screening programmes need a well-developed infrastructure to deliver the programme in an equitable way and to ensure that the anticipated benefits accrue. Quality assurance must also be in place as well as systems to audit the impact of the programme, only then can unanticipated problems be identified and overcome. The need for this is discussed in relation to the cervical and breast cancer screening programmes (*see* Muir Gray & June Austoker, p983) and cardiovascular risk screening (*see* John Robson, p961).

Screening and surveillance often go hand in hand and there may be confusion in separating the objectives of these two activities. Although it is important to make a clear distinction between them, in practice screening may be delivered within the context of surveillance (*see* Astrid Fletcher, p945). For example, although the routine examination of the newborn infant is not a screening examination, it includes screening tests such as the Ortolani-Barlow test to detect hip instability. Similarly, vision and hearing screening are performed within the child surveillance programme (*see* David Hall & Sarah Stewart-Brown, p929).

The importance of informed consent

While there has been much emphasis on uptake of testing as a measure of the success of a screening programme, the importance of informed decision making on the part of the person being screened is a more meaningful, albeit harder to obtain, measure. Paradoxically uptake of testing in a screening programme may fall as informed decision making rises. In one randomised trial of different methods of giving information prenatally about cystic fibrosis, women given extra information were less likely to accept testing[28]. Similarly, the most important determinant of whether a woman accepts antenatal testing for HIV is the midwife she sees rather than the information she receives[29]. The information given to those being screened is a frequently neglected area that needs to be addressed within the framework of quality assurance. Without this, consent cannot be informed. The confidentiality of the information obtained through screening must be safeguarded (*see* Ian Markham, p1011).

Identifying genetic mutations

The identification of genetic mutations, either intentionally or incidentally, raises particularly difficult ethical issues. This debate has mainly centred around screening for haemoglobin disorders and cystic fibrosis, the most common autosomal recessive conditions in the UK. However, it may soon be technically feasible to screen for genetic predisposition to the common multifactorial disorders that make up the major health burden in western countries, such as certain cancers, cardiovascular disease and diabetes. Such tests should not be offered without clear evidence of benefit. However, commercial interests may promote the development of private genetic screening services marketed directly to the public, with the risk that inadequate attention will be paid to the implications for those tested. Commercially available screening initiatives should be subject to the same degree of evaluation as those in the public sector and 'individualising the decision to screen' should be strongly resisted.

Screening programmes that rely on the identification of individuals at high risk, be it through family history or behavioural risk factors, require special consideration (*see* Judith Stephenson, p891). The process of defining high risk is in itself a screening test usually based on history taking. The questions used need to be clearly defined so that those eliciting the history as well as the individuals screened understand their purpose. To date, this approach to screening has been poorly implemented with unsatisfactory results[30].

Tests are now available to identify individuals who carry the abnormal gene for hereditary nonpolyposis colorectal cancer (*see* Mike Robinson & Jack Hardcastle, p807). A recent consensus statement in the US recommended that those affected should have a colonoscopic examination of the whole large intestine every 1–3 years from the age of 25 years with women possibly tested for endometrial cancer[31]. In the US, it has been proposed that carriers of the two main genes for familial breast cancer be offered annual mammography, beginning at 25–35 years[32]. There is little evidence to support this practice and the significance of the cancer predisposing mutations remains uncertain (*see* Paul Pharoah, John Stratton & James Mackay, p823).

Conclusions

Screening programmes have the potential to prevent premature death and disability and to improve quality of life, but they also have the potential for harm. Identifying worthwhile screening programmes, developing the correct strategies, and implementing them effectively is no easy task. A much more critical approach to screening is now being adopted and efforts are being made to ensure that new programmes of proven benefit and which are acceptable to the public, are effectively and equitably implemented in the community. We hope that this issue will stimulate further discussion and debate.

References

1   Wald NJ. Guidance on terminology. *J Med Screen* 1994; **1**: 76
2   Lumley J. Trials and evaluation of screening programs. In: Wilcken B, Webster D. (eds) *Neonatal Screening in the Nineties*. Sydney: 8th International Neonatal Screening Symposium, Australia, 1991; 11–7
3   Standing Advisory Group on Consumer Involvement in the NHS Research and Development Programme. Research: What's in it for me? (Conference report). London: Department of Health, 1998
4   National Screening Committee. First report of the UK National Screening Committee. London: Department of Health, 1998
5   Sherriff R, Best L, Roderick P. Population screening in the NHS: a systematic pathway from evidence to policy formulation. *J Public Health Med* 1998; **20**: 58–62
6   Canadian Task Force on the Periodic Health Examination. *Canadian Guide to Clinical Preventive Health Care*. Ottawa: Canada Communication Group, 1994
7   US Preventive Services Task Force. *Guide to Clinical Preventive Services*. Baltimore: Williams and Wilkins, 1996
8   Selley S, Donovan J, Faulkner A, Coast J, Gillatt D. Diagnosis, management and screening of early localised prostate cancer. *Health Technol Assess* 1997; **1**(2): 1–96
9   Chamberlain JM, Melia J, Moss S, Brown J. The diagnosis, management, treatment and costs of prostate cancer in England and Wales. *Health Technol Assess* 1997; **1**(3): 1–53
10 Prostate cancer screening reduces deaths [news item]. *BMJ* 1998; **316**: 1625

11 Wilson JMG, Jungner G. Principles and practice of screening for disease. Geneva: WHO, 1968

12 Smith L. Time for evidence-based screening? *J R Soc Med* 1998; **91**: 347–8

13 Raffle AE, Alden B, Mackenzie EFD. Detection rates for abnormal cervical smears: what are we screening for? *Lancet* 1995; **345**: 1469–73

14 Woolf SH. Should we screen for prostate cancer? *BMJ* 1997; **314**: 989

15 Rose G. *The Strategy of Preventive Medicine*. New York: Oxford University Press, 1992

16 Wald NJ, Bower C. Folic acid and the prevention of neural tube defects. *BMJ* 1995; **310**: 1019–20

17 Russell LB. *Educated Guesses*. Berkley: University of California Press, 1994

18 Wald NJ, Kennard A. Routine ultrasound screening for congenital abnormalities. *Ann N Y Acad Sci* 1998; **847**: 173–80

19 Dankert-Roelse JE. Screening for cystic fibrosis – time to change our position? *N Engl J Med* 1997; **337**: 997–9

20 Wald NJ, Morris JK. Neonatal screening for cystic fibrosis. *BMJ* 1998; **316**: 404–5

21 US Department of Health and Human Services. Newborn screening for cystic fibrosis: a paradigm for public health genetics policy development. *MMWR Suppl* 1997; **46**: 1–24

22 Altenhofen L, Allhoff PG, Niethard FU. Huftsonographie-Screening im rahmen der U3-Erste erfahrungen. *Z Orthop Ihre Grenzgeb* 1998; **136**: 1–7

23 Parsonnet J, Harris RH, Hack HM, Owen DK. Modelling cost effectiveness of *Helicobacter pylori* screening to prevent gastric cancer: a mandate for clinical trials. *Lancet* 1996; **348**: 150–4

24 Torgerson DJ, Donaldson C. Economic evaluations before clinical trials. *Lancet* 1996; **348**: 687

25 Stewart-Brown S. Screening could seriously damage your health [editorial]. *BMJ* 1997; **314**: 533

26 Haynes RB, Sackett DL, Gibson ES, Johnson AL. Increased absenteeism from work after detection and labelling of hypertensive patients. *N Engl J Med* 1978; **299**: 741–4

27 Streetly A, Grant C, Pollitt RJ, Addison GM. Survey of scope of neonatal screening in the United Kingdom. *BMJ* 1995; **311**: 726

28 Thornton JG, Hewison J, Lilford RJ, Vail A. A randomised trial of three methods of giving information about prenatal testing. *BMJ* 1995; **311**: 1127–30

29 Simpson WM, Johnstone FD, Boyd FM, Goldberg DJ, Hart GJ, Prescott RJ. Uptake and acceptability of antenatal HIV testing: randomised controlled trial of different methods of offering the test. *BMJ* 1998; **316**: 262–7

30 Chrystie I, Sumner D, Kenny A, Banatvala JE. Screening of pregnant women for evidence of current hepatitis B infection: selective or universal? *Health Trends* 1992; **24**: 13–6

31 Burke W, Petersen G, Lynch P *et al*. Recommendations for follow-up care of individuals with an inherited predisposition to cancer I. Hereditary nonpolyposis colon cancer. *JAMA* 1997; **277**: 915–9

32 Burke W, Daly M, Garber J *et al*. Recommendations for follow-up care of individuals with an inherited predisposition to cancer II. BRCA1 and BRCA2. *JAMA* 1997; **277**: 997–1003

33 The National Coordinating Centre for Health Technology Assessment. The Annual Report of the NHS Health Technology Assessment Programme 1998. London: Department of Health, 1998; 1-122

34 Murray J, Cuckle H, Taylor G, Hewison J. Screening for Fragile X syndrome. *Health Technol Assess* 1997; **1**(4): 1–71

35 Pollitt RJ, Green A, McCabe CJ *et al*. Neonatal screening for inborn errors of metabolism: cost, yield and outcome. *Health Technol Assess* 1997; **1**(7): 1–203

36 Seymour CA, Thomason MJ, Chalmers RA *et al*. Newborn screening for inborn errors of metabolism: a systematic review. *Health Technol Assess* 1997; **1**(11): 1–97

37 Snowdon SK, Stewart-Brown S. Preschool vision screening. *Health Technol Assess* 1997; **1**(8): 1–83

38 Davis A, Bamford J, Wilson I *et al*. A critical review of the role of neonatal hearing screening in the detection of congenital hearing impairment. *Health Technol Assess* 1997; **1**(10): 1–176

39 Wald NJ, Kennard A, Hackshaw A, McGuire A. Antenatal screening for Down's syndrome. *Health Technol Assess* 1998; **2**(1): 1–112.

40 Bell R, Petticrew M, Luengo S, Sheldon T. Screening for ovarian cancer: a systematic review. *Health Technology Assess* 1998; **2**(2): 1-84

41 Law J, Boyle J, Harris F, Harkness A, Nye C. Screening for speech and language delay: a systematic review of the literature. *Health Technol Assess* 1998; **2** (9): 1–179

Communication and interpretation of risk

J Richard Eiser

School of Psychology, University of Exeter, Exeter, UK

The 'new genetics' enables people's risk status for many diseases and disorders to be assessed much more accurately than before, yet considerable uncertainty remains over how risk information will be evaluated and acted upon. This paper summarises some of the main themes of psychological research on risk. Risk is traditionally defined in terms of probability. However, people often have difficulty in processing statistical information and may rely instead on simplified decision rules. Decision making under risk is also critically affected by people's subjective assessments of benefits and costs. In the field of genetic risk, such assessments may vary greatly between individuals, reflecting personal and cultural preferences and ethical concerns. The goals of risk communication should, therefore, not be merely the imparting of statistical 'facts' or the reduction of anxiety, but also enabling individuals and their families to make important decisions under conditions of uncertainty.

What is meant by 'risk'?

Risk is a concept that seems deceptively easy to define. To quote *The BMA Guide to Living with Risk* (p 14)[1], the term 'is an expression of the **probability** – the likelihood – that something unpleasant will happen. If the consequence of throwing a six when you roll a dice is that you receive an electric shock, then there is a one-in-six **risk** of being shocked'. Risk, according to this perspective, is a relatively simple numerical concept. This implies that risk is an objectively measurable construct. According to this view, the problems that remain are over how information about risks should be communicated and how ordinary people make decisions on the basis of their own calculations and their interpretations of what they are told. Such decisions by ordinary people can often seem to 'experts' to involve a miscalculation of the risks. For this reason, the term 'subjective risk' is introduced to distinguish ordinary people's estimates from the supposedly more 'objective' estimates made by experts. From the perspective of the person receiving risk information, however, 'correct' or 'objective'

Correspondence to:
Prof J Richard Eiser,
School of Psychology,
University of Exeter,
Exeter EX4 4QG, UK

perception is not a goal in itself, but a means to the end of better decision-making and functioning in a world beset with manifold uncertainties.

In fact, uncertainty is intrinsic not only to the concept of risk but also to any predictions we can make on the basis of risk information. Even where we can calculate precisely that the probability of a given couple having a child with a genetic disorder is one in four, say, it is still a matter of chance whether their **next** child will have the disorder or not. Identification of the genetic basis sets bounds to our uncertainty, but does not eliminate it. Does this merely reflect our incomplete understanding of the underlying causes, or are we observing 'chaotic' effects intrinsic to all biological and environmental systems[2]? Whatever the answer, a more concrete question is whether the risks we are talking about in a given context are at all **controllable**. For instance, a patient with a genetic predisposition for diabetes has no control over the genetic risk as such, but may influence the course and severity of any health consequences by adopting appropriate dietary and exercise habits and complying with medical advice. Statistical calculations of probability in such contexts are less important than their implications for behaviour.

Costs and benefits

Risk does not depend just on the estimation of probability, but on the balance of benefits and costs. From a rationalistic standpoint, there is no reason why any risk should be willingly endured – however slight the chance of a mishap – if no-one expects to derive any benefit from it, or to receive any compensation. It is a truism to say that individuals will evaluate consequences differently, according to their own values and priorities. It is, nonetheless, important to take account of such individual differences which may be both measurable and predictably related to other attitudes. The evaluation of health outcomes, quality of life, *etc.*, bears directly on this question, while obviously being of vital importance to a wide range of other practical and theoretical concerns. If there are sometimes reasons to view probabilistic estimates with caution, we should be even more wary of any suggestion that there is a single 'correct' evaluation of any outcome. In the words of the British Medical Association (p 194–5)[1]:

> '*Health system managers would like to be able to reduce risk assessments to numbers for the purpose of maximizing 'efficiency' and minimizing unnecessary drain on limited resources, but in practice when such complicated issues are concerned the decisions will probably boil down to an individual choice of action based in each case on what the doctor and the patient feel about it all.*'

How are risks interpreted?

The 'psychometric' paradigm

Much work, concerned particularly with public attitudes to new technologies, has required participants to rate heterogeneous sets of hazards (*e.g.* nuclear power, handguns, pesticides), and has then applied factor analytic techniques to identify common dimensions in terms of which these hazards can be differentiated[3]. This research may inform policy-makers of the kind of 'public image' attached to specific technologies in the abstract. However, the implications for how individuals actually make choices between uncertain alternatives are much more tenuous. More relevant is research which asks individuals to estimate the relative risk of different hazards, along response dimensions that allow for comparison with actual risk statistics. For example, people may be asked to estimate incidence or mortality rates for different diseases, or the frequencies of different kinds of accidents. The general picture is that lay people's estimates of such frequencies are reasonable from a **relative** point of view – more probable causes of death or injury tend to be rated overall as more probable than rarer causes – but are poorly calibrated with **absolute** frequencies[4]. In particular, people tend to overestimate the frequency of very rare risks and underestimate the frequency of highly probable ones. Likewise, people may fail to discriminate fully between rarer and more common risks when asked to rate the importance of different causes of death, even when they have been provided with accurate mortality statistics[5].

Biases in risk perception

A substantial body of research in cognitive psychology testifies to the difficulties individuals face in interpreting statistical information[6]. At first, the main thrust of this work was to demonstrate the extent to which statistical principles were violated in human reasoning, although later research emphasised ways in which biases could be behaviourally adaptive and reflect everyday experience[7]. The term 'heuristic' was used to refer to informal rules-of-thumb on which, it was hypothesised, we depend in the place of such principles. For instance, the 'availability heuristic' refers to the tendency to assume that events are more frequent if they can be more easily imagined or remembered. This might lead, among other things, to an overestimation of the likelihood of risks that receive greater media attention. A number of other biases relate to a neglect of base-rate information when drawing inferences about the association between different events or attributes. To take an imaginary example, if we were told that 'depression is the most common reason for GP consultations among vegetarians', we might jump to the conclusion that lack of meat in one's diet makes one prone to depression, without first checking how common depression was among meat-eaters too!

Closely related to this is a tendency to overestimate the extent to which relationships observed in small samples are representative of the larger population. This is not merely a problem for non-experts. The move towards evidence-based medicine is essential, in no small part because few individual doctors can acquire sufficient clinical experience in their own practice to make decisions about the management of less frequently encountered conditions. Yet how ready are most doctors to rely on statistics rather than their own experience? A memorable single case can often seem a firmer basis for judgement. Reasoning about probabilities in the abstract can be difficult for everyone. Concrete examples and interesting case-reports can be appealing precisely because they seem to make decision-making easier.

Optimistic bias

When people are asked to judge their own risk of some disease or mishap compared with that of some average or 'typical' other person, a well-replicated finding is that they rate their chances of avoiding the mishap as better than average[8]. Since people, on average, can't have a 'better than average' risk, this finding is taken as evidence of an 'optimistic bias', also known as 'unrealistic optimism'[8]. This is a very widespread phenomenon, observable for many different kinds of risks. Even individuals in high-risk groups (such as Amsterdam prostitutes and their clients[9]) may show optimism about their personal risk status compared with similar others. Such results appear suggestive of a form of motivated denial, but a number of issues remain to be resolved. One difficulty is that such comparative ratings imply estimates of both one's own risk and that of a (generally) hypothetical comparison person. Some of the effect might be attributable to a tendency to overestimate the unknown other's risk status rather than underestimate one's own.

The implications of such risk ratings for behaviour can also be ambiguous, particularly in studies using correlational designs[10]. A pessimistic self-rating could be taken as a sign of greater concern and, hence, motivation to engage in protective action. This would lead one to expect a negative correlation between optimism and protective health behaviour. Alternatively, those who engage in protective behaviour may be more optimistic about their relative risk, precisely because they believe that their behaviour has reduced their risk. Hence, optimism and protective behaviour could be positively correlated. There is clearly a need for research that clarifies the impact of different kinds of information on estimates of own and other's risk, and whether changes in such estimates lead to changes in behaviour.

Individual differences

There is some evidence that individuals differ in the extent to which they attend to risk information, as opposed to playing down its importance and delaying appropriate action. Janis and Mann[11] distinguished a number of 'cognitive styles', reflecting how individuals react to threatening information when required to make decisions in conflict situations. These include: defensive avoidance; vigilance (careful weighing up of consequences); and hypervigilance (more panicky or obsessive attention to any signs of danger).

A similar distinction is implied by the concept of **monitoring-blunting**. According to Miller[12], individuals differ in the way they respond to threatening information. 'Monitors' seek out high levels of information, while 'blunters' will distract themselves from information and are more likely to suppress or avoid both cognitive and emotional threats. This has been applied to medical contexts, such as reactions to short-term stressors in diagnostic procedures. Monitors are generally seen as vulnerable to stress and anxiety, and may show slower recovery from illness and report greater distress. However, there may be subtypes of more adaptive monitoring, involving watchfulness for possible danger signs without undue anxiety. This accords with the distinction between vigilance and hypervigilance. In the context of screening, such individual differences might help predict the extent to which people are prepared to be vigilant for possible signs of danger, their preparedness to seek further information, and their emotional reactions to any information they receive.

How do we make decisions under uncertainty?

Prospect theory

The research just described shifts the focus away from the question of how risks are 'perceived' to that of how individuals may *use*, or attend to, risk information when making behavioural decisions. Probably the most influential approach in contemporary psychological research on decision-making is **prospect theory**[13]. Classic economic theory implies that people's preferences can be predicted from their estimation of the **likelihood** of relevant outcomes, multiplied by how these outcomes are **evaluated** (this is termed 'subjective expected utility'). Prospect theory asserts that this view is incomplete. In particular, individuals are predicted to be generally **risk-averse** for gains and **risk-seeking** for losses. In other words, granted the choice between a certain, but modest, gain and a less probable but larger gain, people will often opt for the 'sure thing' (avoiding the 'riskier' option). Conversely, when asked to choose between the certainty of a moderate loss on the one hand and, on the other hand, a chance of either escaping scot-free or ending up with an even greater loss, then many will view the riskier gamble as the more attractive option.

This raises a possible question of where tendencies such as risk aversion may 'come from'. In fact, they may not necessarily reflect a specifically **motivational** bias, but may rather be the product of the kind of feedback people receive from making more or less risky choices[14]. The well-known learning principle of **reinforcement** predicts that people will repeat actions that lead to positive outcomes. Hence such action-outcome contingencies will be experienced more frequently. When considering gains, choices that lead only rarely to gains (however large) are less likely (in the short term) to be rewarded and hence repeated than choices associated with certain benefits. Likewise, in the context of losses, riskier choices may, for a while, escape punishment and so will be less likely to be avoided than those that always result in a (smaller) loss. In other words, what appears to be a form of bias can be explained as the acquisition of expectancies based on actual experience.

How can risks be communicated?

Communication and persuasion

Within social psychology, the study of communication and persuasion has been a major field of research. Unfortunately, little of this has been applied specifically to the communication of **risk**. Depending how one draws the boundaries, there is either a vast literature or a tiny one and this, in turn, depends on what definition of risk one adopts – either something tightly tied to notions of probability and expected value or as something vaguely to do with what might happen as a consequence of something else. Although one might anticipate that general principles of attitude change[15] have implications for risk communication, this both needs, and deserves, to be demonstrated.

One classic area of attitude change research, however, deserves brief mention, partly because this comes close to dealing with risk, but also because some well-known findings are frequently over-interpreted. A number of studies on **fear-arousing communications**[16] were, for a long time, interpreted as showing that messages that arouse high levels of fear are **less** effective in changing attitudes and behaviour than those that arouse only moderate fear. Such communications frequently deal with health risks. However, the literature has been critically reviewed by Sutton[17], who argues that many studies fail to include checks of how much fear was actually produced by different messages. Some more extreme messages might be disregarded, not because of their fear content as such, but because they appear less plausible or relevant. According to Sutton, in the better controlled studies higher fear actually produces somewhat more attitude and/or behavioural change than moderate or low fear messages. It should, of course, be stressed that communicating information about a significant risk need not be done in such a way as to arouse fear as an emotional reaction. Indeed, in contexts such as genetic counselling this would seem to be the very opposite of good and ethical practice. Nonetheless, if behavioural change is the aim of a communication, the potential of fear as a motivator should be recognised. (It may often be a reason for individuals either seeking or avoiding screening.)

Words and numbers

With all forms of psychological measurement, care needs to be taken over the wording of questions and the selection of response alternatives presented to respondents[18]. This is especially so when individuals are asked to make estimates of probability or frequency. A number of studies have compared ratings in terms of numerical probabilities with less formal verbal expressions of likelihood[4]. Lichtenstein and Newman[19] asked respondents to identify numerical equivalents, in terms of probability values from 0.01 to 0.99, for various verbal likelihood expressions, including for instance the terms 'likely' and 'unlikely' qualified by the adverbs 'very', 'quite', 'rather' and 'fairly'. Respondents were reasonably consistent in their ranking of the different expressions, but there was variation in the absolute numbers assigned. Expressions of intermediate likelihood showed higher variance, and 'mirror-image' expressions (*e.g.* 'quite likely' *versus* 'quite unlikely') did not yield complementary probabilities (means were 0.79 and 0.11 for these examples).

Later studies[20,21] confirmed the finding of considerable interpersonal variation in the assignment of numerical equivalents to verbal terms. The interpretation of verbal terms can also shown to be context-dependent, that is, influenced by the kinds of events or scenarios being considered. For instance, one study[22] found that lower numerical equivalents were assigned to the **same** verbal expressions when applied to events assumed to happen only rarely, as opposed to more frequently.

In terms of their implications for communication, these findings suggest that verbal expressions of likelihood could easily be misinterpreted. Indeed, **recipients** of such information tend to say that they prefer to be given numerical probabilities, in contexts as diverse as sporting gambles[23] and (hypothetical) treatment prognoses[24]. Paradoxically, however, these studies also showed that the **communicators** of such information preferred to use verbal rather than numerical expressions. This preference for verbal forms was also found when doctors were asked to think aloud when solving a decision task[25]. This suggests that verbal forms of expressions may help decision-makers represent a problem so that a choice can be made, even though they are less precise than numbers.

These studies pose dilemmas for risk communication, especially in clinical settings. The research on cognitive heuristics suggests that people are error-prone in their statistical reasoning. Nonetheless, **if** statistical information is available, this seems to be the kind of information recipients prefer. A possible danger is that this preference may extend to cases where precise statistics are not available, and numerical estimates may be interpreted as more exact than they actually are. On the other hand, there are also dangers in relying on more ambiguous verbal expressions. An obvious one is that a risk that is considered 'extremely unlikely' by one clinician may not be so regarded by another and still less so by the patient even when the numerical probability is known and understood.

Implicit in this is a possibility that merits more direct research attention than it so far seems to have received. Verbal expressions of probability may carry evaluative or gerundive connotations in a way that numerical ones do not. A risk that is described as 'extremely unlikely' is one that can be **justifiable** or **reasonable** to take in order to achieve some goal. A risk that is 'extremely high' is, by implication, *too* high, that is to say **unjustified**. It is a widely held principle in counselling that clients should be helped to make their *own* decisions, rather than pressurised in one direction or another. Nonetheless, the suggestion that words can be better than numbers at capturing the reasoning behind the forming of a choice[25] might also mean that they can **imply** a preference when used communicatively. Perhaps it is very difficult wholly to avoid being directive if verbal expressions are used instead of numbers in risk communication or counselling.

Framing

It is tempting to interpret such evidence as meaning that recipients of information would prefer risk communications to be straightforwardly factual and unadorned. This may indeed be the case, but the same 'facts' can be given different slants, even through the use of numbers rather than verbal expressions. For example, the same treatment could be described as having a 60% chance of success, or a 40% chance of failure. The same diagnostic test could be described as accurate in 95% of cases, or as inaccurate in 5%.

Research on **decision framing**[26] stems from the principle, in prospect theory[13], that 'prospects' (alternative possibilities) are not evaluated as absolute end-states (*i.e.* final balance-sheets), as classic economic models would predict, but as **changes** from some actual or expected comparison standard. In other words, what matters for preferences is not whether an outcome will be 'good' or 'bad', but whether it will be 'better' or 'worse' than some standard. For risk communication, this means that the same information could be interpreted positively or negatively depending on the recipient's prior expectations or some other implicit standard.

This ties in with the concept of risk-aversion and risk-seeking[13], in that the same dilemma can elicit very different preferences depending on whether it is '**framed**' (*i.e.* verbally structured) as a choice between different gains (relative to one standard) or losses (relative to another). There are implications worth exploring here in terms of alternative presentations of messages which focus either on health benefits or avoidance of adverse outcomes. For instance, anti-smoking messages along the lines of 'You **will** feel fitter after you've stopped smoking' (a moderate benefit, presented as certain) may be more appealing than one along the lines of 'Giving up smoking will reduce your **chances** of suffering from lung cancer and other diseases' (uncertain avoidance of a large loss, which needs to be set against the more certain discomfort of withdrawal).

Some questions for future research

It is difficult to overestimate the impact that the 'new genetics' is having on our scientific understanding of disease. The alliance between new investigative methods and a perspective on the aetiology of ill-health constitutes as radical a paradigm shift as anything since, perhaps, the early days of research on hygiene and infection. But how well can the outcomes of this brilliant work be communicated to, and understood by, ordinary people without a biomedical training? And even if the 'facts' can be communicated and understood, where does this leave everyone (the public, patients and health professionals) in terms of addressing issues of value and preference that cannot be so easily defined in precise numerical terms? Psychologists have potentially much to offer in this field, but it is important not to expect either too much, or too little, of us. Psychology is the scientific study of how people think and feel and act. However, people's thoughts and feelings and actions occur within a context that extends much wider than the single individual. If psychological research is this area is to be done well, and well received, in must be firmly based on an appreciation of that context.

The family and cultural context

As soon as we look at the implications of screening information for behaviour, we see that there is more than the individual patient involved. Screening for increased risk of genetic or inherited disorders carries implications for the risk (and/or carrier) status of **other** family members. How are issues of confidentiality to be addressed? What happens if a test shows that one's *sister* could be a carrier? The issue of communication with children and adolescents deserves particular attention. If carrier status is positively identified after one has already become a parent, how and when should children be told about their possible risk status? More broadly, communication and decision-making need to be viewed in their appropriate cultural context. Notions of family roles, attitudes to child-rearing, handicap and termination of pregnancy, for instance, are likely to vary between different social and ethnic groups. Some inherited conditions will also be more prevalent within some such groups than others.

What do the public know or believe about screening?

Communication of genetic risk is unlike much other health communication (for example, concerning BSE, or the health risks of smoking) in that it is typically targeted at specific individuals, and conducted in private. Although other members of the client's family may be brought into the discussion, the extent of their involvement, if any, will vary. The form is much more like that of a clinical consultation than of any public information campaign concerning more familiar health risks. However, it would be a mistake to ignore public attitudes on this issue. The willingness of ordinary members of the public to participate in screening – and even their approval of NHS funding of screening programmes – may depend on what they believe screening involves, how it may benefit patients and/or lead to new treatments being developed.

More generally, we know very little about the general level of public understanding of genetics as it applies to health risks, or about the factors that may facilitate or inhibit societal acceptance of screening for increased risk of genetic or inherited disorders and genetic technology.

Ethical concerns

Although some new technologies may be viewed with suspicion because the underlying science is poorly understood, public opposition to widespread screening for increased risk of genetic or inherited disorders may well depend on more ethical concerns. There is the spectre of eugenics and the removal of 'undesirable' characteristics from the genetic pool. There is the issue of whether parents have the 'right' to risk conceiving a child with a condition likely to need long and expensive medical care. Do we all have the 'right to know' our risk status in terms of any dimensions that are technically identifiable. If so, does our life insurance company have the 'right to know' it too? Science cannot finally resolve such ethical issues, but it can inform the debate. More immediately, the extent of people's ethical concerns in different contexts can itself be studied scientifically.

What outcomes should we be looking for?

Anyone receiving risk information in the context of screening is likely to be faced by problems and decisions of very great significance. Evaluation of any screening programme must look at how such decisions are made. This means that we need appropriate outcome measures which reflect the quality of this **decision process**, many or all of which may need to be systematically developed. This implies a shift of emphasis from much of what has been happening in this area so far. Predominantly[27], such research has relied upon the use of general scales of patient satisfaction, psychological well-being, anxiety or distress, *etc.*, often with a psychiatric flavour. This is not to say that patients' immediate emotional state is unimportant, only that it is, at best, an indirect indicator of what really matters – what patients are **making of** the information they are given. At the other extreme, it is also too restrictive to base one's evaluation only on whether individuals have understood the relevant statistics.

We need to look not just at the interpretation, but at the **use** of information. What impact do screening results have on people's various life choices and aspirations, not just in the immediate aftermath of the news, but over the longer term? The best psychological theory and research in this area seeks to establish a link between how risks are interpreted and the behavioural choices based on these interpretations. Risk information is not 'perceived'. It is **actively** processed by individuals and families with problems to solve and decisions to take.

References

1   British Medical Association. *The BMA Guide to Living with Risk*. London: Penguin, 1990
2   Stewart I. *Does God play Dice? The Mathematics of Chaos*. Oxford: Blackwell, 1989
3   Fischhoff B, Slovic P, Lichtenstein S, Read S, Combs B. How safe is safe enough? A psychometric study of attitudes toward technological risks and benefits. *Policy Sci* 1978; **8**: 127–52
4   Lichtenstein S, Slovic P, Fischhoff B, Layman M, Combs B. Judged frequency of lethal events. *J Exp Psychol Hum Learn Memory* 1978; **4**: 551–78
5   Harding CM, Eiser JR, Kristiansen CM. The representation of mortality statistics and the perceived importance of causes of death. *J Appl Social Psychol* 1982; **12**: 169–81
6   Kahneman D, Tversky A. On the psychology of prediction. *Psychol Rev* 1973; **80**: 237–51
7   Hogarth RM. Beyond discrete biases: Functional and dysfunctional aspects of judgmental heuristics. *Psychol Bull* 1981; **90**: 197–217
8   Weinstein ND. Unrealistic optimism about illness susceptibility: Conclusions from a community-wide sample. *J Behav Med* 1987; **10**: 481–500
9   van der Velde FW, Hooykaas C, van der Pligt J. Risk perception and behavior: Pessimism, realism, and optimism about AIDS-related health behavior. *Psychol Health* 1991; **6**: 23–38
10 Weinstein ND, Nicolich M. Correct and incorrect interpretations of correlations between risk perceptions and risk behaviors. *Health Psychol* 1993; **12**: 235–45
11. Janis IL, Mann L. *Decision Making: a psychological analysis of conflict, choice, and commitment*. New York: Free Press, 1977
12 Miller SM. Monitoring versus blunting styles of coping with cancer influence the information patients want and need about their disease. *Cancer* 1995; **76**: 167–77
13 Kahneman D, Tversky A. Prospect theory: an analysis of decision under risk. *Econometrics* 1979; **47**: 263–91
14 March JG. Learning to be risk averse. *Psycholog Rev* 1996; **103**: 309–19
15 Eagly AH, Chaiken S. *The Psychology of Attitudes*. Orlando, FL: Harcourt Brace Jovanovich, 1993
16 Janis IL, Feshbach S. Effects of fear-arousing communications. *J Abnorm Social Psychol* 1953; **48**: 78–92
17 Sutton SR. Fear-arousing communications: A critical examination of theory and research. In: Eiser JR. (ed) *Social Psychology and Behavioral Medicine*. Chichester: Wiley, 1982; 303–37
18 Schwarz N. Survey research: collecting data by asking questions. In: Semin GR, Fiedler K. (Eds) *Applied Social Psychology*. London: Sage, 1996; 65–90)
19 Lichtenstein S, Newman JR. Empirical scaling of common verbal phrases associated with numerical probabilities. *Psychonom Sci* 1967; **9**: 563–4
20 Budescu DV, Wallsten TS. Consistency in interpretation of probabilistic process. *Organ Behav Hum Decision Processes* 1985; **36**: 391–405
21 Reagan RT, Mosteller F, Youtz C. Quantitative meanings of verbal probability expressions. *J Appl Psychol* 1989; **74**: 433–42
22 Wallsten TS, Fillenbaum S, Cox JA. Base rate effects on the interpretations of probability and frequency expressions. *J Memory Language* 1988; **25**: 571–87
23 Erev I, Cohen BL. Verbal versus numerical probabilities: Efficiency, biases, and the preference paradox. *Organ Behav Hum Decision Processes* 1990; **4**: 1–18
24 Brun W, Teigen K.H. Verbal probabilities: ambiguous, context-dependent, or both? *Organ Behav Hum Decision Processes* 1988; **41**: 390–404
25 Kuipers B, Moskowitz AJ, Kassirer JR. Critical decisions under uncertainty: representation and structure. *Cognitive Sci* 1988; **12**: 177–210
26 Kahneman D, Tversky A. Choices, values, and frames. *Am Psychol* 1984; **39**: 341–50
27 Lerman CE. (ed) Psychological aspects of genetic testing [special issue]. *Health Psychol* 1997; **16**: 1, 3–99

Screening for prostate cancer: the current position

Sue M Moss and **Jane Melia**

Cancer Screening Evaluation Unit, Institute of Cancer Research, Sutton, Surrey, UK

Prostate cancer is a significant and increasing health problem in the UK and elsewhere, and there is considerable interest in the potential for screening. Of the currently available screening tests, measurement of serum levels of prostate specific antigen appears the most promising. However, despite evidence that screening can detect asymptomatic early stage disease, there is, as yet, no evidence that mortality from prostate cancer can be reduced.

There are concerns that screening may result in considerable over-diagnosis of non-progressive or slowly developing disease, and the effectiveness of radical treatment of localised disease, which itself will cause some morbidity, remains a subject of debate. Population screening should not currently be recommended. Randomised controlled trials are in progress to assess the effectiveness of screening, but these will take many years to produce results.

*Correspondence to:
Dr Sue M Moss, Cancer
Screening Evaluation
Unit, Institute of Cancer
Research, Section of
Epidemiology, D Block,
Cotswold Road, Sutton,
Surrey SM2 5NG, UK*

Screening for prostate cancer has been a controversial subject for a number of years. Prostate cancer is of increasing public health importance in view of the ageing of the population and increasing mortality from this cancer. These changes have been accompanied by an increased demand for the earlier detection of prostate cancer through screening on the assumption that earlier treatment reduces mortality. However, the effectiveness of population screening in reducing mortality from prostate cancer remains unproven and must await the outcome of randomised controlled trials currently in progress or planned both in Europe and the US. In the meantime, it is the potential for harm that has led some to question whether even a randomised trial is ethical[1]. The difficulty arises from the recognition that many more men will die with prostate cancer, often undiagnosed as shown by autopsy studies, than will die of the disease, suggesting that the natural history may encompass latent or very slow-growing disease. This is compounded both by the uncertainty surrounding the effectiveness of radical treatment compared with surveillance, and by the morbidity which may be caused by this treatment. In this chapter we address the current knowledge on these issues, and review what are, and should be, the present recommendations on screening for prostate cancer.

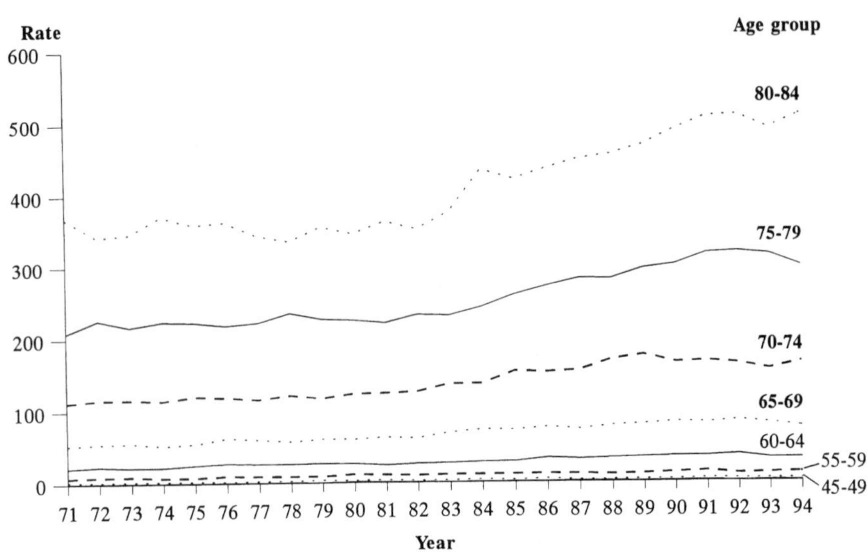

Fig. 1 Mortality rate per 10^5 of prostate cancer in England and Wales presented by age and year, 1971–1994.

The extent of the problem

Mortality rates for prostate cancer have been rising in many countries with white populations during the past few decades[2]. Prostate cancer is now one of the most frequent causes of cancer death in men in the US, with about 41,000 deaths per year[3]. In England and Wales, prostate cancer is the second commonest cause of death after cancer of the lung: in 1994, there were 8,689 deaths from prostate cancer, a mortality rate of 34.0 per 10^5 (30.3 per 10^5 adjusted to the European standard population)[4]. The mortality rate rises steeply with age, with 93% of deaths occurring in men aged over 64 years. During 1971 to 1994, the mortality rate increased in all age groups (Fig. 1).

Prostate cancer is one of the most frequently diagnosed cancers in men both in the US and in England and Wales. There are estimated to be 209,900 American men diagnosed each year[5]. In England and Wales in 1991, there were 13,940 new cases registered, an incidence rate of 55.8 per 10^5 (48.9 per 10^5 adjusted to the European standard population)[6]. Incidence rises steeply with age although less so than mortality. In England and Wales, 88% of new cases occur in men aged over 64 years. From 1971 to 1991, the incidence rate has increased in all age groups (Fig. 2). Incidence rates have also been rising world-wide during the past few decades[2]. In part, this rise may reflect improved ascertainment

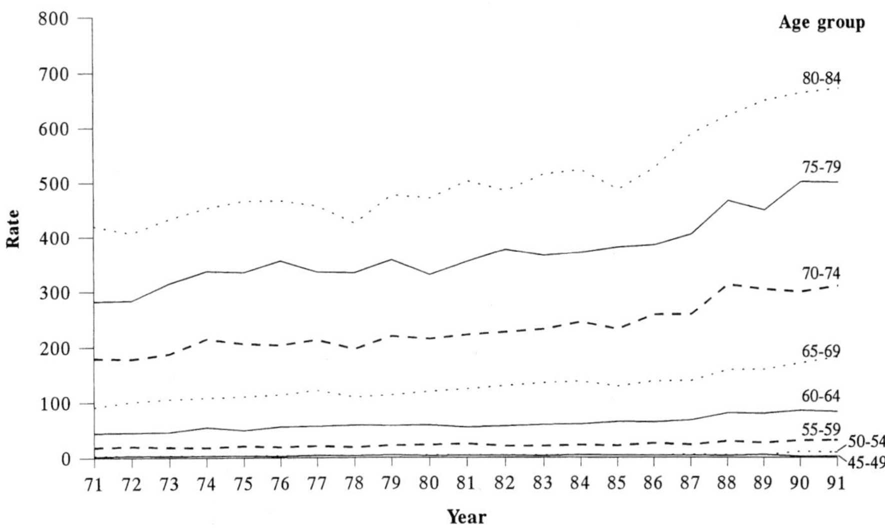

Fig. 2 Rate per 10^5 of newly diagnosed cases of prostate cancer in England and Wales presented by age and year, 1971–1991.

through cancer registries, increased diagnosis due to the use of transurethral prostatectomy and, more recently, screening with prostate specific antigen tests. It is possible, however, that there has also been a true rise in incidence. The 5 year survival rate in men with prostate cancer relative to the general population has been increasing in countries such as US, and England and Wales[7]. As there has been little change in the survival of men with metastatic disease[8], this supports the suggestion that there has been increasing diagnosis of early stage disease. There are no reliable routinely collected data on stage-specific incidence to confirm this.

Screening tests for prostate cancer

Of the three commonly proposed screening tests for prostate cancer – digital rectal examination, transrectal ultrasound, and measurement of serum levels of prostate specific antigen (PSA) – the last of these is currently the most promising, although new markers continue to be identified.

Digital rectal examination

Digital rectal examination has been in use for case finding, or as a screening test for a number of years. The reported sensitivity and specificity are lower than that of PSA[9] and the test may be of limited value in detecting early stage disease[10]. Thus, although its use in combination with PSA may increase the yield and sensitivity of screening slightly, it is likely also to decrease specificity and may be less acceptable as a screening test. Its accuracy is also dependent on the interpretation of the examiner[11]. The use of digital rectal examination can be likened to the addition of clinical examination to mammography; as with the latter, improvements in the accuracy and referral criteria for PSA testing are likely to render the marginal benefit of including digital rectal examination smaller in the future.

Transrectal ultrasound

Transrectal ultrasound has the disadvantage of being a time-consuming and invasive procedure, and is largely now regarded as a secondary diagnostic test rather than an initial screening test; its main use is in the performance of ultrasound guided biopsies.

Prostate specific antigen serum levels

Since the recognition that total PSA values are increased in men with prostate cancer compared with levels in healthy men, considerable work has gone into improving the validity of the test. The aims are firstly to increase the sensitivity and specificity of the test to detect men with cancer, and secondly to distinguish those cancers more likely to progress and to cause morbidity and/or mortality in the lifetime of the man screened. The latter aim is as important as the first in order to avoid considerable over-diagnosis and over-treatment.

Early studies of series of men screened by PSA testing have generally identified a level of total PSA greater than 4 ng/ml as the criteria for further investigation, *i.e.* as the definition of a 'positive screening test'. Further work has concentrated on increasing the specificity, by the identification of additional criteria, particularly for levels in the 4–10 ng/ml range, and improving sensitivity, by identifying additional criteria to be applied when the total PSA is less than 4 ng/ml. The use of age-specific reference levels has been proposed, based on evidence that PSA levels in healthy men increase with age[12]. Other suggested measures include PSA velocity (the rate of change of PSA levels over time)[13], and age-specific PSA velocity[14]. PSA density (serum PSA divided by prostate volume) has also been proposed as a means of distinguishing between prostate cancer and benign prostatic hypertrophy[15].

However, comparisons of PSA levels between studies and over time are potentially hampered by inter-laboratory variation between assays used, with different assays involving different reference levels. In addition, it is now recognised that, in healthy men, the level of PSA may vary in serial samples, with coefficients of variation of 16–24%[16,17], rendering the use of PSA velocity less useful. If the introduction of population screening for prostate cancer were to be considered in the future, reliability of PSA measurements will be of paramount importance.

Currently, the most promising development in PSA measurement is the recognition that the proportion of 'free' PSA, not bound to the two proteins alpha-1-antichymotrypsin and alpha-2-macroglobulin, is lower in men with prostate cancer than in those with benign disease. It has been suggested that the use of free to total PSA ratio may give improved discrimination compared with total PSA when the latter is in the range 4–10 ng/ml[18], with a threshold ratio of 0.15 giving optimum sensitivity and specificity. Again, there is further scope for developing an optimum combination of levels of free and total PSA[19], but the accuracy and repeatability of assays remain crucial[20].

The potential for over-diagnosis

One potential disadvantage of screening is the detection of conditions which are of limited or uncertain relevance to the health and well-being of the man concerned. This includes the detection of non-progressive lesions and the assignment of borderline lesions as malignant. The extent to which routine screening would result in over-diagnosis remains a question of debate. It has been known for many years from autopsy studies that many men at death have undiagnosed prostate cancer, and this has raised concerns that screening might detect a large number of otherwise 'latent' cases. The issue of non-progressive disease is considered here.

One problem with screening for prostate cancer using the PSA test is the possibility that a significant number of the cancers diagnosed might not have caused problems during a man's lifetime, had they been left undetected. This, compounded with the potential morbidity caused by treatment of screen-detected disease, raises concerns about the cost-benefit ratio of screening, even if screening were shown to be effective in reducing mortality from prostate cancer.

The major prognostic factors for prostate cancer at present are stage and histological grade, usually measured by the Gleason score, which is an indicator of malignant potential (Table 1). Several investigators have claimed that the majority of prostate cancers detected by PSA screening are 'clinically significant' and, therefore, that screening will not result in extensive over-diagnosis. For example, in one study of 100 screen-detected

Table 1 Staging prostate cancer by Whitmore-Jewett and TNM classification

Description	Jewett	TNM		
Disease localised to prostate				
Incidental histological finding (TURP)	A	T_1		
Low grade, < 5% specimen	A_1	T_{1a}		
High grade, > 5% specimen	A_2	T_{1b}		
Either identified by needle biopsy or involves both nodes	–	T_{1c}		
Risk recognised clinically	B	T_2		
Tumour confined to 1 lobe	B_1	–		
=1.5 cm: in one lobe with normal prostate on 4 sides	B_{1N}	T_{2a}		
=1.5 cm: :surrounded on 3 sides by normal tissue	B_1	T_{2a}		
> 1.5 cm or tumour in both lobes	B_2	T_{2b}		
Periprostatic disease				
Extension beyond prostate:				
Lateral extension	C_1	T_3	T_4*	
Seminal vesicle extension	C_2	T_3	T_4	
Both	C_3	T_3	T_4	
Distant disease				
Elevated acid phosphatase level only	D_0	T_{1-4}	N_{1-3}[+]	M_{0-1}
Pelvic lymph nodes	D_1	T_{1-4}	N_{0-3}	M_1
Bones, lung, extrapelvic nodal involvement	D_2	T_{1-4}	N_{1-3}	M_0
		T_{1-4}	N_{0-3}	M_1

[+]N_0 no lymph node involvement; N_1 single lymph node, homolateral; N_2 multiple or contralateral lymph nodes; N_3 bulky pelvic lymph nodes; *T_3 penetrates capsule with or without seminal vesicle invasion; and T_4 fixed to periprostatic side wall or adjacent organs.

cases, only 6% were low grade (Gleason score < 5) and 68% had tumour volume > 0.5 ml[21]. However, although PSA testing may be more likely to detect more aggressive disease, the cancer detection rates found in screening series so far suggest that considerable over-diagnosis may still occur. For example, studies from the US have reported detection rates of 3% at initial screen, and of the order of 1% at 6-monthly rescreening[22]. The higher prevalence:incidence ratio indicated by the detection rates at first screen imply a long average preclinical sojourn time and/or the diagnosis of non-progressive disease. However, more information is required on the natural history of prostate cancer to determine whether a latent or non-progressive form exists, or whether this merely represents one end of the distribution of growth rates. At present, it remains unclear what proportion of screen-detected cancers would eventually progress and cause morbidity and/or mortality. Most screening studies reported to date have been based on volunteers or selected populations, and lack information on long-term follow-up[9,22–24]. Results from population-based screening trials, in progress or planned, are needed to provide accurate data not only on detection rates and the prevalence:incidence ratio, but also on what happens to incidence rates in the screened population, both during rescreening and after screening has been completed. Comparison of the cumulative incidence rates in the study and control groups will allow an accurate estimate of the extent of over-diagnosis to be made.

The challenge for future research is to develop methods to differentiate between progressive and non-progressive disease, either by refinements of the PSA test with the use of different measurements or secondary diagnostic tests to determine whether a screen-detected case warrants radical treatment. At present, tumour grade is the best indicator of progression, but the question of whether tumour grade changes over time has not yet been resolved. Data from randomised trials will provide further evidence on the disease natural history.

Treatment issues

One of the prerequisites for the introduction or recommendation of screening is that there should be an available treatment for screen-detected disease. Most prostate cancers detected by routine screening will be localised (Stage T1–T2, Stage A or B; Table 1). Some may be locally extended, and a few may be metastatic. The three main choices of treatment for localised cancer are watchful waiting, radical prostatectomy and external beam radiotherapy. Problems arise with screening due to a lack of evidence regarding the effectiveness of radical treatment, whilst is not clear that there will be any advantage for cancer detected by screening if management is by surveillance only.

Each treatment has advantages and disadvantages. Watchful waiting involves monitoring the progress of the cancer using PSA, digital rectal examination, a record of symptoms, and, where indicated, transrectal ultrasound to monitor local progression as well as bone X-rays and other imaging or biochemical tests. Active treatment is only employed if the cancer appears to progress in stage or to cause symptoms. The advantages are that many men outlive their cancer and die of other causes, so avoiding the side-effects and complications of radical treatment which include incontinence, and impotence. The disadvantages are that some men will go on to develop metastatic disease with all the distress and complications that this will cause. There is also the anxiety associated with the knowledge of having a cancer which is not being treated.

The detailed natural history of untreated prostate cancer remains unclear. Follow-up studies of series of untreated cases provide conflicting results: they are difficult to compare because of different age, stage and grade distributions of the cases, and cannot be readily generalised to cases detected by screening.

Radical prostatectomy involves the removal of the whole prostate gland, without damaging the adjacent neurovascular bundles, by abdominal or perineal surgery. The advantages are that it may provide complete cure of the cancer. The disadvantages are the complications arising from the surgery, the discovery of disease that is not localised and thus may not benefit from surgery, and unnecessary radical treatment of a disease which may never have progressed. Estimates of complication rates vary between studies, but some from the US show 20% of men with non-intermittent incontinence after treatment, over 60% with impotence, and < 1% peri-operative mortality[25,26]. Developments which may help to improve survival or delay progression following radical prostatectomy include: pre-operative endocrine therapy[27]; adjuvant hormone therapy for cases with lesions revised to a more severe stage following surgery[28]; and improved case selection for surgery to identify patients with organ confined disease[29] and to avoid over treatment of insignificant tumours[30].

External beam radiotherapy focuses on the prostate gland plus or minus the seminal vesicles. The advantages are that it can be tolerated by men of varying health and fitness. The disadvantages include complications arising from the procedure, difficulty in monitoring subsequent progress because of damage to surrounding tissues, as well as inaccurate clinical staging and treatment of a disease which might not have been life threatening. Complications include 6.1% with any incontinence, 41% with impotence, 4.5% with urethral stricture, and 2.3% with bowel damage[31]. New developments may well help to improve the outcome of this mode of treatment, including conformal radio-therapy[32,33] downstaging by anti-androgens to reduce the size of the tumour, adjuvant hormone therapy following radiotherapy, and inter-stitial radiotherapy [34].

There are no results available from randomised controlled trials regarding the effectiveness of different treatments. Two trials comparing radical prostatectomy with watchful waiting are now underway in Scandinavia and the US but it will be several years before results become available[8]. In the UK, randomisation of patients into trials of treatment has proved difficult due to patient and clinician preference.

Many non-randomised studies have compared the three modes of treatment but the results are often difficult to interpret because of concerns about biases arising from the selection of patients, and variation in methods and periods of follow-up. One overview of watchful waiting concluded that this was a reasonable choice for some men with grade 1 or 2 clinically localised disease and a life-expectancy of 10 years or less taking co-morbidities into account[35]. Similar conclusions were drawn in a decision analysis comparing the three modes of treatment taking into account a measure for quality of life[36].

Radical prostatectomy or external beam radiotherapy were thought to benefit men aged 65 years or less with moderate to high grade tumours. More recently, a report of cases analysed by 'intention to treat' in the US showed that the survival benefit from radical prostatectomy may have been slightly exaggerated in previous studies which studied only treated patients but, nevertheless, this treatment seem to benefit men even with clinically localised grade 3 tumours[37].

New hopes for the future lie in molecular biology: to identify the cancers that are most likely to progress and would benefit from treatment, and to develop treatments that can specifically target certain functions or points in the cell cycle of the cancer cells. For example, it has recently been shown that the induction of apoptosis by external beam radiotherapy or by hormone therapy may be blocked in patients whose tumours have p53 mutations[38].

Until results of randomised trials become available, clinicians need to help patients make an informed choice of treatment. The current choice of treatment depends mainly on information from clinically based research, as well as personal experience and expertise. The choice varies markedly between countries and between consultants within countries. In the US, radical treatment by prostatectomy is the preferred option whereas in Europe, and Scandinavia, watchful waiting is the first choice[39]. If screening and radical treatment were shown to be effective, countries such as the UK would need considerable extra resources for the management of screen-detected disease.

The effectiveness of screening

Implementation of population screening for prostate cancer requires demonstrable benefit in terms of reducing mortality from prostate cancer. At the present time, this benefit has not been adequately established. The 'gold standard' for demonstrating effectiveness is a randomised controlled trial; other measures, as discussed below, provide supporting but not conclusive information.

It is clear that screening by PSA can detect asymptomatic disease, and current evidence suggests that this will lead to an increasing proportion of earlier stage cancers among screen-detected, as compared with clinically detected, cases. Data on survival indicate an improved prognosis with diagnosis at an early stage; for example, data from the Thames Cancer Registry show 5 year relative survival rates of 72% for localised cases compared with 19% for metastatic cases[8]. However, it cannot be concluded from these findings that screening will necessarily result in a reduction in either the incidence of metastatic disease or mortality from prostate cancer. There are few published data on the survival of prostate cancer cases detected by screening. In any case, comparisons of survival will be affected by lead-time bias, which is the increase in length of survival by the time by which diagnosis is advanced, regardless of any impact on time of death, and by length-bias, which is due to the increased chance of detecting slower-growing cancers which may also have a better prognosis.

A case-control study, in which the history of screening by digital rectal examination in 139 cases of metastatic prostate cancer and matched, disease-free controls was compared, found little apparent effect of screening[40], with a relative risk of 0.9 of metastatic disease in men with one or more screening examinations compared to those with none, after adjustment for racial differences. Again, however, results of such studies need to be interpreted with caution, particularly due to the possible effect of selection bias, whereby those men screened may be at a different underlying risk (either greater or lesser) than those not screened.

It has recently been shown that mortality from prostate cancer in the US has started to fall, and it has been claimed that this may be attributable to earlier diagnosis and screening[41]. However, others have argued that there is no correlation between the size of mortality reduction and either the level of screening or the resulting increased incidence in different states[42].

A true estimate of the effectiveness of screening in reducing mortality from prostate cancer must, therefore, await the results of randomised controlled trials. Trials are currently in progress in the US[43] and Europe[44], although not in the UK.

The financial costs of screening for prostate cancer have not been precisely estimated. Most studies suggest that the cost of detecting one prostate cancer through screening may be less than for other cancers; in one UK pilot study, the cost of detecting one prostate cancer using PSA and digital rectal examination in a general practice setting was estimated to be £1,654[45]. However, in the light of the uncertainties surrounding the effectiveness of screening, the value of the several models which have been developed to estimate the cost-benefit of prostate cancer screening is debatable. All necessarily make assumptions about the natural history of the disease and the effectiveness of treatment which only randomised trials can answer. The financial costs of screening may be offset, in part, by reduced costs of treating metastatic disease. Other 'costs' or disadvantages of screening need to be considered, including the extent of increased morbidity due to over-diagnosis and treatment complications as discussed above, as well as the potential psychological impact of screening. One adverse affect of screening may be increased anxiety, notably among those recalled for further investigation following a positive test, but also at other stages of the screening process. There will also be psychosocial factors associated with the problems of over-diagnosis and the effects of radical treatment. Any man with screen-detected cancer who does not benefit in terms of time of death merely lives longer both with the knowledge of having cancer and with the side-effects of treatment, but, even in those who benefit from screening, these factors must be taken into account.

Guidelines and recommendations

There is increased pressure for guidelines and recommendations on screening for prostate cancer. Organisations which do not currently recommend routine screening include the US Preventive Services Task Force[46], the Canadian Task Force[47], the Cancer Society of New Zealand, the National Health Committee of New Zealand, the Australian Health Technology Advisory Committee[48], the Executive of the Urological Society of Australasia, and the World Health Organization[49]. Two reports commissioned by the National Health Service for England and Wales[8,50] and a summary by the NHS Centre for Reviews and Dissemination[51] also do not support general population screening without evidence from a randomised controlled trial.

In contrast, the American Urological Association and the American Cancer Society[52] have both recommended screening for men aged 50 years and over. The latter proposed annual screening for men with 'average risk', but in the same document recognized that there had been no randomized controlled trial of screening demonstrating a reduction in mortality. In a subsequent revised set of guidelines[5], the American Cancer Society recommended that both the PSA test and digital rectal examination should be offered annually, beginning at age 50 years, to men who have at least a 10 year life expectancy and to younger men who are at high risk. Information should be provided to the men regarding potential risks and benefits of screening.

For a country such as the UK, there are effectively two questions. Should population-based screening for prostate cancer be recommended and introduced nationally? What advice about screening for prostate cancer should be given to individuals consulting their family doctor? The first question is the simplest to answer. Few would argue that there is sufficient evidence on the effectiveness of screening to propose a national policy, with the ethical implications of encouraging participation of healthy men in a programme with no proven benefit and some potential harm. On an individual basis, the solution is less clear. Current recommendations to GPs in this country stress the need to inform men inquiring about PSA testing of the potential benefits and costs of testing, investigation and treatment[51]. Even for the small percentage of men at possible increased risk due to family history, the optimum management is not known.

Recommendations, however, may not always reflect what happens in practice. In the US, a nationwide survey in 1995 showed that 87% of urologists and 76% of primary care physicians 'almost always' requested a PSA test as part of the diagnostic evaluation of men older than 50 years with symptoms suggesting a diagnosis of benign prostatic hypertrophy (BPH)[53]. The proportion of primary care physicians who reported requesting a PSA test as part of health maintenance varied with the age of the patient but was as high as 53% in men aged 80 years or more, most of whom would have a life expectancy of less than 10 years.

In New Zealand, a random survey of 317 family doctors found that about 50% routinely screened some of their male patients aged 50 years or more with PSA and digital rectal examination, including two-thirds of those who reported that they believed the test to be ineffective[54]. About 70% of GPs left the decision about the effectiveness of screening up to their patients and only 5% said that they would refuse to offer a questionable screening test to their patients.

In the UK, a much lower proportion of men are likely to be offered PSA by their family doctor than in the US[8], but the proportion is likely to increase through increasing pressure from the media, public and companies preparing the PSA test kits. In the US, public pressure to be screened is likely to be high.

Conclusions

There is an understandable impatience from urologists in the UK who are unwilling to wait the 10 years or more needed before results from randomised controlled trials of screening become available. However, the potential disadvantages highlighted above mean that evidence from such trials is essential, and that attempts to predict the effect of screening from other data are likely to be subject to bias. The danger is that, if the use of PSA testing continues to increase unchecked, it will become impossible to conduct a randomised trial, either because of the practical difficulty of finding an unscreened control group or because it will no longer be thought ethical to 'deprive' a control group of an intervention thought to be beneficial. The situation will then become akin to that for cervical screening, where evidence of benefit is derived largely from geographical and time trend comparisons, but it is difficult to estimate the magnitude of an effect due to screening.

Acknowledgements

This work was undertaken by the Cancer Screening Evaluation Unit which receives support from the Department of Health; the views expressed in this publication are those of the authors and not necessarily those of the Department of Health.

References

1 Adami H-O, Baron JA, Rothman KJ. Ethics of a prostate cancer screening trial. *Lancet* 1994; **343**: 958–60

2 Coleman MP, Esteve J, Damiecki P, Arslan A, Renard H. *Trends in Cancer Incidence and Mortality*. Lyon: IARC, 1993; 1–806

3 Steimle S. NPCC unifies prostate cancer advocates. *J Natl Cancer Inst* 1997; **89**: 117–8

4 Office for National Statistics. *Mortality Statistics: Cause. England & Wales. 1993 (revised) and 1994. Series DH2 no.21*. London: HMSO, 1996

5 von Eschenbach A, Ho R, Murphy GP, Cunningham M, Lins N. American Cancer Society Guidelines for the early detection of prostate cancer. *Cancer* 1997; **80**: 1805–7

6 Office for National Statistics. *Monitor. Population and Health. Registrations of Cancer Diagnosed in 1991, England and Wales. MB1 96/1*. London: Government Statistical Service, 1996

7 Smart CR. The results of prostate carcinoma screening in the U.S. as reflected in the surveillance, epidemiology, and end results program. *Cancer* 1997; **80**: 1835–44

8 Chamberlain J, Melia J, Moss S, Brown J. Report prepared for the Health Technology Assessment Panel of the NHS Executive on the diagnosis, management, treatment and costs of prostate cancer in England and Wales. *Br J Urol* 1997; **79 (Suppl 3)**: 1–32

9 Mettlin C, Lee F, Drago J. The American Cancer Society National Prostate Cancer Detection Project. Findings on the Detection of Early Prostate Cancer in 2425 men. *Cancer* 1991; **67**: 2949–58

10 Thompson IM, Ernst JJ, Gangai MP, Spence CR. Adenocarcinoma of the prostate: results of routine urological screening. *J Urol* 1984; **132**: 690-2

11 Smith DS, Catalona WJ. Interexaminer variability of digital rectal examination in detecting prostate cancer. *Urology* 1995; **45**: 70–4

12 Oesterling JE, Jacobsen SJ, Chute CG *et al*. Serum prostate-specific antigen in a community-based population of healthy men. Establishment of age-specific reference ranges. *JAMA* 1993; **270**: 860–4

13 Smith DS, Catalona WJ. Rate of change in serum prostate specific antigen levels as a method for prostate cancer detection. *J Urol* 1994; **152**: 1163–7

14 Pearson JD, Carter HB, Metter EJ *et al*. Sensitivity and specificity of age-specific reference ranges for PSA velocity. *Proc Am Urol Assoc* 1995; **153**: 947

15 Benson MC, Whang IS, Pantuck A *et al*. Prostate specific antigen density: a means of distinguishing benign prostatic hypertrophy and prostate cancer. *J Urol* 1992; **147**: 815–6

16 Kadmon D, Weinberg AD, Williams RH *et al*. Pitfalls in interpreting prostate specific antigen velocity. *J Urol* 1996; **155**: 1655–7

17 Stenman UH, Leinonen J, Zhang WM. Problems in the determination of prostate specific antigen. *Eur J Clin Chem Clin Biochem* 1996; **34**: 735–40

18 Akdas A, Cevik I, Tarcan T, Turkeri L, Dalaman G, Emerk K. The role of free prostate-specific antigen in the diagnosis of prostate cancer. *Br J Urol* 1997; **79**: 920–3

19 Bangma CH, Kranse R, Blijenberg BG, Schroder FH. Free and total prostate-specific antigen in a screened population. *Br J Urol* 1997; **79**: 756–62

20 Stamey TA. Some comments on progress in the standardization of immunoassays for prostate-specific antigen. *Br J Urol* 1997; **79**: 49–52

21 Humphrey PA, Keetch DW, Smith DS, Shepherd DL, Catalona WJ. Prospective characterization of pathological features of prostatic carcinomas detected via serum prostate specific antigen based screening. *J Urol* 1996; **155**: 816–20

22 Smith DS, Catalona WJ, Herschman JD. Longitudinal screening for prostate cancer with prostate-specific antigen. *JAMA* 1996; **276**: 1309–15

23 Brawer MK, Chetner MP, Beatie J, Buchner DM, Vessella RL, Lange PH. Screening for prostatic carcinoma with prostate specific antigen. *J Urol* 1992; **147**: 841–5

24 Labrie F, Dupont A, Suburu R *et al.* Serum prostate specific antigen as pre-screening test for prostate cancer. *J Urol* 1992; **147**: 846–52

25 Murphy GP, Mettlin C, Menck H, Winchester DP, Davidson AM. National patterns of prostate cancer treatment by radical prostatectomy: results of a survey by the American College of Surgeons Commission on Cancer. *J Urol* 1994; **152**: 1817–9

26 Wasson JH, Cushman CC, Bruskewitz RC *et al.* A structured literature review of treatment for localized prostate cancer. *Arch Fam Med* 1993; **2**: 487–93

27 Homma Y, Akaza H, Okada K *et al.* Preoperative endocrine therapy for clinical stage A2, B and C prostate cancer: an interim report on short term effects. Prostate Cancer Study Group. *Int J Urol* 1997; **4**: 144–51

28 Ditonno P, Battaglia M, Selvaggi PF. Adjuvant hormone therapy after radical prostatectomy: indications and results. *Tumori* 1997; **83**: 567–75

29 Kupelian P, Katcher J, Levin H *et al.* External beam radiotherapy versus radical prostatectomy for clinical stage T1-2 prostate cancer: therapeutic implications of stratification by pretreatment PSA levels and biopsy Gleason scores. *Cancer J Sci Am* 1997; **3**: 78–87

30 Carter HB, Sauvageot J, Walsh PC, Epstein JI. Prospective evaluation of men with stage T1C adenocarcinoma of the prostate. *J Urol* 1997; **157**: 2206–9

31 Catalona WJ. Management of cancer of the prostate. *N Engl J Med* 1994; **331**: 996–1004

32 Dearnaley DP. Radiotherapy of prostate cancer: established results and new developments. *Semin Surg Oncol* 1995; **11**: 50–9

33 Fukunaga-Johnson N, Sandler HM, McLaughlin PW *et al.* Results of 3D conformal radiotherapy in the treatment of localized prostate cancer. *Int J Radiat Oncol Biol Phys* 1997; **38**: 311–7

34 Grimm P.D, Blasko JC, Ragde H, Sylvester J, Clarke D. Does brachytherapy have a role in the treatment of prostate cancer? *Hematol Oncol Clin North Am* 1996; **10**: 653–73

35 Chodak GW. The role of conservative management in localized prostate cancer. *Cancer* 1994; **74**: 2178–81

36 Fleming C, Wasson JH, Albertsen PC, Barry MJ, Wennberg JE, and the Prostate Disease Patient Outcome Research Team. A decision analysis of alternative treatment strategies for clinically localized prostate cancer. *JAMA* 1993; **269**: 2650–8

37 Lu-Yao GL, Yao S. Population-based study of long-term survival in patients with clinically localised prostate cancer. *Lancet* 1997; **349**: 906–10

38 Grignon DJ, Caplan R, Sarkar FH *et al.* p53 status and prognosis of locally advanced prostatic adenomcarcinoma: a study based on RTOG 8610. *J Natl Cancer Inst* 1997; **89**: 158–65

39 Lange PH. Early detection for prostate cancer? *J Natl Cancer Inst* 1991; **83**: 1199–201

40 Friedman GD, Hiatt RA, Quesenberry Jr CP, Selby JV. Case-control study of screening for prostatic cancer by digital rectal examinations. *Lancet* 1991; **337**: 1526–9

41 Hoeksema MJ, Law C. Cancer mortality rates fall: a turning point for the nation. *J Natl Cancer Inst* 1996; **88**: 1706-7

42 Brawley OW. Prostate carcinoma incidence and patient mortality. The effects of screening and early detection. *Cancer* 1997; **80**: 1857–63

43 Gohagan JK, Prorok PC, Kramer BS, Hayes RB, Cornett JE. The prostate, lung, colorectal, and ovarian cancer screening trial of the National Cancer Institute. *Cancer* 1995; **75**: 1869–73.

44 Auvinen A, Rietbergen JBW, Denis LJ, Schroder FH, Prorok PC, for the International Prostate Cancer Screening Trial Evaluation Group. Prospective evaluation plan for randomised trials of prostate cancer screening. *J Med Screen* 1996; **3**: 97–104

45 Chadwick DJ, Kemple T, Astley JP *et al.* Pilot study of screening for prostate cancer in general practice. *Lancet* 1991; **338**: 613–6

46 US Preventive Services Task Force. Screening for prostate cancer (2nd edn). In: Anonymous *Guide to Clinical Preventive Services*. Baltimore: Williams & Wilkins, 1996; 119–34

47 Canadian Task Force. Canadian guide to clinical preventive health care. In: Anonymous *Canadian Task Force on the Periodic Health Examination*. Ottawa: Canada Communication Group, 1994; 812–23

48 Australian Health Technology Advisory Committee. *Prostate Cancer Screening*. Canberra: Australian Health Technology Advisory Committee, 1996

49 Kuska B. Kiwi conundrum: screening for prostate cancer. *J Natl Cancer Inst* 1997; **89**: 1000

50 Selley S, Donovan J, Faulkner A, Coast J, Gillat D. Diagnosis, management and screening of early localised prostate cancer: a systematic review. *Health Technol Assess* 1997; **1**(2): 1–96

51 NHS Centre for Reviews and Dissemination. Screening for prostate cancer. *Effectiveness Matters* 1997; **2**: 1–4

52 Mettlin C, Murphy GP, Ray P *et al*. American Cancer Society – National Prostate Cancer Detection Project. Results from multiple examinations using transrectal ultrasound, digital rectal examination, and prostate specific antigen. *Cancer* 1993; **71**: 891–8

53 Barry MJ, Roberts RG. Indications of PSA testing. *JAMA* 1977;.**277**: 955–6

54 Morris J, McNoe B. Screening for prostate cancer: what do general practitioners think? *NZ Med J* 1997; **110**: 178–82

Should we be screening for colorectal cancer?

Michael H E Robinson and **Jack D Hardcastle***

*Department of Surgery, City Hospital NHS Trust, Nottingham, UK and *Department of Surgery, University Hospital, Nottingham, UK*

Mass population screening for asymptomatic neoplastic disease is now national policy in the UK for breast cancer and has been established for many years in the early diagnosis of carcinoma of the cervix. Cancer screening is based on the concept that treatment is more effective when the disease is localised and aims to detect it when it is at a less advanced clinico-pathological stage prior to the development of symptoms. Because colorectal cancer develops in benign adenomatous polyps which are often amenable to endoscopic resection, screening may both reduce the incidence of the disease as well as improving outcome from it. Flexible sigmoidoscopy screening focuses mainly on the detection of potentially malignant adenomas, their endoscopic removal producing a decrease in colorectal cancer incidence. It is a promising approach but conclusive data on effectiveness from a Medical Research Council-sponsored multicentre randomised controlled trial will not be available before 2006. Faecal occult blood testing aims to preferentially detect early stage invasive disease. Three randomised controlled trials of faecal occult blood screening show that the disease can be detected earlier in its development leading to reduced mortality from the disease – and that this is achieved at reasonable cost. The Department of Health is currently giving consideration to its national implementation.

Colorectal cancer: the problem

Correspondence to: Mr
Michael H E Robinson,
Consultant Surgeon, City
Hospital NHS Trust,
Hucknall Road,
Nottingham NG5 1PB, UK

After carcinoma of the bronchus, colorectal cancer kills more people than any other malignancy in the developed Western world. Currently, more than 24,000 new cases and 17,000 deaths from the disease are being reported in England and Wales annually[1]. Gender differences in incidence, prognosis and mortality are small. Prognosis is largely determined by the extent of spread of the disease at presentation, corrected 5 year survival figures of 30–40% reflecting that the majority of patients still present with lymph node or distant metastases (Fig. 1)[2]. Slight improvements in survival have been matched by an increasing incidence of the disease in Great Britain, so that death rates have

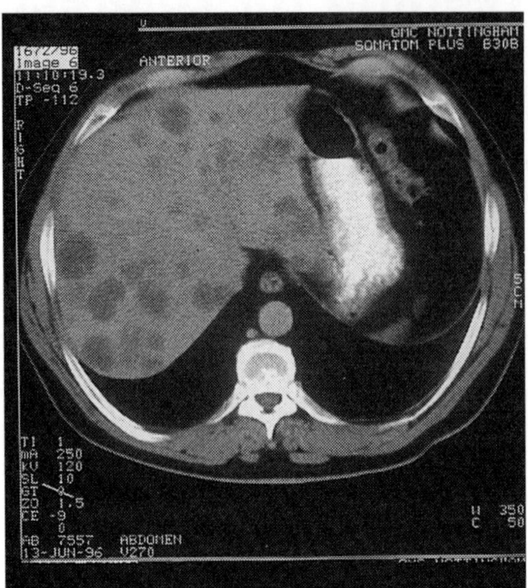

Fig. 1 A CT scan showing multiple liver metastases (from a primary rectal cancer) at initial presentation.

changed little for 40 years. Public health measures to reduce disease incidence require a greater understanding of aetiological (probably largely dietary) factors as well as a willingness by the population to accept changes in life-style. They are unlikely to have any impact for decades. While recent reports of peri-operative radiotherapy[3,4] and chemotherapy[5] are encouraging for Dukes' B and C tumours, currently the most promising potential method for improving disease prognosis would seem to be screening for asymptomatic early stage disease.

Justification for screening

The basis for screening relates to the biology and natural history of the disease. There is widely accepted evidence that most colorectal cancers slowly develop in stepwise fashion from normal mucosa through enlarging adenomatous polyps to localised surgically curable malignancy, eventually culminating in disseminated incurable disease[6,7].

The purpose of screening for colorectal cancer is to reduce mortality from this condition through the early detection of cancers and large adenomas in asymptomatic individuals in the population. Treatment of confirmed cases of cancer may lead to improved cure rates for colorectal cancer and, as a result of the detection of large adenomas, a reduction in its incidence.

Certain screening tests aim primarily to detect early stage invasive disease (e.g. faecal occult blood screening) with treatments leading to improvements in colorectal cancer cure rates. This is analogous to breast cancer screening by the mammographic detection of early breast cancers. Other screening tests (*e.g.* flexible sigmoidoscopy screening) focus mainly on the detection of potentially malignant adenomas, their endoscopic removal producing a decrease in colorectal cancer incidence. This is similar to screening for cervical cancer through Pap smear detection of premalignant cervical neoplasia.

The incidence of colorectal cancer increases exponentially with age, those over 50 years old making up only 37% of the population yet accounting for 95% of cases and more than 96% of deaths[1]. To be cost-effective, screening needs to be applied to this older age group ('average risk') unless other risk factors for colorectal cancer apply.

Issues of cost-effectiveness

The issue of cost-effectiveness, and the way that information is presented, is critical. It is often said that 'the most expensive treatment is one that doesn't work'. In this era of evidence-based medicine, this might be extended to 'the most expensive treatment is one that hasn't been shown to work'.

Effectiveness

Effectiveness of a cancer screening programme must be measured by its ability to reduce disease-specific mortality and morbidity. (However, it is also important to understand that, since colorectal cancer – like breast cancer – accounts for only 2% of all deaths, any reasonable reduction in disease-specific mortality will not impact on overall mortality.) Because of selection, length and lead-time biases, effectiveness can only reliably be measured in the setting of a randomised controlled trial with reduction in disease-specific mortality as the end-point.

Presentation of data – theory

Effectiveness data may be presented in different ways[8]. A doctor may want to know about the relative reduction in mortality or the absolute reduction in mortality expressed in percentage terms. The number of deaths prevented each year through screening (absolute reduction in real terms) may, however, be more meaningful. The public may understand more clearly the number of people that need to be screened (of which they may be one) to prevent a single colorectal cancer death. They may also wish to know what chance they have of coming to harm as a consequence of screening in relation to their chance of benefiting from screening.

Presentation of data – example

An example of this presentation of data in terms of the number needed to treat or the number that need to be harmed to produce the desired outcome is given in relation to a Swedish randomised controlled trial of short-course pre-operative radiotherapy in patients with rectal cancer[3,4]. In the control group not receiving radiotherapy there were 150 local recurrences in 557 patients treated (27%). In the treated group only 63 of 553 patients (11%) developed local recurrence. This could be presented as a 58% (*i.e.* [27%–11%]/27%) relative reduction in local recurrence rate or a 16% (i.e. 27%–11%) absolute reduction[3]. Alternatively, 6 individuals need to be treated with radiotherapy to prevent one person developing local recurrence: this is the number needed to treat, calculated as the inverse of the absolute reduction in local recurrence. Because 235 (43%) patients undergoing preoperative radiotherapy suffered one or more complications compared with 182 (33%) in the surgery only group, 53 (235–182) additional patients suffered a complication to prevent local recurrence in 87 (150–63). Therefore, approximately one person needed to be harmed for every two in whom local recurrence was prevented by radiotherapy: this is the number needed to be harmed. Clearly, these estimates will be affected by the desired outcome chosen and the definition of 'harm'. However, they are an important development in the presentation of research data to the public at large and in the presentation of risk and benefit to individual patients.

Costs

However it is presented, effectiveness has to be measured against the costs that are incurred in producing the benefit. These have to be acceptable to both the population and, particularly, the government that serves it. Costs are usefully presented in terms of the cost per cancer detected; the cost per life or year of life saved; or the cost per quality-adjusted-life year (QALY) saved. The increasingly open debate about rationalising (or rationing!) health care has rightly led to a greater emphasis on health economics[9].

Potential screening tests

A screening test should be inexpensive, rapid and simple and is not intended to be diagnostic, those with positive tests requiring further evaluation[10]. The use of symptom questionnaires is ineffective because colorectal symptoms are common and poorly predictive and because the presence of symptoms may signify more advanced disease[11]. Digital rectal examination will detect no more than 10% of cancers while rigid sigmoidoscopy will adequately visualise only the distal 16 cm[12] allowing detection of, at most, 40% of all colorectal cancers. The method is further disadvantaged by the fact that it is unpleasant and inconvenient. However, a recent case-control study of the efficacy of screening sigmoidoscopy in the setting of regular health checks has shown a significant 70% reduction in death from rectosigmoid (but not colon) cancer[13].

Flexible sigmoidoscopy

Following a simple enema, fibreoptic flexible sigmoidoscopy allows direct examination of the distal 30–60 cm where 70% of cancers and large adenomas are found. Though more costly, it is better tolerated than rigid sigmoidoscopy and yield is significantly greater[12]. A small case-control study of flexible sigmoidoscopy screening found a 79% (95% CI 48–92%) reduction in the risk of dying from cancer distal to the splenic flexure[14]. Furthermore, the economic and logistic problems of population screening by this means may be offset by training nurse or family doctor endoscopists[15]. The case for once-only flexible sigmoidoscopy·screening has been well argued by Atkin et al[16]. It centres around a number of key points. Firstly, the aim is detection and subsequent removal of adenomatous polyps. This should lead to a reduction in colorectal cancer incidence and, therefore, mortality. Secondly, the relatively high cost of the test is offset by the fact that it is carried out once only (because of its high sensitivity and the long sojourn time of the adenoma-carcinoma sequence). Thirdly, evidence that single small (< 1 cm) tubular adenomas in the left colon are not predictive of increased risk of subsequent colon cancer[17] means fewer individuals will need to undergo colonoscopy which is relatively expensive. It is currently being evaluated in a UK multicentre randomised controlled trial. Early data from this study suggest compliance with flexible sigmoidoscopy of 45%; and that 6% of subjects will need to progress to colonoscopy[18]. However, incidence and mortality results from this important trial will not be available until about 2006.

Colonoscopy

Colonoscopy is the gold standard for assessment of large bowel mucosa but it is a labour-intensive, expensive examination with a serious complication rate (perforation and haemorrhage) of 0.2%[19]. While probably not suitable as a screening tool, it is the means of surveillance of choice for high-risk patients, particularly those with long-standing ulcerative colitis and those from hereditary non-polyposis syndrome kindreds, where proximal lesions predominate. The ability to carry out snare polypectomy at the same time as diagnosis makes it particularly suited as the secondary investigation of subjects with positive faecal occult blood tests.

Double contrast barium enema

Though less sensitive than colonoscopy[20], it is safer and cheaper. However, it is invasive and requires mechanical bowel preparation. Few studies have evaluated it as a screening test. Mathematical models have suggested that it may be a very cost-effective means of screening[21], but there are no published trial data to support this and we are unaware of any current trials.

Faecal occult blood tests

Introduction: In 1971, Greegor reported twelve cases of 'silent' colon cancer detected by the use of guaiac impregnated slides[22]. Since then,

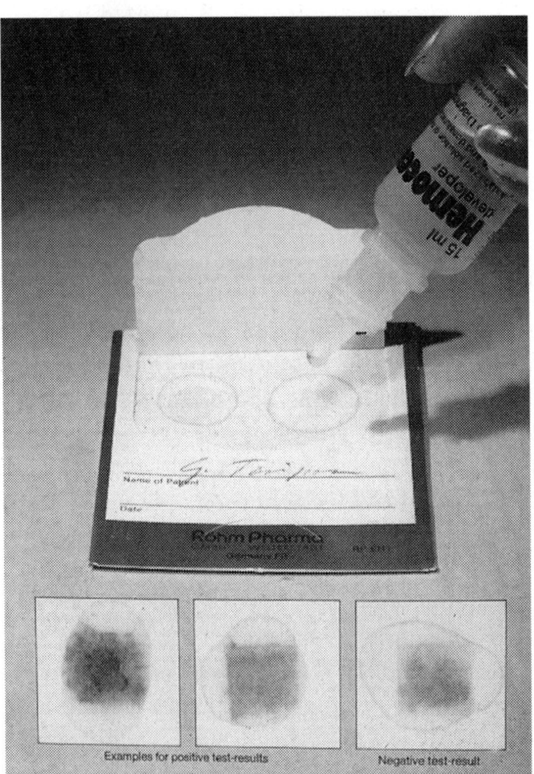

Fig. 2 Developing a Haemoccult test card. A blue colour reaction denotes a positive test result.

guaiac-based faecal occult blood tests, in particular Haemoccult® (SmithKline Diagnostics, San Jose, CA, USA), have become the most widely evaluated means of population screening for colorectal cancer (Fig. 2). The test detects the peroxidase-like activity of haematin in faeces. A significant drawback is the interference from ingested animal haemoglobin and from certain vegetables (broccoli, cauliflower, parsnip) containing naturally occurring peroxidases. While normal blood loss from the gastro-intestinal tract is approximately 1 ml per day, Haemoccult will detect losses of 10 ml per day or more in 67% of cases[23]. Because of substantial overlap between normal and pathological bleeding, this allows for reasonable test sensitivity without resulting in large numbers of false positive results and hence low specificity. By specifically detecting human haemoglobin, immunological tests avoid the problem of dietary interference and are potentially more sensitive[24]. False-positive reactions from upper gastro-intestinal tract bleeding (because of rapid digestion of haemoglobin in the stomach and small bowel) are also less likely although this may be offset by higher detection rates of innocent perianal bleeding. These immunological tests are being simplified and warrant further investigation.

Trial: *(a) Compliance, positive rate and yield.* Several studies and programmes around the world to evaluate screening with Haemoccult confirm its potential. In the controlled studies[25-30], 60–90% of the population offered screening faecal occult blood tests completed at least one while 38–60% accepted every invitation. There were similar rates of positive reactions for unrehydrated slides (1.0–2.3%), similar predictive values for all neoplasia (22–58%), for cancer (5–18%) and a significant shift towards Dukes' stage A cancers (21–26% in the group offered

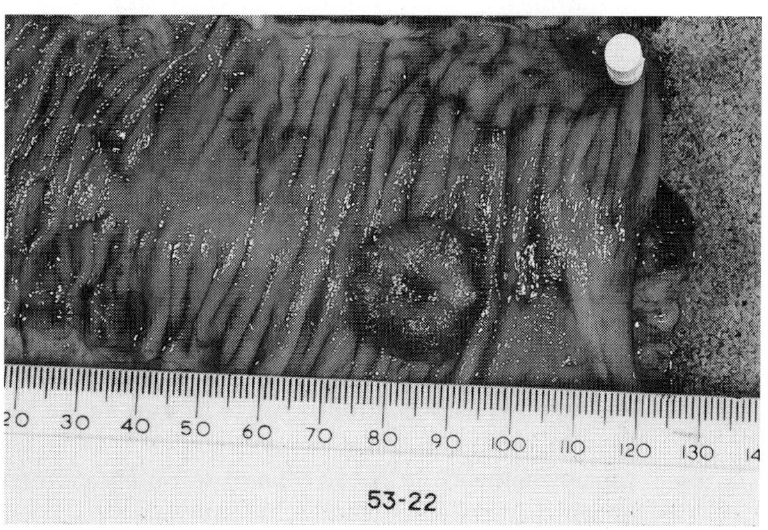

Fig. 3 A small screen-detected Dukes' stage A colonic cancer. Note the traces of blood on the specimen.

screening *versus* 9–13% in the control group for the European studies). Sensitivity can only be measured indirectly by assessing the proportion of cancers presenting in the interval between tests and is estimated at 46–81%, the rectum and caecum being the sites where cancers are most likely to be missed[31]. All data indicate an improved sensitivity for cancers after rehydration (addition of a drop of water to the slide before development) but, because of loss of specificity when the tests are rehydrated (positive rate 6.1–10.2%)[25,28], this practice is probably not cost-effective. Complete evaluation of the colon is necessary in patients with positive faecal occult blood tests and has been achieved in more than 90% of cases within the trials. To maintain these high levels outside a trial setting, physician as well as patient education and clear guidelines as to investigation of individuals with positive test results will be needed. The centrally administered model of screening, so successful for breast cancer screening, is likely to be the best way to ensure such programme efficiency.

(b) Mortality. (i) Case control studies. However, while these parameters are encouraging, screening can only be judged by its ability to reduce disease-specific mortality at a reasonable cost. In the last 5 years, a number of studies have reported mortality reduction with faecal occult blood screening. Six well-designed case-control studies from countries with established regional or national screening programmes (two from the US, two from Japan and one each from Germany and Italy[32–36a]), have shown a 31–60% reduction in the risk of dying from colorectal cancer in those screened (Table 1). They are, however, subject to selection bias. *(ii) Randomised controlled trials.* The strongest evidence for effectiveness comes from the three randomised controlled trials which have reported mortality data, demonstrating a 15–33% statistically significant reduction in mortality[25–27]. In Nottingham, UK,[26] and Funen, Denmark[27], the trial design was similar and a meta-analysis of these two trials found a 16% (95% CI: 6–25) reduction in mortality from screening. The data from the Nottingham trial can be used to illustrate the different ways in which effectiveness can be presented. A 15% relative reduction in mortality is also an absolute reduction in mortality of one death per 10,000 person years of screening[26]. Alternatively, 1254 individuals have to be offered screening (or 746 individuals have to accept screening) to prevent one colorectal cancer death while one person is sufficiently harmed by colonoscopy to require surgery for every ten colorectal cancer deaths prevented.

(c) Incidence: Any effect on disease incidence as a result of polypectomy will require prolonged follow-up to be seen. In the Minnesota study[25] at 17 year follow-up, there is a non-significant 20% reduction in colorectal cancer incidence in those offered screening compared with the control group (J Mandel, personal communication). Though none of the other

Table 1 Case control studies of colorectal cancer screening using faecal occult blood test

Author	Population	FOBT	Exposure	Results (including odds ratio)	Conclusions
Hiwatashi et al 1993[36a]	Residents of 3 municipalities in which FOBT was available from 1983–90 *Cases:* 28 deaths before 3/91 with access to screening *Controls:* population matched for sex, age + residential	Immunological	Having at least one screen within 3 years of diagnosis of the case as noted in records of the Miyagi Cancer Society	FOBT within 3 years of diagnosis; adjusted OR 0.24 (0.08–0.76)	Screening is effective although selection bias is possible
Wahrendorf et al 1993[34]	Population with access to annual FOBT *Cases:* 522 CRC deaths aged 55–75 years, 372 analysed *Controls:* age-matched, 5 from each case's GP or gynaecologist	Haemoccult	Screening history within the 6 months to 3 years prior to diagnosis of case as noted in files of referring GP or gynaecologist	FOBT performed on asymptomatic individuals 6–36 months prior to diagnosis Women: 0.43 (0.27–0.68) Men: 0.92 (0.61–1.75); very low rate of acceptance of screening by men	Screening is effective in women
Selby et al 1993[32]	Members of HMO *Cases:* 486 CRC deaths *Controls:* 727 matched for age, sex, date of entry to plan; included history of polyps + CRC	Haemoccult	Screening history in 5 years prior to diagnosis of case	FOBT within 1 yr: 0.73 (0.50–1.05) FOBT within 2 yr: 0.76 (0.55–1.03) FOBT within 5 yr: 0.69 (0.52–0.91)	Findings consistent with 25–30% reduction in risk due to screening
Lazovich et al 1995[35]	Members of HMO Offered biennial FOBT since 1983, without prior diagnostic sigmoidoscopy or adenomatous polyps *Cases:* 236 CRC deaths between 1986–91 *Controls:* 457 matched for birth year, sex, year of HMO enrolment HMO, excluded history of chronic bowel disease or CRC before diagnosis of case	Haemoccult	FOBT performed in absence of gastro-intestinal symptoms Examination of time between screening + reference date (date of clinical suspension of CRC) and site of screening (home or office)	Ever scr.: 0.72 (0.51–1.02) Home scr.: 0.71 (0.50–1.00) Office scr.: 0.95 (0.67–1.36) $\leq$ 74: 0.65 (0.44–0.97) $\geq$ 75: 0.98 (0.49–1.96) Screened $\leq$ 3 years before reference date: 0.87 (0.63–1.22)	44% of cases + 76% of controls with positive FOBT had limited diagnostic work-up Small benefit possible
Saito et al 1995[33]	Residents of a district in which FOBT was offered from 1986. *Cases:* 193 CRC deaths *Controls:* 577 controls matched for age and sex	Immunological	Screening history in 5 years prior to diagnosis of case	FOBT within 1 yr: 0.40 (0.17–0.92) FOBT within 2 yr: 0.41 (0.20–0.82) FOBT within 3 yr: 0.48 (0.25–0.92)	
Zappa et al 1997[36]	Residents of a district in which FOBT was offered 2 yearly from 1982 *Cases:* 206 CRC deaths before 1991 *Controls:* 1030 matched for age and sex	Haemoccult		Adjusted odds ratio Ever screened: 0.60 (95%, CI 0.4–0.9). Screened within 3 years of diagnosis: 0.84 (95% CI 0.3–0.9)	

FOBT, faecal occult blood test; CRC, colorectal cancer; HMO, health maintenance organisation; scr., screened.

trials are sufficiently mature, it is encouraging that the adenoma yield is high in all studies. While more than 90% of prevalent adenomas are smaller than 1 cm, 63% of those detected by screening in Nottingham (8/1000 screened) have been larger than 1 cm[26].

Costs of screening

Even if screening is shown to be effective, the magnitude of the effect must be sufficiently great to justify the cost to the nation. The cost per cancer detected by Haemoccult in the Nottingham study has been estimated at less than £2700[37], a figure which compares favourably with the costs of cancer detection by cervical smear or mammography. Recent data on cost per year of life saved in the same study[38] also compare well with similar data on mammographic screening. Mathematical models have provided estimates of cost-effectiveness and cost-benefit. Ransohoff has suggested that it would cost $1200 million to screen the American population over the age of 50 years[39]. The US Congress Office of Technology Assessment has constructed a model of the cost-effectiveness of annual faecal occult blood test screening in a population from the age of 65 years using data and assumptions that were unfavourable towards screening. They found that it would prevent approximately 23,000 cases of colorectal cancer and provide 45,000 added years of life to that population of 2.1 million. They estimated a cost of $35,000 per year of life gained, again similar to the costs of breast cancer screening[40]. Two other distinct models of the cost-effectiveness of colorectal cancer screening have been produced with differing assumptions built in[21,41]. Both publish estimates of the cost per life-year saved from screening by FOB testing alone, FOB testing with flexible sigmoidoscopy, colonoscopy and barium enema – with costs varying greatly according to the interval between screening. Estimated cost for annual FOB testing is about $15,000 compared to $80,000 for annual barium enema or $170,000 for annual colonoscopy, per life-year saved. Extending the interval for barium enema and colonoscopy to 5 yearly reduces the cost to a quarter of that for annual examination. Atkin estimated the cost per cancer prevented by once-only flexible sigmoidoscopy at $12,500[16]. With a projected gain of 7 years of life per case, their equivalent cost is less than $2000 per life-year saved – at least an order of magnitude less than the other screening modalities. This figure clearly requires verification.

Risks of screening

The risks of physical harm and psychological morbidity associated with colorectal cancer screening have, until recently, received scant attention. Two reports, both based on prospectively collected data from the

Nottingham trial, suggest that there is little objectively measured psychological harm due to the screening process[42]. Similarly physical harm is limited. There is no evidence that inappropriate reassurance from a falsely negative test worsens the outlook, nor that cancers are being diagnosed and treated that would not have presented during the patient's remaining lifetime. However, a tangible harm arising from screening were seven major complications from colonoscopy (rate = 0.5%) adding to morbidity but not mortality[43].

Should we be screening for colorectal cancer?

While Canada and most European countries have made no recommendations on colorectal screening, five national US expert groups have suggested annual faecal occult blood testing and 3–5 yearly flexible sigmoidoscopy for their population over 50 years. These recommendations have been recently unified[44].

The available evidence for faecal occult blood test screening is now compelling – in terms of effectiveness and cost. Indeed, there is little to choose between the data on mammographic screening for breast cancer and faecal occult blood test screening for colorectal cancer. The former has been implemented as a national screening programme in the UK since the 1980s, while the latter is currently under consideration by the UK Department of Health. There is compelling evidence of effectiveness and cost-effectiveness of screening in reducing colorectal cancer mortality. However, implementation of such a programme (even if based only on biennial FOB testing) will require substantial investment in developing the existing endoscopic infrastructure; and in the training of sufficient numbers of skilled colonoscopists. Antagonists would argue that screening is inappropriate. This is based on the arguement that substantial resources are diverted away from needy symptomatic patients (e.g. long waiting lists for hip replacements) towards the 'worried well'.

The future

Results from a trial investigating the effectiveness of once-only flexible sigmoidoscopy in reducing the incidence of colorectal cancer will not be available until the year 2006.

Research into alternative serum, faecal or urine markers, possibly genetic[45], of the disease is required. Appropriate immunological faecal occult blood tests require assessment in representative populations. Since most interval cancers are left-sided, adding flexible sigmoidoscopy to Haemoccult screening may increase sensitivity and specificity for cancer detection. Furthermore, flexible sigmoidoscopy allows for detection of a much higher proportion of potentially malignant adenomas which are mainly located in the left colon. Therefore, the two tests are complementary and combine a modality aiming to detect early cancers (and large adenomas secondarily) throughout the colon, with another, the emphasis of which is to detect large adenomas (and carcinomas secondarily) mainly in the left colon.

Virtual colonoscopy (reconstruction of the colon based on 3D computed tomography) is now a realistic possibility. Advantages are that there is no need for sedation; the examination is non-invasive and, therefore, more acceptable; and it may be possible to 'subtract' the stool from the image, thereby abolishing the need for bowel preparation. Finally, like flexible sigmoidoscopy screening, a once-only examination should suffice. Disadvantages are the radiation dosage (though this is no greater than that needed for barium enema) and cost. However, the cost of hardware and software will fall while scan/reconstruction times are now less than 10 min for the most powerful systems.

Individuals with a family history of colorectal cancer

For this group, the most pressing need is to develop methods which accurately quantify an individual's risk of subsequent cancer. Genetic markers may be useful in this respect. Although theoretically attractive, genetic testing of individuals with a positive family history may not achieve a high sensitivity because of the large number of potential mutations that can occur in sporadic colorectal cancer. There is no evidence to support screening of those with a positive family history. Furthermore, it is unlikely that a randomised trial would be considered ethical or feasible given the current widespread, albeit haphazard, surveillance.

Screening may then be tailored according to individual risk either by changing the age at which screening starts, the frequency of testing or finally by employing more sensitive tests, either alone or in combination. The converse of this may be the identification of individuals with a particularly low risk of the disease who do not need to be screened at all. At present, practice throughout the UK varies widely with very large numbers of individuals undergoing too frequent too extensive investigation[46]. National guidelines to support consistent practice are urgently needed.

Conclusions

- Colorectal cancer is a major public health problem accounting for 17,000 deaths in England and Wales each year. This represents 12% of all deaths from malignancy, more than breast and cervical cancer combined.

- Faecal occult blood screening has been shown to significantly reduce mortality and is cost-effective.

- Flexible sigmoidoscopy screening is a promising alternative or adjunct to faecal occult blood screening but conclusive data from trials will not be available before 2006.

- Facilities for colonoscopy and flexible sigmoidoscopy within the UK would need to be strengthened if screening was introduced.

- There is no evidence to support screening of those with a positive family history.

- The evidence for the benefits of faecal occult blood screening from the Haemoccult trials is now strong. What remains to be seen is whether there is a public and political will to support its implementation nationally.

References

1   Office of Population Censuses and Surveys. *Mortality Statistics by Cause. England and Wales 1992*. Series DH2, No 20. London: HMSO, 1995

2   Stower MJ, Hardcastle JD. The results of 1115 patients with colorectal cancer treated over an 8-year period in a single hospital. *Eur J Surg Oncol* 1985; **11**: 119–23

3   Swedish Rectal Cancer Trial. Improved survival with preoperative radiotherapy in resectable rectal cancer. *N Engl J Med* 1997; **336**: 980–7

4   Swedish Rectal Cancer Trial. Initial report from a Swedish multicentre study examining the role of preoperative irradiation in the treatment of patients with resectable rectal carcinoma. *Br J Surg* 1993; **80**: 1333–6

5   IMPACT. Efficacy of adjuvant fluorouracil and folinic acid in colon cancer. *Lancet* 1995; **345**: 939–44

6   Fearon ER, Vogelstein B. A genetic model for colorectal tumourigenesis. *Cell* 1990; **61**: 759–67

7   Morson BC. Evolution of cancer of the colon and rectum. *Cancer* 1974; **34**: 845–9

8   Abbasi K. Headlines: more perilous than pills? *BMJ* 1998; **316**: 82

9   Smith R. Rationing health care: moving the debate forward. *BMJ* 1996; **312**: 1553–4

10 Wilson JMG, Jungner G. *Principles and Practice of Screening for Disease*. WHO: Geneva 1968 (Public Health Papers No 34)

11 Farrands PA, Hardcastle JD. Colorectal screening by a self-completion questionnaire. *Gut* 1984; **25**: 445–7

12 Marks G, Boggs HW, Castro AF, Gathright JB, Ray JE, Salvati E. Sigmoidoscopic examinations with rigid and flexible sigmoidoscopes in the surgeon's office: a comparative prospective study of effectiveness in 1012 cases. *Dis Colon Rectum* 1979; **22**: 162–8

13 Selby JV, Friedman GD, Quesenberry CP, Weiss NS. A case-control study of screening sigmoidoscopy and mortality from colorectal cancer. *N Engl J Med* 1992; **326**: 653–7

14 Newcomb PA, Norfleet RG, Storer BE, Surawicz TS, Marcus PM. Screening sigmoidoscopy and colorectal cancer mortality. *J Natl Cancer Inst* 1992; **84**: 1572–5

15 Maule WF. Screening for colorectal cancer by nurse endoscopists. *N Engl J Med* 1994; **330**: 183–7

16 Atkin WS, Cuzick J, Northover JM, Whynes DK. Prevention of colorectal cancer by once-only sigmoidoscopy. *Lancet* 1993; **341**: 736–40

17 Atkin WS, Morson BC, Cuzick J. Long-term risk of colorectal cancer after excision of rectosigmoid adenomas. *N Engl J Med* 1992; **326**: 658

18 Atkin WS, Hart AR, Edwards R *et al*. Uptake, yield of neoplasia and adverse effects of flexible sigmoidoscopy screening. *Gut* 1998; **42**: 560–5.

19 Macrae FA, Tan KG, Williams CB. Towards safer colonoscopy: a report on the complications of 5000 diagnostic or therapeutic colonoscopies. *Gut* 1983; **24**: 376–83

20 Rex DK, Rahmani EY, Haseman JH, Lemmel GT, Kastor S, Buckley JS. Relative sensitivity of colonoscopy and barium enema for detection of colorectal cancer in clinical practice. *Gastroenterology* 1997; **112**: 17–23

21 Eddy DM. Screening for colorectal cancer. *Ann Intern Med* 1990; **113**: 373–84

22 Greegor DH. Occult blood testing for detection of asymptomatic colon cancer. *Cancer* 1971; **28**: 131–4

23 Stroehlein JR, Fairbanks VF, McGill BD, Go VLW. Haemoccult detection of faecal occult blood quantitated by radioassay. *Am J Dig Dis* 1976; **21**: 841–4

24 Robinson MHE, Marks CG, Farrands PA, Bostock K, Hardcastle JD. Screening for colorectal cancer with an immunological faecal occult blood test: 2 year followup. *Br J Surg* 1996; **83**: 500–1

25 Mandel JS, Bond JH, Church TR *et al*. Reducing mortality from colorectal cancer by screening for fecal occult blood. *N Engl J Med* 1993; **328**: 1365–71

26 Hardcastle JD, Chamberlain JO, Robinson MHE *et al*. Randomised controlled trial of faecal occult blood screening for colorectal cancer. *Lancet* 1996; **348**: 1472–7

27 Kronborg O, Fenger C, Olsen J, Jorgensen OD, Sondergaard O. Randomised study of screening for colorectal cancer with faecal-occult-blood test. *Lancet* 1996; **348**: 1467–71

28 Kewenter J, Brevinge H, Engaras B, Haglind E, Ahren C. Results of screening, rescreening and follow-up in a prospective randomised study for detection of colorectal cancer by faecal occult blood testing. Results for 68,308 subjects. *Scand J Gastroenterol* 1994; **29**: 468–73

29 Winawer SJ, Flehinger BJ, Schottenfeld D, Miller DG. Screening for colorectal cancer with fecal occult blood testing and sigmoidoscopy. *J Natl Cancer Inst* 1993; **85**: 1311–8

30 Faivre J, Arveux P, Milan C, Durand G, Lamour J, Bedenne L. Participation in mass screening for colorectal cancer: results of screening and rescreening from the Burgundy study. *Eur J Cancer Prev* 1991; **1**: 49–55

31 Thomas WM, Hardcastle JD, Jackson J, Pye G. Chemical and immunological testing for faecal occult blood: a comparison of two tests in symptomatic patients. *Br J Cancer* 1992; **65**: 618–20

32 Selby JV, Friedman GD, Quesenberry CP, Weiss NS. Effect of fecal occult blood testing on mortality from colorectal cancer: a case-control study. *Ann Intern Med* 1993; **118**: 1294–7

33 Saito H, Soma Y, Koeda J *et al*. Reduction in risk of mortality from colorectal cancer by fecal occult blood screening with immunochemical hemagglutination test. A case-control study. *Int J Cancer* 1995; **61**: 465–9

34 Wahrendorf J, Robra BP, Wiebelt H, Oberhausen R, Weiland M, Dhom G. Effectiveness of colorectal cancer screening: results from a population-based case-control evaluation in Saarland, Germany. *Eur J Cancer Prev* 1993; **2**: 221–7

35 Lazovich DA, Weiss NS, Stevens NG, White E, McKnight B, Wagner EH. A case-control study to evaluate efficacy of screening faecal occult blood. *J Med Screen* 1995; **2**: 84–9

36 Zappa M, Castiglione G, Grazzini G *et al*. Effect of faecal occult blood testing on colorectal cancer mortality: results of a population-based case-control study in the district of Florence, Italy. *Int J Cancer* 1997; **73**: 208–10

36a Hiwatashi N, Morimoto T, Fukao A *et al*. An evaluation of mass screening using faecal occult blood test for colorectal cancer in Japan. *Jpn J Cancer Res* 1993; **84**: 1110–12

37 Whynes DK, Walker AR, Chamberlain JO, Hardcastle JD. Screening and the costs of treating colorectal cancer. *Br J Cancer* 1993; **68**: 965–8

38 Whynes DK, Neilsen A, Walker AR, Hardcastle JD. Randomised controlled trial of faecal occult blood screening for colorectal cancer: an economic analysis. *Health Econ* 1998; In press

39 Ransohoff DF, Lang CA. Screening for colorectal cancer. *N Engl J Med* 1991; **325**: 37–41

40 Wagner JL, Herdman RC, Wadhwa S. Cost effectiveness of colorectal cancer screening in the elderly. *Ann Int Med* 1991; **115**: 807–17

41 Byers T, Gorsky R. Estimates of costs and effects of screening for colorectal cancer in the United States. *Cancer* 1992; **70**: 1288–95

42 Parker MA, Robinson MHE, Chamberlain JO, Hardcastle JD. The psychological risks of faecal occult blood screening for colorectal cancer. Submitted

43 Robinson MHE, Hardcastle JD, Chamberlain JO *et al*. The risks of screening: data from the Nottingham randomised controlled trial of faecal occult blood screening for colorectal cancer. Submitted

44 Winawer SJ, Fletcher RH, Miller L *et al*. Colorectal cancer screening: clinical guidelines and rationale. *Gastroenterology* 1997; **112**: 594–640

45 Sidransky D, Tokino T, Hamilton SR *et al*. Identification of *ras* oncogene mutations in the stool of patients with curable colorectal cancer. *Science* 1992; **256**: 102–5

46 Scholefield JH, Johnson AG, Shorthouse AJ. Current surgical practice in screening for colorectal cancer based on family history criteria. *Br J Surg* 1998; **85**: 1543–6

Screening for breast and ovarian cancer: the relevance of family history

Paul D P Pharoah* †, **John F Stratton**† ‡ and **James Mackay**† §

*Department of Community Medicine, †CRC Human Cancer Genetics Group, ‡WellBeing Ovarian Cancer Research Centre and §Department of Oncology, University of Cambridge, Cambridge, UK

The recent identification of two breast and ovarian cancer susceptibility genes – BRCA1 and BRCA2 – has received a lot of publicity. Public and professional expectations of the availability and utility of genetic testing have been raised and the importance of a family history of breast cancer overemphasised. In this chapter, we examine the significance of a family history of breast or ovarian cancer in determining individual risk. A strategy for management is proposed, based on stratifying women with such a history into three different categories of risk for breast cancer: high, moderate and low. Some of the more controversial aspects of screening for breast and ovarian cancer are reviewed, including the issue of management of women who are at increased risk of these cancers by virtue of a family history, genetic predisposition, or both. There is a need for further research to clarify the most appropriate management of those at moderate risk of developing these cancers. A management strategy for women at high risk is proposed. We believe that adoption of this strategy will strengthen consistent information giving from primary to tertiary care.

The recent identification of the breast and ovarian cancer susceptibility genes *BRCA1* and *BRCA2* has fostered an unrealistic expectation that genetic tests will become readily available, together with an assumption that identifying women who carry a mutation in one of these genes will be of benefit to them. The importance of a family history of breast and ovarian cancer has been overemphasised, with many women seeking medical attention because they perceive themselves to be at substantial risk of inherited breast cancer. It is possible to identify women at increased risk of breast or ovarian cancer through a positive family history, as well as women who are at very high risk because they carry an alteration in one of the known breast cancer susceptibility genes. However, the most appropriate way of managing that risk is less clear.

In this paper, familial breast and ovarian cancer risks are reviewed, together with the evidence for the effectiveness of different strategies to manage that risk. We propose a strategy, based on existing evidence, for

Correspondence to:
Dr J Mackay, Consultant
in Cancer Genetics,
Department of Oncology,
Box 193, Addenbrooke's
Hospital, Cambridge
CB2 2QQ, UK

Table 1 Relative risk (95% CI) of breast cancer by age of subject and age of affected relative

Age of affectedrelative	Age of subject		
	< 50 years	≥ 50 years	All ages
	Any first degree relative		
< 50 years	3.3 (2.8,3.9)	1.8 (1.6,2.0)	2.3 (2.2,2.5)
≥ 50 years	1.8 (1.5,2.2)	1.7 (1.5,2.0)	1.8 (1.6,2.0)
All ages	2.4 (2.2,2.7)	1.9 (1.8,2.0)	2.1 (2.0,2.2)
	Mother		
< 50 years	2.5 (1.6,3.8)	1.7 (1.1,2.6)	2.0 (1.7,2.4)
≥ 50 years	1.6 (1.1,2.3)	1.7 (1.2,2.4)	1.7 (1.5,2.0)
All ages	2.2 (1.9,2.6)	1.8 (1.6,2.1)	2.0 (1.8,2.1)
	Sister		
< 50 years	3.3 (2.1,4.5)	1.8 (1.2,2.4)	2.7 (2.4,3.2)
≥ 50 years	3.0 (1.4,4.6)	1.9 (1.1,2.7)	2.0 (1.7,2.4)
All ages	3.0 (2.5,3.5)	2.0 (1.8,2.3)	2.3 (2.1,2.4)
	Any second degree relative		
All ages	1.7 (1.4,2.0)	1.6 (1.3,2.0)	1.5 (1.4,1.6)

managing women at increased risk of breast and ovarian cancer because of family history.

Breast cancer

Incidence and mortality

Breast cancer is the commonest cancer in women in westernised countries, and is responsible for 20% of all female cancers. In the UK, around 1 in 12 women will develop breast cancer at some time in their life. In the UK in 1991, there were 34,500 women newly diagnosed with the disease and around 14,000 deaths. Breast cancer is rare in women in their teens or early twenties, but the incidence rises with age, so that most cases occur in postmenopausal women (80%). About 15% of women with breast cancer have a family history of the disease and 5% of all cases may be caused by cancer predisposition genes. The prevalence of cancer predisposition genes is higher in young women diagnosed with breast cancer. For example a mutation in BRCA1 will be found in about 10% of women with breast cancer diagnosed before the age of 40 years.

Familial breast cancer

In this paper, we consider two main types of breast cancer: **genetic** breast cancer, which occurs in women with an alteration in a breast cancer susceptibility gene which has been inherited through the germline (this is synonymous with **inherited** breast cancer); and **sporadic** breast cancer, which occurs in women with no such predisposition. **Familial** breast cancer occurs in women who have a relative with breast cancer, and includes either sporadic or genetic breast cancer. This is because familial clustering of breast cancer may occur by chance, or as a consequence of increased genetic susceptibility, or shared environmental or lifestyle risk factors.

All women with a family history of breast cancer are at increased risk of breast cancer themselves. However, the extent of that risk will vary according to the nature of the family history, specifically which relative was affected, their age at diagnosis, the number of relatives affected, as well as the age of the woman concerned. The relative risks associated with different family histories have been summarised in a recent systematic review and meta-analysis (Table 1)[1]. However, the risk categories described in most studies are simple, being usually based on single factors. The risks associated with more complex histories are difficult to establish. For example, it is difficult to estimate with any precision the risk of breast cancer in a 40 year old woman with three sisters, whose mother and oldest sister developed breast cancer at the age of 65 and 51 years, respectively.

Genetic breast cancer

Epidemiological studies suggest that much of the familial clustering of breast cancer is due to the inheritance of dominant predisposing genes. The risks of breast cancer associated with these genes vary. Some, such as the BRCA genes, are associated with an absolute life-time risk of breast cancer of 70% or more, while others, such as some alleles of *HRAS1*, are associated with a life-time risk of 15%. Three major breast cancer susceptibility genes have now been identified: *BRCA1*, *BRCA2* and *p53*. *BRCA1* and *BRCA2* are between them responsible for the majority (84%) of families with 4 or more members affected with either breast cancer before 60 years of age or ovarian cancer[2]. Germline mutations in *p53* are rare and account for a tiny proportion of breast cancer cases (< 1%)[3]. The proportion of smaller families, that is those with only two or three affected members, which are due to *BRCA1* or *BRCA2* mutations is still unclear, but may be considerably lower. Population frequencies of the known breast cancer susceptibility genes are given in Table 2.

Table 2 Population frequencies of known breast cancer susceptibility genes

Gene	Population carrier frequency
BRCA1 mutation	0.006%
BRCA2 mutation	0.006%
HRAS1 rare allele	6%
AT mutation	1%

Breast and ovarian cancer risks

The risk of breast cancer in women with mutations in *BRCA1* has been estimated indirectly from data collected on linkage families[4,5], as well as directly for women carrying one of the three Ashkenazim founder mutations (Table 3)[6]. The risk of breast cancer conferred by *BRCA2* seems to be similar[7], but the risk of ovarian cancer is much lower. Estimates of risk using linkage families are likely to be too high, while so-called direct estimates from a highly select population with 3 common founder mutations may be too low. It is, therefore, likely that the true risk lies somewhere between these two estimates.

Table 3 Breast and ovarian cancer risks associated with mutations in BRCA1

Age (years)	Cumulative breast cancer risk % (95% CI)	Cumulative ovarian cancer risk % (95% CI)	Reference
50	51 (25–67)	23 (5–38)	Ford *et al*[2]
70	85 (51–95)	63 (25–82)	
50	33 (23–44)	7 (2–14)	Streuwing *et al*[4]
70	56 (40–73)	16 (6–28)	

Mutations in more common genes, such as *HRAS1,* have been shown to confer a moderately increased risk of breast cancer. The so called 'rare' alleles of *HRAS1*, which are associated with an increased risk of breast cancer, are present in about 6% of the population. Because they are so common in comparison to *BRCA1*, the attributable risk is estimated at 9%, over twice as much as for *BRCA1*. Other candidate 'low risk' breast cancer genes for which there is already some evidence include the ataxia-telangiectasia gene and the vitamin D receptor gene.

Breast cancer screening

There are several potential methods for primary prevention, *i.e.* reducing the likelihood of developing breast cancer, including chemoprevention, prophylactic mastectomy and lifestyle modification, but discussion of these options is outside the scope of this article. Possible methods for early detection (secondary prevention) include breast self-examination, clinical breast examination and regular mammography.

Good evidence for the effectiveness of breast self-examination is lacking. The results of observational studies have been conflicting[8–10], and preliminary results from a randomised controlled trial failed to show benefit[11]. Approximately 10% of breast cancers may be detected by clinical examination alone. Expert panels have suggested that clinical examination provides a useful adjunct to mammography in women at very high risk of breast cancer[12].

The mainstay of early detection of breast cancer is regular screening of the breasts by mammography. Before considering the merits of mammography in those at high risk, the arguments for and against mammographic screening in women of average (or population) risk need to be rehearsed and interpreted with respect to women at increased risk. We will, therefore, review the contentious issues around screening in general, before discussing the role of mammography in those at high risk.

The UK National Breast Screening Programme offers three yearly mammography to women between the ages of 50 and 64 years. Women over the age of 64 years can continue screening if they specifically request it. The effectiveness of mammography for women aged 50–69 years of general population risk has been confirmed by several randomised controlled trials. Meta-analyses of these trials have shown that mammography will produce a relative reduction in breast cancer mortality of around 30% in these women[13]. The absolute reduction in risk is, however, small and it has been argued that the high financial costs of a screening programme outweigh the marginal clinical benefit[14,15]. The effectiveness of mammographic screening in younger women is controversial. A US National Cancer Institute workshop concluded that there was no proof of benefit for women under the age of 50 years[16], though evidence of benefit in women aged 40–49 years is mounting[17] and some groups, including the American Cancer Society, recommend screening for women aged 40–49 years. Even if the relative risk reduction were the same as in older women, the absolute benefit would be considerably reduced because breast cancer is less common in this age group.

The potential harm caused by mammographic screening includes the false reassurance of women with a false negative mammogram, the adverse effects of unnecessary investigation of false positives and a potential increased cancer risk associated with early and repeated radiation exposure[18]. In true positives, there is the possibility of adverse effects arising from methods used to confirm a presumptive positive screening result. In small lesions detected by mammography, diagnosis is usually confirmed by fine needle aspiration or core biopsy, and this may result in the seeding of cancer cells along biopsy needle tracks[19,20]. Thus, a tumour which may otherwise have remained localised could be inadvertently spread. Factors such as these have been suggested to explain the reduced mortality benefit seen in the most recent screening trials[21].

Perhaps the most serious concern is the generation of false positive results. About 5% of women screened will have a mammographic abnormality, of whom only 10–20% will subsequently be found to have cancer[22]. A positive or suspicious mammogram inevitably leads to further studies or interventions including fine needle biopsy or open biopsy, all of which have an associated morbidity. In addition, until given the 'all clear', the fear and anxiety that go hand in hand with a possible diagnosis of cancer may be considerable in women with a false positive screening test.

The issues discussed above relate to women of general population risk, but the benefit:harm ratio may be quite different in women at increased risk because of family history. Various authors have argued that because women with a family history are at greater risk it is likely that the absolute benefit will be greater[12,14,23,24]. This is likely to be true if the performance of the screening test is the same in high risk and average risk women. There is, in addition, the possibility of greater harm from mammography in some groups. For example, some genetic alterations may increase susceptibility to ionising radiation, though many experts believe the benefit of early detection will outweigh the risk[12]. It has also been assumed that because the prevalence of cancer will be higher in a high risk group, the problem of false positives will be lessened, but no research data are available to confirm this. The biology of familial breast cancer is likely to differ from that of non-familial disease and subtle changes in little understood areas such as the screening–treatment interface could substantially alter the benefit:harm ratio.

In the absence of randomised controlled trial data, it is difficult to make firm recommendations on the value of mammography in women under the age of 50 years with a family history of breast cancer. There is an urgent need to institute a study to evaluate accurately the efficacy and cost-effectiveness of mammographic screening in this group of women.

Proposed management

Given the lack of evidence for benefit of mammography in women at increased risk of breast cancer, we do not believe it is appropriate to offer all women who have a family history of breast cancer mammographic screening outside that currently offered through the National Breast Screening Programme. We propose that women with such a history be classified into one of three groups according to the

Table 4 Criteria for breast cancer risk stratification

High risk group

1   Breast/breast ovarian families with 4 or more relatives on the same side of the family affected at any age.
2   Breast cancer (only) families with three affected relatives average age of diagnosis < 40 years.
3   Breast/ovarian cancer families with three affected relatives, average age at diagnosis of breast cancer < 60 years.
4   Families with one member with both breast and ovarian cancer.

Moderate risk group

1   One first degree female relative with breast cancer diagnosed under 40 years or 1 first degree male relative with breast cancer diagnosed at any age, or one first degree paternal female relative with breast cancer diagnosed under 60 years, or
2   Two first or second degree relatives with breast cancer diagnosed under 60 years on the same side of the family, or
3   Three first or second degree relatives with breast cancer at any age on the same side of the family, or
4   A first degree relative with bilateral breast cancer diagnosed under 60 years.

Low risk group

1   Women with a family history of breast cancer not fulfilling the criteria for the other two groups.

magnitude of their risk and managed accordingly. The criteria used to stratify women into the three risk groups are given in Table 4. Broadly similar schemes are in use by many centres throughout the UK, the EC and Australia.

High risk group. Women in the high risk group are from families with a 20% or greater chance of breast cancer that is caused by a mutation in *BRCA1*. The probability that any individual in the family has a mutation will depend on her relationship to affected family members. The management of women in this group is best carried out under expert guidance and we recommend referral to a specialist cancer genetics clinic. Expert management would include a discussion of the advantages and disadvantages of instituting mutation searching, the advantages and disadvantages of direct genetic testing in unaffected individuals, and an examination of the available screening and treatment options. Most tertiary centres offer similar advice. There are no UK studies comparing different management strategies in terms of outcome.

Moderate risk group. Women in this category are at substantially increased risk of developing breast cancer below the age of 50 – at least 3 times the population risk – because of a positive family history, but are less likely to be carrying a mutation in one of the known breast cancer susceptibility genes. Given the lack of evidence of benefit for screening

Table 5 Proposed management of women at moderate risk of breast cancer

Age (years)		Management
< 30		No mammography
30–34	Youngest affected first degree relative diagnosed age 40+ years	No mammography
30–34	Youngest affected first degree relative diagnosed age ≤ 39 years	Annual mammography from 5 years before the age of diagnosis of the youngest affected relative
35–49		Annual mammography
50 and over		Mammography every 18 months

for women in this group, no intervention should be offered outside the context of a research study. There has been much discussion about the most appropriate study design: a randomised controlled trial of screening *versus* no screening in women at high risk would be ideal, but this solution has been considered unworkable because most patients, having been accurately informed of their increased risk, will not accept a no-screen option and, therefore, it would not be possible to assemble a large enough control group to make any conclusions reached significant. A proposal to carry out a national observational study with complete mammographic, surgical and pathological data collection is currently under discussion. A suggested management that could be evaluated by such a study is given in Table 5.

Because precise estimation of risk for minor degrees of family history is difficult, any categorisation according to family history will be crude. Thus, some women falling outside the moderate risk criteria (*i.e.* they fall into the low risk group) will still have a risk of breast cancer three times greater than that of the general population. However, making great efforts to estimate risk precisely is inappropriate because the most appropriate intervention (if any) for this group of women is not yet clear.

Low risk group.   Women in this category are at increased risk of breast cancer because of a positive family history which falls outside the criteria for the moderate risk group. Their relative risk is less than 3 times that for the general population. We do not believe that there is sufficient evidence to warrant mammography before the age of 50 years, but women in this group should be encouraged to enter the National Breast Screening Programme when appropriate.

Ovarian cancer

Ovarian cancer is the most common of the gynaecological malignancies, but is relatively rare compared to breast cancer. There are around 4,500 new cases per year in England and Wales. For the general population, the lifetime probability of developing ovarian cancer is 1 in 70 and the lifetime risk of death from ovarian cancer is approximately 1 in 120. Clinical staging of ovarian cancer is by the International Federation of Obstetrics and Gynaecology classification, which sub-divides ovarian cancer into four major groups according to the extent of tumour spread at presentation. The four stages are: Stage I, growth limited to one or both ovaries; Stage II, growth limited to one or both ovaries with pelvic extension; Stage III, growth involving one or both ovaries with intraperitoneal metastases outside the pelvis; and Stage IV, growth involving one or both ovaries with distant metastases.

Familial ovarian cancer

For the majority of women with a single affected first degree relative with ovarian cancer their risk of developing ovarian cancer is small. Their lifetime risk of developing ovarian cancer up to the age of 70 years is approximately 4%, equivalent to a relative risk of 3.1 (95% CI = 2.6–3.7). However, for women with more than one relative with ovarian cancer, the relative risk is 11.7 (95% CI = 5.3–25.9), which is equivalent to a lifetime risk of 14%[25]. This lifetime risk will be higher if the two cases are first degree relatives of the proband. Certain other women may also be at a higher risk of ovarian cancer, such as those with a first degree relative with ovarian cancer and a breast cancer which has occurred under the age of 50 years, or two relatives with breast cancer diagnosed before 60 years on the same side of the family and who are first degree relatives, *i.e.* breast/ovarian cancer families. Women from some hereditary non-polyposis colorectal cancer (HNPCC) families, where a first degree relative has ovarian cancer, may also have a higher risk compared to women with only a single affected first degree relative with ovarian cancer.

Genetic ovarian cancer

Approximately 5–10% of ovarian cancers are inherited and three distinct hereditary patterns have been identified: ovarian cancer alone; ovarian and breast cancer; and ovarian and colon cancer in HNPCC families. In most families affected with the breast and ovarian cancer syndrome or site-specific ovarian cancer, genetic linkage has been found to the BRCA1 locus on chromosome 17q21[26–28]. The lifetime risk for developing ovarian cancer in patients harbouring germ-line mutations in BRCA1 is significantly increased over the general population and confers an ovarian cancer risk of up to 63% by age 70 years (Table 3)[2,4].

Ovarian cancer screening

As for breast cancer, methods of primary prevention, such as prophylactic oophorectomy, are available, but discussion of these is outside the scope of this article.

Currently available screening strategies for ovarian cancer consist of transvaginal ultrasound and measurement of serum levels of CA125, a protein secreted by many ovarian cancers. The efficacy of these in reducing mortality has not been demonstrated in randomised trials and there are several characteristics of ovarian cancer which suggest that the benefit of screening may be limited. Although ovarian cancer demonstrates a variety of different stages at presentation similar to other carcinomas, the natural history of the condition is not well understood. It is not clear how ovarian cancers progress from early stage disease to advanced disease over a period of time. While this may be true in the majority of cases, there is evidence to suggest that many ovarian cancers may present *de novo* as advanced disease[29,30].

For a screening programme to be successful, not only is it necessary to detect disease at an early stage, but, more importantly, early treatment should be more effective than treatment of advanced disease whilst taking into account lead time bias. There is some doubt whether this is true for ovarian cancer. There have been documented cases of primary peritoneal cancer developing following prophylactic oophorectomy[31]. Similarly, a subset of early stage tumours appear to undergo a rapid downhill course despite adequate treatment. At the other end of the spectrum, women with apparently advanced disease at initial presentation, achieve optimal clearance of tumour at surgery and are cured of their cancer. This would suggest that there are differences in the biology of the cancer, that affect prognosis regardless of stage at presentation[32].

Ultrasound. While ultrasound is effective at picking up ovarian abnormalities, it is poor at distinguishing benign from malignant pathology. In an early observational study of transabdominal ultrasound, 326 of 5,479 (5.9%) screened women subsequently underwent laparotomy[33]. Ovarian cancer was found in 9, but only 5 of these were primary cancers of the ovary. Some improvement in specificity can be obtained by using transvaginal sonography (TVS), colour Doppler flow imaging and a morphologic index. A screening trial of TVS yielded persistently abnormal scans in 1.4% of asymptomatic, postmenopausal women. Of these lesions, 90% were found to be benign at follow-up surgery[34]. Both these studies were carried out in women of average risk, and it has been suggested that the false positive rate would be reduced if women at high risk were screened. However, in a study of both transabdominal and transvaginal sonography in self-referred women with a first- or second-degree relative with ovarian cancer, abnormalities requiring surgical exploration were found in 3.8% of screened women, of whom only 10% found to have ovarian cancer (5 of 6 had stage I disease)[35]. Five additional cases of cancer not detected by screening (3 ovarian and 2 peritoneal) were reported 2–44 months after the last ultrasound.

CA125.   CA125 is a protein secreted by many ovarian cancers. Rising levels in women with previously undetectable or normal levels following treatment for ovarian cancer are a good indicator of recurrent disease, often preceding clinical evidence of recurrence by a period of 6 months. Unfortunately CA125 is not specific for ovarian cancer and levels are raised in many physiological and benign conditions such as pregnancy, menstruation, endometriosis and pelvic inflammatory disease. Perhaps more importantly, however, is the fact that, although 90% of women with ovarian cancer (stage 2 or greater) have elevated levels of CA125, only 50% of women with stage 1 disease have levels above the normal range.

The sensitivity of CA125 for the detection of ovarian cancer has been determined in two case-control studies using serum banks[36,37]. For CA125 levels of ≥ 35 U/ml, sensitivity was estimated to be 20–57% for cases occurring within the first 3 years of follow-up, with a specificity of 95%. In a prospective cohort study of 9,320 postmenopausal women, 49 cancers were identified[38]. One and five years following screening, a serum CA125 concentration of at least 30 U/ml was associated with a relative risk (95% CI) of cancer of 35.9 (18.3, 70.4) and of 14.3 (8.5, 24.4), respectively. At a CA125 concentration of 100 U/ml, the relative risks were 204.8 (79.0, 530.7) and 74.5 (31.1, 178.3), respectively. Women with CA125 levels below 30 U/ml had risks of 0.13 (0.03, 0.58) and 0.54 (0.32, 0.91), respectively.

In a screening programme using CA125 and based on 22,000 postmenopausal women, those with elevated CA125 levels (reference value of 30 U/ml) were examined subsequently with transabdominal ultrasound. Eleven of 19 cases of ovarian cancer occurring in this cohort were detected, an estimated sensitivity of 58% at the two year follow-up and a specificity of 99.9%[39]. Three of the 11 cancers detected through screening were stage I. Another study of postmenopausal women using both CA125 and ultrasound obtained a specificity of 97.6% for CA125 levels of 35 U/ml[40].

As previously discussed, screening women at higher risk because of family history may yield greater absolute benefit. In one study of 386 women with a first-degree relative or multiple second degree relatives with ovarian cancer using ultrasound and CA125, 15 women underwent exploratory laparotomies, 10 as a result of abnormal ultrasound findings alone, 3 as a result of abnormal CA125 levels and ultrasound findings, and 2 women because of rising CA125 levels. No cancer was identified in any of these women, one of whom sustained unrecognised small bowel damage requiring further surgery[40].

Proposed management

The population incidence in the UK of ovarian cancer for women over the age of 45 years is 40/100,000 women/year. To screen this population and ensure a minimum of 1 diagnosis of ovarian cancer for every 10 laparotomies performed on the basis of a positive screen, the required specificity of the screening test is 99.6%. The only way of achieving this is by the sequential combination of CA125 with ultrasonography. To maintain the same positive predictive value in women who have a 4–5-fold increased risk, *i.e.* women with an affected first degree relative, the required specificity is 98%. For women with a BRCA1 mutation who have a lifetime risk of approximately 45% the specificity required is 93%.

Given the lack of evidence on the efficacy of screening the general population for early ovarian cancer – either with regular ultrasound, regular tumour marker measurement or a combination of the two – and the uncertainty surrounding possible biological differences between genetic and sporadic ovarian cancer, the most attractive scientific solution would be the institution of a randomised trial of screening versus no-screening in the high risk population. As with breast cancer, a randomised controlled trial has been considered unfeasible because most patients, having been informed of their increased risk, will not accept a no-screen option.

The second most attractive option is a single arm screening study aiming to collect all the data necessary to make as accurate an analysis as possible of screening performance in this high risk group, and then compare screening performance in this group with performance including projected mortality reduction in the ongoing randomised

Table 6 Eligibility criteria for the UKCCCR National Familial Ovarian Cancer Screening Study

An eligible woman must be over 25 years of age and a first degree relative of an affected member of an 'at risk' family. At risk families are defined by the following criteria:

1. Two or more first degree relatives[a] with ovarian cancer.

2. One first degree relative with ovarian cancer and one first degree relative with breast cancer diagnosed under 50 years of age.

3. One first degree relative with ovarian cancer and two first or second degree relatives[b] with breast cancer diagnosed under 60 years of age.

4. An affected individual with one of the known ovarian cancer predisposing genes

5. Three first degree relatives with colorectal cancer with at least one diagnosed before the age of 50 years and at least one first degree relative with ovarian cancer.

[a]A first degree female relative is mother, sister or daughter.
[b]A second degree female relative is grandmother, grand-daughter, aunt or niece.

population studies. Such a study is the UKCCCR National Familial Ovarian Cancer Screening Study. The eligibility criteria for this study, given in Table 6, define a cohort of women at increased risk of ovarian cancer. The proposed management of this cohort is annual ultrasound and CA125 measurement. In this collaborative study, collection and analysis of family history data will be performed in the CRC Human Cancer Genetics Research Group in Cambridge, and collection and analysis of the screening data will be performed in the Ovarian Cancer Screening Unit in St Bartholomew's Hospital, London. The clinical care of the patient remains with the local clinician, although the study team are happy to advise with interpretation of abnormal findings. Further details of this study may be obtained from the corresponding author.

Key points for clinical practice

- Any woman with a relative with breast cancer has an increased risk of developing breast cancer. The magnitude of that increased risk depends on the number of relatives with breast or ovarian cancer, the type of relatives affected, the ages at which cancer is diagnosed and the age of the 'at risk' individual.

- Two high penetrance breast/ovarian cancer genes have been identified and genetic testing is available in some genetic centres for a small number of families.

- The recent high profile genetic advances in breast and ovarian cancer have raised unrealistic public and professional expectations of genetic testing.

- The efficacy of mammographic screening of women at average risk between 50 and 69 years has been proven in several randomised studies, but the effectiveness of mammographic screening in women below 50 years of age remains controversial.

- Women at moderate risk of breast cancer should only be offered annual mammography from the age of 35 years within the context of an evaluable research study.

- Women at significant risk of ovarian cancer should be offered annual ultrasound and CA125 measurement within the UKCCCR National Familial Ovarian Cancer Screening Study.

- Women with a family history of breast or ovarian cancer which falls outside the proposed criteria should receive an understandable accurate and supportive explanation, and not be offered regular or one-off investigation.

- Adoption of the proposed management strategy strengthens consistent information given from primary to secondary to tertiary care.

Acknowledgements

PDPP and JM are funded by the Cancer Research Campaign. JFS is a WellBeing Clinical Research Fellow.

References

1   Pharoah PDP, Day NE, Duffy S, Easton DF, Ponder BAJ. Family history and the risk of breast cancer: a systematic review and meta-analysis. *Int J Cancer* 1997; **71**: 800–9
2   Ford D, Easton DF, Stratton M *et al*. Genetic heterogeneity and penetrance analysis of the *BRCA1* and *BRCA2* genes in breast cancer families. *Am J Hum Genet* 1998; **62**: 676–89
3   Borresen AL, Andersen TI, Garber J *et al*. Screening for germ line TP53 mutations in breast cancer patients. *Cancer Res* 1992; **52**: 3234–6
4   Ford D, Easton DF, Bishop DT, Narod SA, Goldgar DE, Breast Cancer Linkage Consortium. Risks of cancer in BRCA1 mutation carriers. *Lancet* 1994; **343**: 692–5
5   Bishop DT, Cannon-Albright LA, McLellan T, Gardner EJ, Skolnick MH. Segregation and linkage analysis of 9 Utah breast cancer pedigrees. *Genet Epidemiol* 1988; **5**: 151–69
6   Streuwing JP, Hartge P, Wacholder S *et al*. The risk of cancer associated with specific mutations of BRCA1 and BRCA2 among Ashkenazi Jews. *N Engl J Med* 1997; **336**: 1401–8
7   Easton DF, Steele L, Fields P *et al*. Cancer risks in two large breast cancer families linked to BRCA2 on chromosome 13q12-13. *Am J Hum Genet* 1997; **61**: 120–8
8   Foster RSJ, Lang SP, Costanza MC, Worden JK, Haines CR, Yates JW. Breast self-examination practices and breast cancer stage. *N Engl J Med* 1978; **299**: 265–70

9 Greenwald P, Nasca PC, Lawrence CE. Estimated effect of breast self-examination and routine physician examinations on breast cancer mortality. *N Engl J Med* 1978; **299**: 271–3

10 Newcomb P, Weiss N, Storer B. Breast self-examination in relation to the occurrence of advanced breast cancer. *J Natl Cancer Inst* 1991; **83**: 260–5

11 Thomas DB, Gao DL, Self SG *et al.* Randomized trial of breast self-examination in Shanghai: methodology and preliminary results. *J Natl Cancer Inst* 1997; **89**: 355–65

12 Burke W, Daly M, Garber J *et al.* Recommendations for follow-up care of individuals with an inherited predisposition to cancer. II. BRCA1 and BRCA2. *JAMA* 1997; **277**: 997–1003

13 Kerlikowske K, Grady D, Rubin SM, Sandrock C, Ernster VL. Efficacy of screening mammography: a meta-analysis. *JAMA* 1995; **273**: 149–54

14 Wright CJ, Barber Mueller C. Screening mammography and public health policy: the need for perspective. *Lancet* 1995; **346**: 29–32

15 Jatoi I, Baum M. Screening for breast cancer, time to think – and stop? *Lancet* 1995; **346**: 436–7

16 Fletcher SW, Black W, Harris R, Rimer BK, Shapiro S. Report of the international workshop of screening for breast cancer. *J Natl Cancer Inst* 1993; **85**: 1644–56

17 Feig SA. Increased benefit from shorter screening mammography intervals for women ages 40–49 years. *Cancer* 1997; **80**: 2035–9

18 John EM, Kelsey JL. Radiation and other environmental exposures and breast cancer. *Epidemiol Rev* 1993; **1993**: 157–62

19 Harter LP, Curtis JS, Ponto G, Craig PH. Malignant seeding of the needle track during stereotaxic core needle breast biopsy. *Radiology* 1992; **185**: 713–4

20 Roussel F, Dalion J. The risk of tumoral seeding in needle biopsies. *Acta Cytol* 1989; **33**: 936–9

21 Watmough DJ, Bhargava S, Memon A, Syed F, Roy S, Sharma P. Does breast cancer screening depend on a wobbly hypothesis? *J Public Health Med* 1997; **19**: 375-379.

22 Baines CJ, McFarlane DV, Miller AB. Sensitivity and specificity of first screen mammography in 15 NBSS centers. *J Can Assoc Radiol* 1988; **39**: 273–6

23 Hoskins JF, Stopfer JE, Calzone CA. Assessment and counseling for women with a family history of breast cancer: a guide for clinicians. *JAMA* 1995; **273**: 577–85

24 Vasen HFA. Screening in breast cancer families: is it useful? *Ann Med* 1994; **26**: 185–90

25 Stratton JF, Pharoah PDP, Smith SK, Easton D, Ponder BJ. A systematic review and meta-analysis of family history and risk of ovarian cancer. *Br J Obstet Gynae*col 1997; **105**(5): 493–499

26 Miki Y, Swensen J, Shattuck-Eidens D *et al.* A strong candidate for the Hq linked breast and ovarian cancer susceptibility gene BRCA1. *Science* 1994; **266**: 66–71

27 Easton DF, Bishop DT, Ford D, Crockford GP. Genetic linkage analysis in familial breast and ovarian cancer: results from 214 families. The Breast Cancer Linkage Consortium. *Am J Hum Genet* 1993; **52**: 678–701

28 Steichen-Gersdorf E, Gallion H, Ford D, Girodet C, Easton D, DiCioccio R. Familial site-specific ovarian cancer is linked to BRCA1 on 17q12-21. *Am J Hum Genet* 1994; **55**: 870–5

29 Bell DA, Scully RE. Early *de novo* ovarian carcinoma. A study of fourteen cases. *Cancer* 1994; **73**: 1859–64

30 Scully RE, Bell DA, Abu-Jawdeh GM. Update of early ovarian cancer and cancer developing in benign ovarian tumours. In: Sharp F, Mason P, Blackett T, Berek J. (eds) *Ovarian Cancer*. London: Chapman & Hall Medical, 1995; 139–44

31 Tobacman JK, Tucker MA, Kase R, Greene MH, Costa J, Fraumeni JF. Intra-abdominal carcinomatosis after prophylactic oophorectomies in ovarian-cancer-prone families. *Lancet* 1982; **ii**: 795–797.

32 Pecorelli S, Odicino F, Tessadrelli A. Primary and interval debulking surgery for advanced disease. In: Sharp F, Blackett T, Leake R, Berek J. (eds) *Ovarian Cancer*. London: Chapman & Hall Medical, 1996; 105–9

33 Campbell S, Bhan V, Royston P. Transabdominal ultrasound screening for early ovarian cancer. *BMJ* 1989; **299**: 1363–7

34 DePriest PD, van Nagell JR, Gallion HH *et al.* Ovarian cancer screening in asymptomatic postmenopausal women. *Gynaecol Oncol* 1993; **51**: 205–9

35 Bourne TH, Campbell S, Reynolds KM *et al.* Screening for early familial ovarian cancer with transvaginal ultrasonography and colour blood flow imaging. *BMJ* 1993; **306**: 1025–9

36 Zurawski VR, Orjaseter H, Andersen A *et al*. Elevated serum CA 125 levels prior to diagnosis of ovarian neoplasia: relevance for early detection of ovarian cancer. *Int J Cancer* 1988; **42**: 677–80

37 Helzlsouer K, Bush TL, Alberg AJ *et al*. Prospective study of serum CA-125 levels as markers of ovarian cancer. *JAMA* 1993; **269**: 1123–6

38 Jacobs IJ, Skates S, Davies AP *et al*. Risk of diagnosis of ovarian-cancer after raised serum ca-125 concentration – a prospective cohort study. *BMJ* 1996; **313**: 1355–8

39 Jacobs I, Davies AP, Bridges J *et al*. Prevalence screening for ovarian cancer in postmenopausal women by ca125 measurement and ultrasonography. *BMJ* 1993; **306**: 1030–4

40 Einhorn N, Sjovall K, Knapp RC *et al*. Prospective evaluation of serum CA 125 levels for early detection of ovarian cancer. *Obstet Gynaecol* 1992; **80**: 14–8

Prenatal screening for chromosome abnormalities

Lyn Chitty

Department of Clinical Genetics, Institute of Child Health, London, UK

An abnormal chromosome complement (aneuploidy) contributes significantly to fetal loss during pregnancy, as well as to perinatal morbidity and mortality. The contribution of chromosomal abnormalities to fetal loss decreases as pregnancy continues with an estimated 50% of first trimester spontaneous abortions due to chromosomal abnormalities, but only 5% of stillbirths (after 28 weeks). Prenatal screening for aneuploidy (in particular Down syndrome) can be undertaken using maternal serum biochemistry, fetal ultrasound or a combination of both. In this chapter the advantages and disadvantages of screening programmes currently in use, or undergoing evaluation, will be reviewed.

An abnormal chromosome complement (aneuploidy) contributes significantly to fetal loss during pregnancy, as well as to perinatal morbidity and mortality. The contribution of chromosomal abnormalities to fetal loss decreases as pregnancy continues with an estimated 50% of first trimester spontaneous abortions due to chromosomal abnormalities, but only 5% of stillbirths (after 28 weeks)[1]. In early pregnancy a wide range of chromosomal anomalies are detected, but as pregnancy progresses fewer types are found, as many affected fetuses are not viable beyond the first trimester. Although fetuses affected with trisomy 21 (Down syndrome) are viable, there is fetal loss among this group so that prevalence declines with increasing gestational age. This early fetal loss must be taken into consideration when evaluating prenatal screening for Down syndrome[2]. Combined data from two multicentre studies based on amniocentesis at 16–20 weeks' gestation have shown that the prevalence of trisomy 21 is about 30% higher at this stage of pregnancy than at birth[3,4]. Data from fetal karyotyping at 9–14 weeks have also demonstrated a 48–50% higher prevalence of trisomy 21 in the first trimester than at birth[5,6].

Major abnormalities found later in pregnancy include trisomies 13, 18 and 21, sex chromosomal anomalies and structural re-arrangements. It has been estimated that aneuploidy accounts for about 5–7% of infant and childhood deaths and 10% of developmental delay[1]. These

Correspondence to:
Dr Lyn Chitty, Dept of Clinical Genetics, Institute of Child Health, 30 Guilford Street, London WC1N 6EH, UK

estimates are derived from information obtained in developed countries in the mid 1970s. Future estimates will depend on the proportion of older mothers in the population, as the prevalence of aneuploidy increases with advancing maternal age, as well as on the extent of prenatal screening and subsequent termination of pregnancies complicated by aneuploidy.

Trisomy 21 (Down syndrome) is the most common chromosomal abnormality associated with significant risk of long-term morbidity. It occurs with an estimated prevalence at birth of 1.21/1000 livebirths. Trisomies 18 and 13, which are usually lethal either *in utero* or within the first year of life, occur less frequently: 0.15 and 0.08 per 1000 births, respectively[1]. Most prenatal screening programmes are designed to detect Down syndrome, but will, in addition, identify sex chromosome anomalies which may be associated with infertility and some with varying degrees of developmental delay.

The National Down Syndrome Cytogenetic Register has recorded data on the majority of cases of Down syndrome diagnosed both pre- and postnatally in England and Wales from the beginning of 1989. The number of cases reported each year has increased from 1066 in 1989 to 1281 in 1996, despite a decrease in the annual number of births from 688,000 to 650,000 over the same period[7]. This has been attributed to an increase in the number of older mothers and to an increase in the proportion of cases diagnosed prenatally (from 30% to 56%), many of which would have aborted spontaneously. Similar data were reported from Western Australia, where an increase in serum screening and prenatal detection of Down syndrome pregnancies was accompanied by a fall in prevalence at term, but an overall increase in the number of cases detected[8].

In most clinical situations, screening is performed to identify that proportion of the population who may benefit from further investigation or diagnostic tests, so that the presence of, or potential to develop, a condition amenable to treatment or prevention, can be detected. The primary objective of prenatal screening for aneuploidy is to allow parents the choice of whether to continue with a seriously affected pregnancy or to have the pregnancy terminated. It is, therefore, primarily directed at secondary, rather than primary prevention. Additional benefits of prenatal screening[10] include parental re-assurance that the baby is normal and, for those who opt to continue with an affected pregnancy, the opportunity to adjust to this information before the baby is born[10]. On the other hand, disadvantages of screening include the risk of fetal loss following invasive diagnostic procedures, as well as the anxiety caused, following false positive results and the false re-assurance given to women with a false negative result.

Prenatal screening for aneuploidy (in particular Down syndrome) can be undertaken using maternal serum biochemistry, fetal ultrasound or a combination of both. In this chapter the advantages and disadvantages of screening programmes currently in use, or undergoing evaluation, will be reviewed.

The detection rate (sensitivity) refers to the proportion of affected pregnancies identified through screening and the false positive rate, the proportion of unaffected pregnancies screened positive. The false positive rate provides a measure of the possible rate of invasive testing in unaffected pregnancies. The potential benefit, in terms of the number of affected fetuses identified, must, therefore, be weighed against the risk of loss of normal pregnancies as a consequence of amniocentesis. Conventionally, a false positive rate of about 5% is accepted. Depending on the demographic characteristics of the population, this results in women with a risk greater than 1 in 250 to 1 in 300 being offered amniocentesis[11]. This means that women with a lower risk are not offered amniocentesis but have a small residual risk of an affected pregnancy. This risk of false re-assurance from screening needs to be considered in relation to the risk of harm to normal pregnancies following an invasive diagnostic test.

Screening based on maternal age

The risk of having a baby with Down syndrome increases with increasing maternal age. The risk at birth for a woman of 25 years is around 0.74–0.85 per 1000 births, at 35 years 2.6–3.08 per 1000 and at 45 it is as high as 33.08–47.1 per 1000[1]. Screening on the basis of maternal age alone achieves a maximal detection rate of about 26% for Down syndrome and 30% for the other major autosomal trisomies. In practice, the detection rate is considerably less as many women (up to 50%) decline amniocentesis. As the majority of affected pregnancies occur in younger women, this screening approach is highly ineffective and, in the UK, it has largely been replaced by programmes combining maternal age and biochemical markers in maternal serum, measured in the second trimester of pregnancy. More recently, developments in ultrasound as well as measurement of biochemical markers during the first trimester have increased the number of screening strategies available based on various combinations of maternal age, serum markers and ultrasound findings. There is currently much debate as to the most effective approaches for screening for aneuploidy, and practice varies across the country. A recent survey revealed that, in the UK, second trimester serum screening is predominant, although a few maternity units still screen on the basis of maternal age alone, while some are beginning to screen in the first trimester using nuchal translucency measurement (Maclachlan, personal communication).

Table 1 Screening for Down syndrome: performance for selected combinations of maternal age and serum markers

Detection rate based on:	Menstrual dates		Ultrasound scan	
Marker(s)	Detection rate* (%)	OAPR*	Detection rate* (%)	OAPR*
Age alone	30	1:130	30	1:130
Age plus				
AFP	36	1:110	37	1:105
hCG/free β-hCG	49	1:80	51	1:75
Oestriol	41	1:95	49	1:80
Inhibin A	44	1:90	44	1:90
AFP, hCG	54	1:70	59	1:65
AFP, hCG, oestriol	59	1:65	69	1:55
AFP, hCG, inhibin A	64	1:60	68	1:55
AFP, hCG, oestriol,inhibin A	67	1:55	76	1:50

Data from Wald et al[20,85,86].

*Detection rates and the odds of being affected given a positive result (OAPR) have been estimated for a 5% false positive rate.

AFP, alpha-fetoprotein; hCG = human chorionic gonadotrophin.

Serum markers in the second trimester

The association between low maternal serum alpha-fetoprotein and fetal aneuploidy was first reported by Merkatz *et al* in 1983, who noted a very low maternal serum alpha-fetoprotein level in a woman who gave birth to a child with trisomy 18. Since then, many serum markers for aneuploidy have been identified, which, in combination, can achieve detection rates in excess of 60% and are considerably better than screening based on maternal age alone[12]. However, the performance of serum markers is highly dependent on gestational age. As up to 40% of reported menstrual dates are inaccurate, ultrasound is used to estimate gestational age, to improve test performance (Table 1). The effect of gestational age is most marked for serum analytes that show significant change in level with gestational age, for example, the change is smaller for oestradiol than for inhibin A (Table 1). Maternal weight, insulin dependent diabetes, multiple pregnancy and ethnic origin may also influence maternal serum levels and affect test performance. These need to be taken into consideration when estimating risk. Other factors, such as smoking, parity, serum levels in previous pregnancies and assisted conception have a minimal or unknown effect[12]. The level of each serum marker is expressed as a multiple of the median for that gestational age. A computer algorithm, which includes maternal age, is used to derive a risk estimate. In pregnancies with Down syndrome, alpha-fetoprotein and oestriol are lower and human chorionic gonadotrophin higher, than expected. Although discrimination is sufficient for most units to offer screening from 15–22 weeks, the optimum gestational age for screening is 16–18 weeks for most serum markers, when the discrimination between normal and affected pregnancies is greatest.

Using a different algorithm, second trimester serum screening can also be used to identify pregnancies at increased risk of trisomy 18, as levels of human chorionic gonadotrophin are low[13]. The use of the three serum markers (alpha-fetoprotein, oestriol and human chorionic gonadorophin), in combination with maternal age, and a mid-trimester risk cut-off of 1 in 100, has been estimated to detect about 60% of affected fetuses for a false positive rate of about 0.2%[13,14]. Trisomy 18 occurs about 8 times less frequently than Down syndrome[1] and does not confer the same degree of long-term morbidity, because the majority of cases die *in utero*. Of those alive at birth, only about 10% will survive for as long as a year and longer survival is rare[15,16]. Screening for trisomy 18 alone cannot, therefore, be justified, but the available data suggest that extending Down syndrome screening to include trisomy 18 could yield a high detection rate with only a small increase in false positive rate[13,14,17].

In the UK, the most commonly used second trimester serum markers include alpha-fetoprotein, human chorionic gonadotrophin and oestriol in combination with maternal age. A significant improvement in maternal serum screening can be made by the addition of dimeric inhibin-A. This additional marker improves the estimated performance of second trimester serum screening for Down syndrome by around 7%[18] to between 68–75 %[19,20]. Table 1 summarises the estimated detection rates of Down syndrome using a combination of maternal age and the various markers currently in clinical use, given a 5% false positive rate. These estimates have been borne out in clinical practice, with detection rates of between 48–91% (mean 70%) reported for the 'triple' test (alpha-fetoprotein, oestriol and human chorionic gonadotrophin) and of 50–70% (mean 66%) for the 'double' test (alpha-fetoprotein and human chorionic gonadotrophin (Table 2)[12]. Examples are given in Table 2, where only those studies where screening was offered to all women are shown, together with observed and estimated detection rates, taking spontaneous fetal loss into account. Direct comparison of these studies is limited by the different criteria used for screening, variable cut off levels, and differences in the age distribution of the antenatal population. In a comprehensive review of Down syndrome screening, Wald reported that uptake of serum screening ranged from 67–92%[12]. The amniocentesis rate in those pregnancies identified at increased risk was around 80%, and about 90% of parents elected to have the pregnancy terminated following a confirmed diagnosis of Down syndrome. However, local demographic variation, particularly with respect to maternal age, has significant economic implications for screening. A study of regions in England and

Table 2 Screening for Down syndrome: results of selected serum screening programmes in current practice

Author	Country	Number screened	Risk given as 1 in:	% with positive screen test	% uptake of amnio-centesis	Detection rate % Observed	Detection rate % Estimated at term
MSAFP, hCG and oestriol							
Haddow1992[72]	USA	25,207	250	3.8	7.9	60	54
Wald 1992[73]	UK	12,603	250	4.1	77	48	42
Pescia 1993[74]	Switzerland	7,039	350	5.9	97	69	63
Piggot 1994[75]	UK	6,990	250	3.0	80	73	67
Goodburn 1994[76]	UK	25,359	200	4.1	86	75	70
MSAFP and hCG							
Dawson1993[77]	UK	8,414	300	3.5	85	50	44
Beekhuis 1993[78]	The Netherlands	2,099	250	7.3	79	83	79
Spencer 1993[79]	UK	8,317	300	5.3	89	69	63

Adapted from Wald et al[12].
MSAFP, maternal serum alpha-fetoprotein; hCG = human chorionic gonadotrophin.

Wales showed that, for a fixed risk cut-off level of 1 in 250, the detection rate could vary from 55–70% for false positive rates of 4.4–8.8%[11].

There are disbenefits, including economic and opportunity costs, as well as benefits in any screening programme. For serum screening, economic costs include the cost of the biochemical assays (which will vary depending on the analytes measured), ultrasound, diagnostic testing (usually amniocentesis), and counselling. The measurable clinical costs include the number of unaffected fetal losses, which occur as a result of the diagnostic test. More intangible costs include those due to unnecessary parental anxiety as well as to the acquisition of unanticipated information at the time of definitive diagnostic testing, such as discovering a sex chromosome anomaly in the fetus. The benefits, in clinical terms, include giving parents the opportunity to avoid having a child with a significant handicap and, in economic terms, avoiding the life-time costs of caring for a person with Down syndrome. The balance of these costs depends on a number of factors, including the risk cut-off level used, the proportion of the population taking up the offer of screening, the number of screen positive women who elect to have an invasive diagnostic procedure, and the number with a positive result who have their pregnancy terminated. Wald *et al*[12] estimated that, using the double test and taking all these factors into account, the cost of avoiding a Down syndrome birth was around £27,500 and the unaffected fetal loss rate around 0.63% per 100,000 term pregnancies. In a detailed comparison of the various combinations of tests which could be used, they estimated that, for a detection rate of 65%, the quadruple test (alpha-fetoprotein, oestriol, beta-human chorionic gonadotrophin and inhibin A) was the most cost effective.

Serum markers in the first trimester

All serum markers used in the second trimester have been evaluated for use in the first and early second trimester. Only free beta-human chorionic gonadotrophin and pregnancy associated plasma protein A have been shown to significantly differentiate between Down syndrome and normal pregnancies (Table 3). In an international multicentre study, free beta-human chorionic gonadotrophin was found to be elevated, and pregnancy associated plasma protein-A reduced, in affected pregnancies. These two markers, in combination with maternal age, identified an estimated 62% of Down syndrome pregnancies for a 5.5% false positive rate[21].

Factors discussed above in relation to second trimester serum screening, such as gestational age and maternal weight, also influence first trimester test performance. Based on the limited data available, Wald *et al*[12] have estimated that first trimester serum screening is less effective and less cost effective than biochemical screening in the second trimester, with a lower detection rate and higher cost of the diagnostic procedure (which would be chorionic villus sampling at this gestation).

Urinary metabolites

Human chorionic gonadotrophin, its subunits and metabolites are also raised in maternal urine in Down syndrome pregnancies[22–25]. Early studies have shown that, when combined with maternal age, urinary

Table 3 Screening for Down syndrome in first trimester using serum biochemical markers with maternal age[21, 88–90]

Maternal age combined with	Detection rate (%) for 5% false positive rate
Pregnancy associated plasma protein-A	44–66
Free beta-human chorionic gonadotrophin	9–38
Alpha-fetoprotein	18–32
Total human chorionic gonadotrophin	32
Dimeric inhibin-A	31
Oestriol	30
Free beta-human chorionic gonadotrophin + pregnancy associated plasma protein-A	62

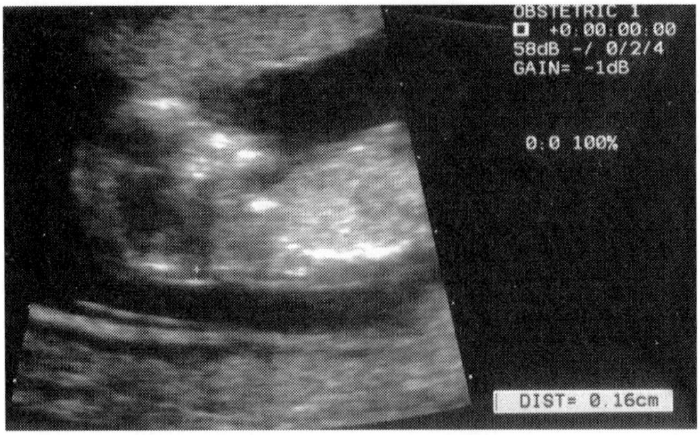

Fig. 1 Ultrasound image showing an 11 week fetus with a normal nuchal translucency measurement marked by the two small crosses. The fetal head is on the left.

beta-core human chorionic gonadotrophin, may be a useful marker in both first and second trimesters, with predicted detection rates varying from 41–80% for a 5% false positive rate[22]. However, not all studies have produced such encouraging results in either the first or second trimester[25]. The potential advantages of urinary biochemistry include cost and ease of collection, but disadvantages include the need to correct for dilution, as well as variation in reported efficacy. With the move towards community based antenatal care, urinary markers are potentially useful, but further prospective study in a routine clinical setting is required to assess their performance in primary screening.

Sonographic markers in the first trimester

Variation in fetal heart rate pattern, a reduced crown rump length and an increased nuchal translucency measurement have been associated with aneuploidy in the first trimester, however, only the latter has been shown to be of use in screening[26,27]. Nuchal translucency describes the maximum thickness of the subcutaneous translucency between the skin and the soft tissue overlying the cervical spine of the fetus (Fig. 1). Bronshtein *et al*[28] first reported the association of increased nuchal translucency thickness with fetal aneuploidy in 1989. It has been variously defined as nuchal translucency[29], simple hygroma[30] and cystic hygroma[31]. Since these early reports, there have been many studies describing the value of this sign in screening for aneuploidy, in particular Down syndrome. Based on published series, the average detection rate for Trisomy 21 is 77% and, for all karyotypic abnormalities, 67%. However, the sensitivities ranged from 0–88% for a false positive rate of 2.6–9.9% (Table 4). There were also other differences between studies reported in the literature, with the prevalence of Down syndrome

Table 4 Screening performance of nuchal translucency scanning

	Gestational age (weeks)	Nuchal thickness (mm)	Reported detection rate (%)		False positive rate (%)	Total population (n)
			Trisomy 21	All aneuploidies		
High risk or mixed populations						
Nicolaides 1994[52]	10–13	≥ 3	84	72	4.4	1,273
Szabo 1995[44]	9–12	≥ 3	88	92	2.6	1,380
Comas 1995[80]	9–13	≥ 3	57	47	9.9	481
Brambati 1995[40]	8–15	≥ 3	?	30	3.2	1,819
Pandya 1995[42]	10–14	≥ 2.5	77	77	6.9	20,804
Kornman 1996[37]	13	≥ 3	0	0	2.7	484
Snijders 1996[26]	10–14	95th	86	87	6.0	42,619
Theodoropoulos 1998[87]	10–14	Var	91	95	4.9	3,550
Orlandi 1997[81]	9–13	Var		57	5.8	744
Unselected populations						
Bewley 1995[35]	8–14	≥ 3	33	40	6.0	1,368
Szabo 1995[44]	9–12	≥ 3	100	100	0.9	2,100
Hafner 1995[82]	10–13	≥ 2.5	50	73	0.9	1,972
Kornman 1996[37]	13	≥ 3	67	67	4.8	439
Pandya 1995[19]	10–13	≥ 2.5	75	76	3.4	1,763
Bower 1995[83]*	8–13	≥ 3	45	53	6.3	2,566
Economides 1998[84]	11–14	Var	79	65		2,281

Adapted from Chitty and Pandya 1997[27].

*Includes Bewley et al 1995[35].

Var = variable cut-off depending on gestational age.

ranging from 12–88%, presumably reflecting differences in maternal age distribution (with many studies describing selected populations) as well as in the definition of abnormal nuchal translucency. The prevalence of trisomies has been shown to increase with maternal age (as might be expected), as well as with increasing nuchal translucency thickness[29,32,33].

There is relatively little information on the use of nuchal translucency measurements to screen for aneuploidy in unselected obstetric populations, although similar performance to that observed in high risk populations was reported following its introduction into two maternity units providing routine antenatal care[34]. Other 'routine screening' studies have reported detection rates of between 40–100% (mean 62%) for Down syndrome, and 33–100% (mean 70%) for all aneuploidies (Table 4). Some of these studies have been criticised for the high rate of failure (18%) to obtain a nuchal translucency measurement[35–37]. This partly reflects gestational age at measurement, since the success of nuchal measurement is greater with increasing gestational age[38], and improves considerably after 11 weeks. It has been suggested that 11 weeks is the optimum time for nuchal translucency screening, as chorionic villus sampling (the diagnostic test of choice in the first trimester) is not recommended until at least 10–11 weeks' gestation in view of the risk of procedure-related limb anomalies[39]. It would, therefore, seem unreasonable to offer screening earlier.

Nuchal translucency size varies with gestational age[38,40–42]. In a multientre screening study at 10–14 weeks of gestation based on 20,804 pregnancies, 164 fetuses with chromosomal abnormalities were detected[42]. Risk estimates for trisomy 21 were derived based on the degree of deviation in nuchal translucency from the normal median for gestation. Using this with maternal age, a 78% detection rate for trisomy 21 was predicted for a 5% false positive rate. Others have used different statistical approaches to take account of this variation with gestational age by using multiples of the expected median (as with serum screening)[43].

Specific points must be addressed before implementing a first trimester screening programme based on nuchal translucency measurement. Identifying and measuring the nuchal translucency takes time, sonographers require training and screening programmes must be audited[26,34]. Pandya and colleagues[34] reported the successful implementation of such a programme in two maternity units without a requirement for additional staff or machines. However, costs will vary between units depending on workload, availability and type of ultrasound machines, and training requirements. Although there is considerable variation (Table 4), overall the detection rate using nuchal translucency does not appear to be significantly greater than that reported for second trimester serum screening. Furthermore, an increased miscarriage rate has been reported in pregnancies with an increased nuchal translucency[33,35,44]. In one study, 11.8% of 70 fetuses with an increased nuchal translucency measurement who were known to have Down syndrome aborted spontaneously between chorionic villus sampling and termination of pregnancy[45].

Combined serum and sonographic screening in the first trimester

Recently it has been suggested that combining ultrasound with two serum biochemical markers and maternal age, between 10–14 weeks' gestation, may further improve detection rates. In an Australian study, a combination of free beta-human chorionic gonadotrophin, nuchal translucency measurement and maternal age identified 87.5% of Down syndrome pregnancies for a 14% false positive rate in a high-risk population. They estimated that, in routine use, a 71% detection rate could be achieved for a 7% false positive rate[46]. Using published data, Wald and Hackshaw[47] predicted an 80% detection rate for a 5% false positive rate using nuchal translucency measurement combined with free beta-human chorionic gonadotrophin and pregnancy associated plasma protein-A. While this appears to be better than maternal age with nuchal translucency or serum markers alone (63% and 62%, respectively, for a 5% false positive rate), these estimates need to be confirmed in practice.

Sonographic markers in the second trimester

The majority of maternity units in the UK offer an ultrasound scan at 16–20 weeks to examine fetal anatomy. At this stage, major and minor abnormalities may be detectable that are associated with aneuploidy. However, the performance of these 'markers' for aneuploidy in screening is uncertain. Studies from tertiary referral centres suggest that most fetuses with trisomy 13, 77–100% of fetuses with trisomy 18 and 33–50% of fetuses with Down syndrome have significant sonographic signs which may be detected by a second trimester scan[48–52]. The risk of chromosomal abnormality rises with increasing numbers of sonographic abnormalities in the fetus[53] and, when multiple abnormalities are present, the overall risk may be as high as 35%[54]. There are limited data on the detection of aneuploidy using ultrasound alone (without maternal serum biochemistry) in low risk pregnancies. In a retrospective survey of all low risk pregnancies in Vienna, ultrasound examination between 16–20 weeks detected 22% of aneuploid fetuses (trisomy 21, 11.8%; trisomy 18, 22%; and trisomy 13, 67%)[55]. Before serum screening became widely practised in the UK, two studies of routine second trimester ultrasound screening reported 9 of 34 (26%) fetuses with an abnormal karyotype identified through sonographic abnormality[56,57].

The association of minor but relatively common sonographic abnormalities (including choroid plexus cysts, mild pyelectasis, nuchal thickening, echogenic bowel and mild ventriculomegaly; Table 5) with aneuploidy has not been fully assessed in unselected populations. The majority of reported studies are based on selected populations and do not allow for known risk factors such as maternal age or serum markers. A good example is choroid plexus cysts which are cystic (or anechoic) areas in the choroid plexus, readily visualised in the fetal brain, and were first identified in 1984 when they were described as a benign transient finding[58]. Many subsequent studies have shown an association of choroid plexus cysts with trisomy 18. The estimated risk of aneuploidy in a fetus with isolated choroid plexus cysts varies from 1:30 to 1:477[59]. If the data from unselected populations are pooled, the risk is about 1–2:100[60]. Published results are difficult to interpret and compare as the populations are often not defined and may include both low and high

Table 5 Summary of estimates of screening performance of minor sonographic markers in the second trimester

Sonographic marker	Mean %aneuploidy detection rate (range)	Mean % false positive rate (range)
Nuchal fold 6 mm	38 (8–83)	1.3 (0–9.4)
Femoral length (observed:expected)	34 (13–68)	5.9 (2–56)
Humeral length (observed:expected)	37 (24–56)	5.3 (4–15)
Mild renal pelvic dilations	19 (6–25)	2.4 (1.6–2.8)
Echogenic bowel	11 (6–12)	0.7 (0.6–2.2)

Data from review of literature.

risk pregnancies. The mean prevalence of aneuploidy in fetuses with isolated choroid plexus cysts is 1 in 194 (0.59%) in studies reporting unselected pregnancies, 1 in 92 (1.07%) in those reporting selected populations and 1 in 43 (2.3%) in those where the population is not clearly defined[10]. Similar problems are encountered when assigning risk for the other minor sonographic markers. The wide variation in the management of pregnancies with such markers reflects clinical uncertainty. In some UK maternity units, karyotyping is offered when one of these minor sonographic markers is identified, while in others the findings are not documented nor are they mentioned to parents (Machlachan, personal communication, 1997).

Prior risk based on maternal age and serum markers, may be modified by the presence or absence of minor sonographic markers[61]. Based on a detailed search for specific sonographic markers in pregnancies at high risk for Down syndrome, detection rates of 73–92.8% and specificities of 86.7–96% have been reported[62,63]. In one[64], a detailed search, taking an average of 45 min, was made and prior risk reduced by 50% if no markers were found, and increased by 45% if they were. However, the time required precludes its routine use. By including only nuchal fold thickening, pyelectasis and humeral length, the false positive rate decreased to 6.7% but the detection rate remained at 87%. As the data were derived from tertiary centres, the generalisability of these findings is uncertain.

Using second trimester ultrasound markers of aneuploidy for screening is problematic since minor sonographic markers are common and are found in at least 5% of fetuses. Although it is reasonable to conclude that the presence of a minor sonographic marker increases the risk of aneuploidy, assignment of that risk following its identification in an otherwise low risk fetus is fraught with difficulty.

Which screening strategy for Down syndrome should be adopted?

There is no doubt that second trimester maternal serum screening can effectively detect around 60% of Down syndrome fetuses. Recent data have demonstrated that, in the first trimester, nuchal translucency measurement, particularly in combination with serum markers, may be equally effective. Although there may be some advantage, both social, medical and economic, in the early identification of pregnancies at increased risk of aneuploidy, there are also disadvantages. Earlier screening will identify up to 32% of fetuses destined to miscarry spontaneously[5]. Whilst this also applies to a lesser extent when screening at 16 weeks[65], earlier screening will expose more parents to the need to make difficult decisions about the termination of a pregnancy which might otherwise have miscarried spontaneously. Understanding the reason for the pregnancy loss may be helpful for parents, but this benefit must be carefully weighed against potential harm which may result from making parents choose to terminate a wanted pregnancy which might have been lost spontaneously. When using nuchal translucency measurement, there is some evidence, as discussed earlier, that this does occur[66]. Furthermore, these women may be labelled as being at increased risk for aneuploidy, and thus more likely to undergo karyotyping in future pregnancies. This would not have been so had the pregnancy ended in a spontaneous miscarriage. Another consideration in any first trimester screening programme is that invasive testing is required earlier. Currently this is done by chorionic villus sampling, which may carry an increased procedural related loss rate when compared with routine second trimester amniocentesis[67]. In addition, analysis of chorionic villi is more labour intensive and more expensive than amniocentesis, and it is also less accurate[67,68].

Data from the National Down Syndrome Cytogenetic Register show that the proportion of cases of Down syndrome diagnosed prenatally now exceeds that diagnosed postnatally[7]. The contribution of the various prenatal screening techniques has changed with time, reflecting the evolution of tests. In 1989, maternal age alone was the indication for testing in 78% of cases, but by 1996 had fallen to 22%[7]. Over the same period, the proportion detected through serum screening rose from 6% to 37%, and through ultrasound from 13% to 38%. First trimester ultrasound appears to have made a significant impact since 1994. The rise in prenatally diagnosed cases (92% of which were aborted in 1989–1993) was accompanied by a fall in the numbers of affected live births and a fall from 1.1 in 1989 to 0.9 in 1993 in the number per 1000 total live births in England and Wales[69]. Although these data are encouraging, a major problem is the availability of multiple screening tests. In the UK this is resulting in serial screening (first trimester ultrasound followed by second trimester serum screening and then second trimester ultrasound). This is likely to lead to an increase in the number of false positive results and invasive procedures as well as costs, both financial and clinical, secondary to the procedure-related loss of normal fetuses. Two studies have demonstrated that the positive predictive value of second trimester biochemical screening falls when first trimester nuchal translucency measurements are introduced[37,70]. The use of second trimester 'marker scans' following an increased risk on serum screening should be discouraged. There is some debate as to what proportion of fetuses with Down syndrome have a sonographic marker in the second trimester, but some estimates are as low as 44%[71]. The use of ultrasound to modify risk estimates based on serum screening, may, therefore, serve to decrease the sensitivity of the first screening test.

In the UK, a review of screening policies for Down syndrome has been identified as a priority. In a recently published report[12], commissioned by the NHS Standing Group on Health Technology, it was recommended that screening be organised from about 35 centres throughout the UK, with specialised training available for health professionals involved in this programme. In order to avoid the *ad hoc* introduction of serial or multistep screening, it was concluded that second trimester serum markers (either the triple or quadruple tests) should be used for screening until the results of further evaluation of first trimester serum and ultrasound markers become available.

References

1   Hook EB. Chromosome abnormalities: prevalence, risks and recurrence. In: Brock DJH, Rodeck CH, Ferguson-Smith MA. (eds) *Prenatal Diagnosis and Screening*. Edinburgh: Churchill Livingstone, 1998; 351–92

2   Palomaki GE, Neveux LM, Haddow JE. Can reliable Down's syndrome detection rates be determined from prenatal screening intervention trials? *J Med Screen* 1996; **3**: 12–7

3   Hook EB, Cross PK, Regal RR. The frequency of 47,+21, 47,+18, and 47,+13 at the uppermost extremes of maternal ages: results on 56,094 fetuses studied prenatally and comparisons with data on livebirths. *Hum Genet* 1984; **28**: 211–20

4   Ferguson-Smith MA, Yates JRW. Maternal age specific rates for chromosomal aberrations factors influencing them: report of a collaborative European study on 52,965 amniocenteses. *Prenat Diagn* 1984; **4**: 5–44

5   MacIntosh MCM, Wald NJ, Chard T *et al*. The selective miscarriage of Down's syndrome from 10 weeks of pregnancy. *Br J Obstet Gynaecol* 1996; **103**: 1171–2

6   Snijders RJM, Sebire NJ, Nicolaides KH. Maternal age and gestational age-specific rates for chromosomal defects. *Fetal Diagn Ther* 1995; **10**: 349–55

7   Mutton D, Ide RG, Alberman ED. Trends in prenatal screening diagnosis of Down's Syndrome: England and Wales 1989–97. *BMJ* 1998; **317**: 922–3

8   O'Leary P, Bower C, Murch A, Crowhurst J, Goldblatt J. The impact of antenatal screening for Down syndrome in Western Australia: 1980–1994. *Aust N Z J Obstet Gynaecol* 1996; **36**: 385–8

9   Chitty LS, Barnes CA, Berry C. Continuing with pregnancy after a diagnosis of lethal abnormality: experience of five couples and recommendations for management. *BMJ* 1996; **313**: 478–80

10 Chitty LS, Chudleigh P, Wright E, Campbell S, Pembrey ME. The significance of choroid plexus cysts in an unselected population: the results of a multicentre study. *Ultrasound Obstet Gynecol* 1998; **12**: 1–7

11 Huang T, Watt HC, Wald NJ. The effect of differences in the distribution of maternal age in England and Wales on the performance of prenatal screening for Down's syndrome. *Prenat Diagn* 1997; **17**: 615–21

12 Wald NJ, Kennard A, Hackshaw A, McGuire A. Antenatal screening for Down's syndrome. *J Med Screen* 1997; **4**: 181–246

13 Hackshaw AK, Kennard A, Wald NJ. Detection of pregnancies with trisomy 18 in screening for Down's syndrome. *J Med Screen* 1995; **2**: 228–9

14 Palomaki GE, Haddow JE, Knight GJ *et al.* Risk-based screening for trisomy 18 using alphafetoprotein, unconjugated oestriol and human chorionic gonadotrophin. *Prenat Diagn* 1995; **15**: 713–23

15 Goldstein H, Nielson ICG. Rates and survival in individuals with trisomy 13 and 18. *Clin Genet* 1988; **27**: 59–61

16 Carter PE, Pearn JH, Bell J, Martin W, Anderson NG. Survival in trisomy 18. Life tables for use in genetic counselling and clinical paediatrics. *Clin Genet* 1985; **17**: 59–61

17 Barkai G, Goldman B, Ries L, Chaki R, Zer T, Cuckle H. Expanding multiple marker screening for Down's syndrome to include Edward's syndrome. *Prenat Diagn* 1993; **13**: 843–50

18 Cuckle HS, Holding S, Jones R, Groome NP, Wallace EM. Combining inhibin A with existing second-trimester markers in maternal serum screening for Down's syndrome. *Prenat Diagn* 1996; **16**: 1095–100

19 Spencer K, Wallace EM, Ritoe S. Second-trimester dimeric inhibin-A in Down's syndrome screening. *Prenat Diagn* 1996; **16**: 1101–10

20 Wald NJ, Densem JW, George L *et al.* Inhibin-A in Down's syndrome pregnancies: revised estimate of standard deviation. *Prenat Diagn* 1997; **17**: 285–90

21 Wald NJ, George L, Smith D, Densem JW, Petterson K. Serum screening for Down's syndrome between 8 and 14 weeks of pregnancy. *Br J Obstet Gynaecol* 1996; **103**: 407–12

22 Spencer K, Aitken DA, Macri JN, Buchannan PD. Urine free beta hCG and beta core in pregnancies affected by Down syndrome. *Prenat Diagn* 1996; **16**: 605–13

23 Kellner LH, Canick JA, Palomaki GE *et al.* Urinary markers: a new approach to screening for Down syndrome in the second trimester. *Am J Hum Genet* 1996; **59**: A41

24 Isozaki T, Palomaki GE, Bahado-Singh RO, Cole LA. Screening for Down syndrome pregnancy using B-core fragment: prospective study. *Prenat Diagn* 1997; **17**: 407–13

25 Macintosh MCM, Nicolaides KH, Noble P, Chard T, Gunn L, Iles R. Urinary B-core hCG: screening for aneuploidies in early pregnancy (11–14 weeks' gestation). *Prenat Diagn* 1997; **17**: 401–5

26 Snijders RJM, Johnson S, Sebire NJ, Noble PL, Nicolaides KH. First-trimester ultrasound screening for chromosomal defects. *Ultrasound Obstet Gynecol* 1996; **7**: 216–26

27 Chitty LS, Pandya PP. Ultrasound screening for fetal abnormalities in the first trimester. *Prenat Diagn* 1997; **17**: 1269–81

28 Bronshtein M, Rottem S, Yoffe N, Blumenfeld Z. First-trimester and early second-trimester diagnosis of nuchal cystic hygroma by transvaginal sonography: diverse prognosis of the septated from the nonseptated lesion. *Am J Obstet Gynecol* 1989; **161**: 78–82

29 Nicolaides KH, Azar G, Byrne D, Mansur C, Marx K. Fetal nuchal translucency: ultrasound screening for fetal trisomy in the first trimester of pregnancy. *BMJ* 1992; **304**: 867–9

30 Johnson MP, Johnson A, Holzgreve W *et al.* First-trimester sample hyroma: cause and outcome. *Am J Obstet Gynecol* 1993; **168**: 156–61

31 Shulman LP, Emerson DS, Felker RE, Phillips OP, Simpson JL, Elias S. High frequency of cytogenic abnormalities in fetuses with cystic hygroma diagnosed in the first trimester. *Obstet Gynecol* 1992; **80**: 80–2

32 Pandya PP, Brizot ML, Kuhn P, Snijders RJM, Nicolaides KH. First trimester fetal nuchal translucency thickness and risk for trisomies. *Obstet Gynecol* 1994; **84**: 420–3

33 Pandya PP, Kondylios A, Hilbert L, Snijders RJM, Nicolaides KH. Chromosomal defects and

outcome in 1,105 fetuses with increased nuchal translucency. *Ultrasound Obstet Gynecol* 1995; **5**: 15–9

34 Pandya PP, Goldberg H, Walton B *et al.* The implementation of first trimester scanning at 10–13 weeks' gestation and the measurement of fetal nuchal translucency thickness in two maternity units. *Ultrasound Obstet Gynecol* 1995; **5**: 20–5

35 Bewley S, Roberts LJ, Mackinson AM, Rodeck CH. First-trimester fetal nuchal translucency: problems with screening the general populations 2. *Br J Obstet Gynaecol* 1995; **102**: 386–8

36 Kornan LP, Morssink JR, De Wolf BTHM, Heringa MP, Mantingi A. Nuchal translucency cannot be used as a screening test for chromosomal abnormalities in the first trimester of pregnancy in a routine ultrasound practice. *Prenat Diagn* 1996; **16**: 797–805

37 Thilaganathan B, Slack A, Wathen NC. Effect of first-trimester nuchal translucency on second-trimester maternal serum biochemical screening for Down's syndrome. *Ultrasound Obstet Gynecol* 1997; **10**: 261–4

38 Roberts LJ, Bewley S, Mackinson AM, Rodeck CH. First trimester fetal nuchal translucency: problems with screening the general population 1. *Br J Obstet Gynaecol* 1995; **102**: 381–5

39 Firth H. Chorionic villus sampling and limb deficiency – cause or coincidence? *Prenat Diagn* 1997; **17**: 1313–30

40 Brambati B, Cislaghi C, Tului L *et al.* First-trimester Down's syndrome screening using nuchal translucency: a prospective study in patients undergoing chorionic villus sampling. *Ultrasound Obstet Gynecol* 1995; **5**: 9–14

41 Pajkrt E, Bilardo CM, Van Lith JMM, Mol BWJ, Bleker OP. Nuchal translucency measurement in normal fetuses. *Obstet Gynecol* 1995; **86**: 994–7

42 Pandya PP, Snijders RJM, Johnson SP, De Lourdes Brizot M, Nicolaides KH. Screening for fetal trisomies by maternal age and fetal nuchal translucency thickness at 10 to 14 weeks of gestation. *Br J Obstet Gynaecol* 1995; **102**: 957–62

43 Biagiotti R, Periti E, Brizzi L, Vanzi E, Cariati E. Comparison between two methods of standardisation for gestational age differences in fetal nuchal translucency measurement in first-trimester screening for trisomy 21. *Ultrasound Obstet Gynecol* 1997; **9**: 248–52

44 Szabo J, Gellen J, Szmere G. First-trimester ultrasound screening for fetal aneuploidies in women over 35 and under 35 years of age. *Ultrasound Obstet Gynecol* 1995; **5**: 161–3

45 Hyett JA, Sebire NJ, Snijders RJM, Nicolaides KH. Intrauterine lethality of trisomy 21 fetuses with increased nuchal translucency thickness. *Ultrasound Obstet Gynecol* 1996; **7**: 101–3

46 Scott F, Wheeler D, Sinosich M, Boogert A, Anderson, Edelman D. First trimester screening using nuchal translucency free beta human chorionic gonadotrophin and maternal age. *Aust NZ J Obstet Gynecol* 1996; **36**: 381–4

47 Wald NJ, Hackshaw AK. Combining ultrasound and biochemistry in first-trimester screening for Down's syndrome. *Prenat Diagn* 1997; **17**: 821–9

48 Nyberg DA, Resta RG, Luthy DA, Hickok DE, Mahoney DS, Hirsch JH. Prenatal sonographic findings of Down syndrome: review of 94 cases. *Obstet Gynecol* 1990; **76**: 370–7

49 Benaceraff BR, Miller MA, Frigoletto FD. Sonographic detection of fetuses with trisomies 13 and 18: accuracy and limitations. *Am J Obstet Gynecol* 1988; **158**: 404–9

50 Benaceraff BR, Gelman R, Frigoletto FD. Sonographic identification of 2nd trimester fetuses with Down syndrome. *N Engl J Med* 1987; **317**: 1371–6

51 Benaceraff BR. The second-trimester fetus with Down syndrome: detection using sonographic features. *Ultrasound Obstet Gynecol* 1996; **7**: 147–55

52 Hill LM. The sonographic detection of trisomies 13, 18 and 21. *Clin Obstet Gynecol* 1996; **39**: 831–50

53 Nicolaides KH, Snijders RJM, Gosen CM, Berry C, Campbell S. Ultrasonographically detectable markers of fetal chromosomal abnormalities. *Lancet* 1992; **340**: 704–7

54 Rizzo N, Pittalis MC, Pilu G, Orsini LF, Porolo A, Bovicelli L. Prenatal karyotype on malformed fetuses. *Prenat Diagn* 1990; **10**: 17–23

55 Bernaschek G, Kolankaya A, Stuempflen I, Deutinger MT, Deutinger J. Chromosomal abnormalities: how much can we predict by ultrasound examination in low-risk pregnancies? *Am J Perinatol* 1996; **13**: 259–63

56 Chitty LS, Hunt GH, Moore J, Lobb MO. Effectiveness of routine ultrasonography in detecting fetal structural abnormalities in a low risk population. *BMJ* 1991; **303**: 1165–9

57 Shirley IM, Bottomley F, Robinson VP. Routine radiographer screening for fetal abnormalities by ultrasound in an unselected low risk population. *Br J Radiol* 1991; **65**: 565–9

58 Chudleigh P, Pearce JM, Campbell S. Prenatal diagnosis of transient cysts of the choroid plexus. *Prenat Diagn* 1984; **4**: 135–7

59 Snijders RJM. Isolated choroid plexus cysts: should we offer karyotyping? *Ultrasound Obstet Gynecol* 1996; **8**: 223–4

60 Chitty LS. Choroid plexus cysts: the need for further study. *Ultrasound Obstet Gynecol* 1994; **4**: 444–5

61 Drugan A, Johnson MP, Reichler A, Hume Jr RF, Itskovicz-Eldor J, Evans MI. Second-trimester minor ultrasound anomalies: impact on the risk of aneuploidy associated with advanced maternal age. *Obstet Gynecol* 1996; **88**: 203–6

62 Vintzileos AM, Egan JF. Adjusting the risk for trisomy 21 on the basis of second-trimester ultrasonography. *Am J Obstet Gynecol* 1995; **172**: 837–44

63 Benaceraff BR, Nadel A, Bromley B. Identification of second trimester fetuses with autosomal trisomy by use of a sonographic scoring index. *Radiology* 1994; **193**: 135–40

64 Vintzileos AM, Campbell WA, Guzman ER, Smullian JC, McLean DA, Ananth CV. Second-trimester ultrasound markers detection of trisomy 21: which markers are best? *Obstet Gynecol* 1997; **89**: 941–4

65 Nicolaides KH, Sebire NJ, Snijders RJM. Down's syndrome screening with nuchal translucency. *Lancet* 1997; **349**: 438

66 Hyett JA, Sebire NJ, Snijders RJM, Nicolaides KH. Intrauterine lethality of trisomy 21 fetuses with increased nuchal translucency thickness. *Ultrasound Obstet Gynecol* 1993; **7**: 101–3

67 Alfirevic Z, Gosden C, Neilson JP. Chorionic villus sampling vs amniocentesis for prenatal diagnosis. In: Neilson JP, Crowther CA, Hodnett ED, Hofmeyr GJ. (eds) *Pregnancy and Childbirth Module of the Cochrane Database of Systematic Reviews* 1997

68 Hahnemann JM, Vejerslev LO. Accuracy of cytogenetic findings on chorionic villus sampling (CVS) – diagnostic consequences of CVS mosaicism and non-mosaic discrepancy in centres contributing to euromic 1986–1992. *Prenat Diagn* 1997; **17**: 801–20

69 Alberman E, Mutton D, Ide R, Nicholson A, Bobrow M. Down's syndrome births and pregnancy terminations in 1989 to 1993: preliminary findings. *Br J Obstet Gynaecol* 1995; **102**: 445–7

70 Kadir RA, Economides DL. The effects of nuchal translucency measurement on second-trimester biochemical screening for down's syndrome. *Ultrasound Obstet Gynecol* 1997; **9**: 244–7

71 Rotmensch S, Liberati M, Bronshtein M *et al*. Prenatal sonographic findings in 187 fetuses with Down syndrome. *Prenat Diagn* 1997; **17**: 1001–9

72 Haddow JE, Palomaki GE, Knight GJ. Prenatal screening for Down's syndrome with use of maternal serum markers. *N Engl J Med* 1992; **327**: 588–93

73 Wald NJ, Kennard A, Densem JW, Cuckle HS, Chard T, Butler L. Antenatal maternal serum screening for Down's syndrome: results of a demonstration project. *BMJ* 1992; **305**: 391–4

74 Pescia G, Dao MH, Wekhs D. Le triple depistage del la trisomie 21: resultats prospecifs de 7039 evaluations. *Rev Med Suisse Romande* 1993; **113**: 277–80

75 Piggot M, Wilkinson P, Bennett J. Implementation of an antenatal screening programme for Down's syndrome in two districts (Brighton and Eastbourne). *J Med Screen* 1994; **1**: 45–9

76 Goodburn SF, Yates JRW, Raggatt PR. Second trimester maternal serum screening using alpha-fetoprotein, human chorionic gonadotrophin and unconjugated oestriol: experience of a regional programme. *Prenat Diagn* 1994; **14**: 391–402

77 Dawson AJ, Jones G, Matharu MS *et al*. Serum screening for Down's syndrome. *Br J Obstet Gynaecol* 1993; **100**: 875–7

78 Beekhuis JR. Maternal serum screening for fetal Down's syndrome and neural tube defects. A prospective study performed in the north of The Netherlands. 1993; (Abstract)

79 Spencer K, Carpenter P. Prospective study of prenatal screening for Down's syndrome with free beta human chorionic gonadotrophin. *BMJ* 1993; **307**: 764–9

80 Comas C, Martinex JM, Ojuel J *et al*. First-trimester nuchal edema as a marker of aneuploidy. *Ultrasound Obstet Gynecol* 1995; **5**: 26–9

81 Orlandi F, Damiani G, Hallahan TW, Krantz DA, Macri JN. First-trimester screening for fetal aneuploidy: biochemistry and nuchal translucency. *Ultrasound Obstet Gynecol* 1997; **10**: 381–6

82 Hafner E, Schuchter K, Philipp K. Screening for chromosomal abnormalities in an unselected population by fetal nuchal translucency. *Ultrasound Obstet Gynecol* 1996; **6**: 330–3.

83 Bower SJ, Chitty L, Bewley S *et al*. First-trimester Down's syndrome screening using nuchal translucency: a prospective study in patients undergoing chorionic villus sampling. *Proceeding of the British Congress Obstetrics and Gynaecology, Dublin 3 1995*

84 Economides DL, Whitlow BJ, Kadir R, Lazanakis M, Verdin SM. First trimester sonographic detection of chromosomal abnormalities in an unselected population. *Br J Obstet Gynaecol* 1998; **105**: 58–62

85 Wald NJ, Densem JW, Smith D, Klee GG. Four marker screening for Down syndrome. *Prenat Diagn* 1994; **14**: 707–16

86 Wald NJ, Densem JW, George L, Muttukrishna S, Knight PG. Prenatal screening for Down syndrome using inhibin-A as a serum marker. *Prenat Diagn* 1996; **16**: 143–53

87 Theodoropoulos P, Lolis D, Papageorgiou C, Papaionnou S, Planchouras N, Makrydinas G. Evaluation of first-trimester screening by nucahal translucency and maternal age. *Prenat Diagn* 1998; **18**: 133–8

88 Wald NJ, Kennard A, Hackshaw AK. First trimester serum screening for Down syndrome. *Prenat Diagn* 1995; **15**: 1227–40

89 Casals E, Fortuny A, Grudzinskas JG, Suzuki Y, Teisner B, Comas C *et al*. First trimester biochemical screening for Down syndrome with the use of PAPP-A, AFP and β-hCG. *Prenat Diagn* 1996; **16**: 405–410

90 Bizot ML, Snijders RMJ, Bersinger NA, Kuhn P, Nicolaides KH. Maternal serum pregnancy-associated plasma protein A and fetal muchal translucency thickness for the prediction of fetal trisomies in early pregnancy. *Obstet Gynecol* 1994; **84**: 918–22.

Screening for cystic fibrosis and its evaluation

Mark F Wildhagen, Leo P ten Kate* and J Dik F Habbema

*Department of Public Health, Erasmus University, Rotterdam, The Netherlands and *Department of Human Genetics, Vrije Universiteit, Amsterdam, The Netherlands*

Cystic fibrosis (CF) is a recessively inherited disorder for which screening has been proposed. A number of different screening strategies have been suggested, including prenatal, preconceptional, school and neonatal carrier screening, as well as screening of newborns to identify affected infants. We discuss the advantages and disadvantages of these strategies, and identify gaps in knowledge relevant to decisions to introduce a screening programme for cystic fibrosis. Screening to identify carriers during the newborn period or among school age children is inadvisable, mainly on psychosocial and cost-effectiveness grounds. Although early diagnosis of CF may improve prognosis, current scientific evidence is not sufficient to support screening newborns to identify affected infants. Of the remaining two options, prenatal screening has a practical advantage because of existing facilities, while with screening before conception all reproductive options are, in principle, open to detected carrier couples. If adequate pre- and post-test counselling can be provided, both two types of screening could be introduced.

Correspondence to:
Mark F Wildhagen MSc, Department of Public Health, Faculty of Medicine, Erasmus University Rotterdam, PO Box 1738, 3000 DR Rotterdam, The Netherlands

Cystic fibrosis (CF) is a recessively inherited disorder for which screening has been proposed. There is widespread agreement that individuals with a family history of CF should be offered genetic testing as they are at increased risk of being a carrier (Table 1)[1]. Direct experience of CF in a family member may make decisions regarding carrier testing more informed and less abstract. Partners of affected individuals and of known carriers should also be offered genetic testing, as these couples are at increased risk of having a child with CF. However, the role of population-based testing of couples who are not known to be at high risk, either in early pregnancy or before conception, and of neonatal patient screening is less clear and is the subject of review in a number of countries. Recently, a consensus development panel of the US National Institutes of Health has recommended that genetic testing for CF be offered to couples currently planning a pregnancy, and to couples seeking prenatal care, in addition to adults with a positive family history of CF and to partners of people with CF[1]. In this article, current knowledge regarding screening for CF will be reviewed and the implications for policy assessed.

Table 1 Probability of being a CF gene carrier for relatives of an affected individual

Proband	Probability (%)
Brother/sister	67
Aunt/uncle	51
First cousin	26
First cousin once removed	14
Second cousin	8

Natural history

Cystic fibrosis (CF), first described in the medical literature in the 1930s[2,3], is characterised by recurrent lower respiratory tract infections resulting in chronic suppurative lung disease, and pancreatic insufficiency[4,5]. It is associated with a shortened life span and impaired quality of life and requires lifelong medical care, as well as extensive support from relatives and friends, which may interfere with the normal daily life of both affected individuals and their relatives[6,7].

Meconium ileus occurs in 10–20% of newborns with CF and may be the earliest clinical manifestation of the condition[4,8]. Most affected individuals need daily physiotherapy, repeated courses of antibiotics to treat pulmonary infections, as well as lifelong enzyme supplementation and a high energy diet. Affected adult males almost always have azoospermia, but reduced fertility also occurs in women[9,10].

There have been considerable advances in the medical care of individuals with CF, including recombinant human DNase which reduces the viscosity of purulent airway secretions, heart-lung transplantation, and home therapy[5,11–14]. Current research in gene therapy may soon progress to the point of widespread clinical use. While these advances may improve the length and quality of life, for most affected individuals CF remains a disorder associated with reduced life expectancy. In the US, median survival is 31.1 years for men and 28.3 years for women[5], while in the UK, the median life expectancy of children with cystic fibrosis born in 1990, assuming continuous progress in survival in years to come, is estimated to be 40 years[15].

Genetics and prevalence

Cystic fibrosis is one of the most common recessively inherited disorders in Caucasian populations. Affected individuals (or homozygotes) have a CF gene mutation present on both chromosomes 7, but this is present on only one chromosome 7 of carriers (or heterozygotes), who are not affected by the disorder and are healthy. Couples in which both partners are carriers have a 1 in 4 risk with each pregnancy of having an affected child. Without screening, the existence of a carrier within the family is often only revealed following the clinical diagnosis of an affected infant. More than 80% of affected infants are born in families with no prior family history[16].

The prevalence of CF carrier status varies widely across different racial and ethnic groups, being very common among people in Northern Ireland (carrier prevalence 1 in 21 and birth prevalence 1 in 1807) and relatively rare among Hawaiian Orientals (carrier prevalence 1 in 150 and birth prevalence 1 in 90,000)[17,18]. In the US and UK, the carrier prevalence is about 1 in 25, and, in The Netherlands around 1 in 30[19,20]. There are suggestions that a high frequency of carriers reflects past or present genetic advantage[21,22], for example the gene may protect against typhoid fever which was a major killer in the past[23].

The gene responsible for CF was identified in 1989[24-26]. This gene, called the cystic fibrosis transmembrane conductance regulator (CFTR) gene, codes for a protein that regulates a low-conductance chloride channel[27]. Many, although not all, of the clinical manifestations of CF can be explained by the lack of this function. Soon after the CF gene was cloned, it was realised that screening for carriers would be possible through direct mutation detection.

Since 1989, a large number of mutations in the CFTR gene have been discovered, some of which have been detected in only one family. Currently more than 800 mutations have been identified (CF Genetic Analysis Consortium, *http://www.genet.sickkids.on.ca/cftr/*), the most common of which is the ΔF508 mutation, a three-base deletion in the gene. This mutation, together with a further 6–10 non-ΔF508 mutated genes, account for more than half of the population variation in CF mutations world-wide (Table 2).

Table 2 Most frequent mutations in the CFTR-gene

	Northern Europe (%)	Northern America (%)	World (%)
ΔF508	70.3	66.1	66.0
G542X	2.1	2.2	2.4
G551D	1.7	2.0	1.6
N1303K	1.0	1.2	1.3
1717-1G→T	0.8	0.4	0.6
R553X	0.8	0.9	0.7
W1282X	0.6	2.3	1.2
621+1G→T	0.5	1.5	0.7
A455E	0.2	0.3	0.1
R1162X	0.2	0.2	0.3
14–16 other mutations	2.3	2.7	2.2
Total	80.2	79.9	77.3

Source: CF Genetic Analysis Consortium[99]

Screening and screening tests

CFTR mutations can be detected by PCR analysis of material obtained by a mouthwash or bloodspot[28]. With the mouthwash procedure there is no need for medical supervision of sample collection. The mouthwash procedure has, theoretically, an almost perfect sensitivity and specificity, apart from laboratory errors[28]. This relatively simple detection of CFTR mutations makes it possible to consider introducing a screening programme for carriers of the cystic fibrosis gene, where the primary aim is to assess carrier status and counsel couples whose members are both carriers of a CF gene mutation[29,30]. These couples can then be offered prenatal diagnosis by chorion villus sampling or amniocentesis.

Because of the large number of mutations in the CFTR gene it is not feasible to test all individuals for all possible mutations. However, if individuals are tested with a panel of probes consisting of the mutations from Table 2, approximately 80% of the carriers and 64% (80% of 80%) of the carrier couples can be detected. Because of the imperfect test sensitivity, couples with one test-positive and one test-negative partner have an (increased) risk of 1 in 484 of having an affected child, compared to a 1 in 2500 baseline risk[31]. However, these individuals cannot be offered prenatal diagnosis.

New methods of DNA testing, for example allele specific oligonucleotide (ASO) and denaturing gradient gel electrophoresis (DGGE), use a combination of probes in one panel. These have a high sensitivity, for example over 90% for ASO and 98% for DGGE per individual in The Netherlands. This means that more carrier couples can be detected, but, on the other hand, the costs of the screening will increase also since these tests are rather expensive at the moment.

Screening strategies

Several screening strategies for cystic fibrosis have been suggested[32–35]. Of these, prenatal, preconceptional, school and neonatal screening can be considered for general population screening.

Screening couples before conception and in early pregnancy

For high risk couples, screening before conception (preconceptional screening) has several potential advantages over screening in early pregnancy (prenatal screening), including the option not to have children, time to adjust to the information presented and time to make decisions about prenatal diagnosis, with potentially less anxiety[36,37].

Other reproductive options available as a consequence of preconceptional screening include the use of artificial insemination with screened donor sperm, screened egg cell donation or pre-implantation diagnosis. However, the effectiveness of preconceptional screening is uncertain, since at present there is no routinely available opportunity to screen all couples who are not yet pregnant but may intend to become so in the near future. In view of this, a preconceptional consultation centre has been proposed as a new health service provision[38]. Alternatively, couples planning to become pregnant may consult their general practitioner.

Several strategies and definitions for prenatal and preconceptional carrier screening exist, and these can be distinguished with regard to the testing process and the information process[31,32,39,40]. Among the strategies are stepwise screening, where one partner (usually the woman) is screened first, and only the partners of those found to be carriers will be offered screening. One disadvantage of the approach is that it generates anxiety in women identified as carriers. However, this anxiety appears to be short-lived and disappears among women whose partners test negative[41]. In stepwise screening, three test outcomes are possible: both partners are test-positive (++ couples), one partner is test-positive and the other test-negative (+– couples), and one partner is test-negative and the other is not tested (–? couples).

Another strategy is couple screening, where the couple is treated as an entity. Both partners submit a sample simultaneously and, if both are identified as carriers, the couple is designated as being at high risk and reported as positive. In contrast, couples in which one partner is tested positive and one negative are designated negative although their risk of an affected infant is higher than the prior risk for the general population. One of the arguments for couple screening is that unnecessary anxiety, due to identifying couples of mixed carrier status, can be avoided by simply treating all couples not at high risk as negative. This caused concern among geneticists as it was felt that the results of all genetic testing should be made available to those tested and not withheld[42]. A compromise has been to make the results available on request rather than routinely. Early experience from pilot studies in The Netherlands shows that almost all couples want both partners to be tested and to obtain individual results (L Henneman, unpublished data).

Since stepwise screening also aims at the couple, the terminology 'stepwise' and 'couple' can be confusing. For this reason, the terms single-entry two-step (SETS) couple screening and double-entry two-step (DETS) couple screening have been proposed (Fig. 1)[31]. In these strategies, both partners submit a sample. In single-entry two-step screening, one partner is tested first (first step) and if he/she is identified as a carrier the second partner is tested. The first partner is tested for the ΔF508 and other frequent mutations, while the second partner is tested

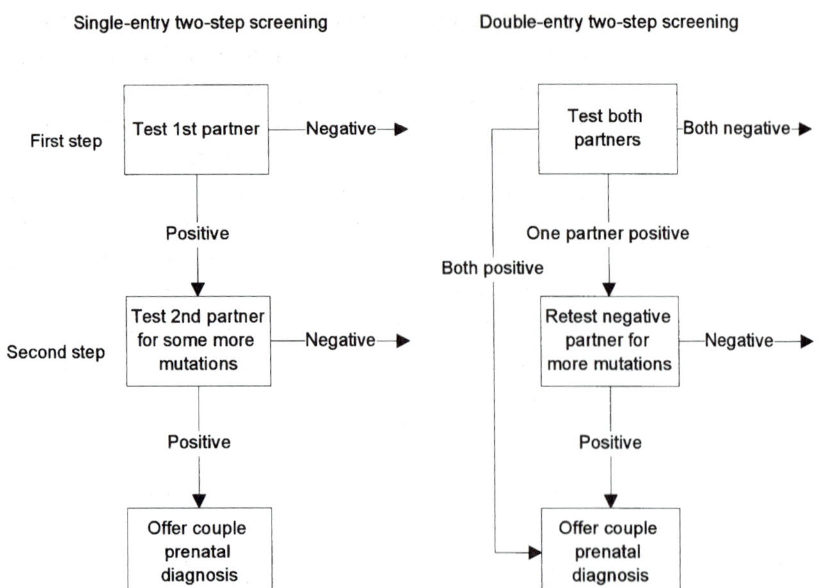

Fig. 1 Single-entry two-step (SETS) screening and double-entry two-step (DETS) CF screening

for a larger number of less common mutations (second step). In double-entry two-step couple screening, both partners are tested for the ΔF508 and other frequent mutations (first step), and the test-negative partner of an identified carrier is tested for a larger number of less common mutations (second step). The advantage of DETS over SETS is that the remaining risk in couples with two negative partners (– – couples) in the DETS strategy is significantly lower than in couples with one test-negative partner and one individual that is not tested (–? couples) in the SETS strategy. On the other hand, approximately 5% of couples identified in the DETS approach will comprise one test positive partner and one test negative partner, compared with 2.5% for single-entry two-step screening. For these couples, the risk is not reduced with the current test sensitivities, but is higher than the risk in the general population[31].

Screening for carriers in the neonatal period or at school age

Screening school aged children for recessive conditions is feasible, and pilot projects have been conducted to screen for thalassaemia carriers in Italy, for Tay-Sachs disease carriers in Canada, and for CF carriers in Australia and Canada[43–46]. Although, from a community-genetic perspective, school screening may offer an opportunity for teaching genetics, this has been questioned[47]. One problem is the difficulty in maintaining confidentiality of test results. Furthermore, there is concern that because school screening takes place in a rather unstable stage of life, this might lead to stigmatisation[48].

Since a blood sample, stored as a dried blood spot, is obtained from all newborns and tested for phenylketonuria and congenital hypothyroidism, it would be easy to include screening for CF carriers in the existing neonatal metabolic screening programme. Identification of newborn carriers provides an opportunity to test both parents with a view to ascertaining previously unrecognised high risk couples and extend their future reproductive choices. Obviously, as the average family has less than two children, detected carrier couples can use this knowledge of being carrier only for about one child on average. However, there are several problems with this approach. It may be a disadvantage to combine routine screening for conditions for which effective treatments are available with screening for carriers of genetic conditions.

Another disadvantage of identifying carriers as newborns or school children, is that this information only becomes relevant to the carrier when they are of reproductive age, some 10–30 years later. Considerable efforts would be required to retain this information and this would be helped by a computer database or an individual health-passport. Furthermore, it is most likely that the current screening tests will be obsolete in 10–30 years as new screening methods and new insights in the disease process will have emerged.

Cascade testing

Specific to genetic diseases is the possibility of testing relatives and offspring of affected patients and known carriers – this is termed cascade testing. The advantage of cascade testing is that the relatives or offspring of the affected individual have a higher-than-average risk of being carriers (Table 1). In addition, as discussed earlier, contact with an affected relative and hence greater familiarity with the implications of being affected, may allow more informed choices about screening and reproduction to be made than are possible for the general population.

A disadvantage of cascade testing is that it will not identify the majority of carrier couples since more than 80% of affected infants are born in families without a prior history of the disease[16]. It cannot, therefore, be considered an effective screening strategy. Holloway and Brock[49,50] estimated that 4–13% of all carriers in Scotland would be detected by cascade testing, which would result in 8–24% of all carrier couples being detected, compared with more than 50% detection through prenatal screening[31]. Brock[50] concluded that cascade testing should only be considered in combination with general population screening.

Neonatal patient screening

In 1968, Schutt and Isles reported excessive albumin in the meconium of patients with meconium ileus due to CF[51]. This made neonatal screening for cystic fibrosis patients a possibility[52,53]. In 1979 Crossley *et al* reported that immunoreactive trypsin (IRT) was raised in the serum of children with cystic fibrosis[54]. Since newborn screening using a dried blood-spot assay for IRT has a higher sensitivity than meconium albumin and because it was widely believed that early diagnosis would improve outcome, newborn screening programmes were developed in Europe, the USA and Australia. The sensitivity of the IRT test (85.7%) and the specificity (99.8%) are improved by testing for the ΔF508 mutation in high-risk bloodspots (sensitivity 95.2%, specificity 99.9%), but false positives are still possible[55]. Therefore, the diagnosis is confirmed by a sweat test[56].

The rationale for newborn screening to identify affected infants has been questioned. It has been argued that evidence is lacking that an early diagnosis will substantially improve outcome for the patient. While the findings of several studies have suggested that patients with CF who are diagnosed early, *i.e.* before the onset of clinical pulmonary involvement, have a better prognosis than those whose diagnosis was made when pulmonary symptoms developed[57–65], all of these studies have some methodological problems.

The only randomised controlled trial, funded by the National Institutes of Health, started in 1985 in Wisconsin, USA[66]. A total of 650,341 newborns were recruited, and allocated to either newborn screening or no screening. Dried blood spots were tested for the 325,170 recruited newborns allocated to no screening but the results were withheld until these infants reached 4 years of age. In the screening arm of the trial, infants who screened positive received a sweat test and confirmed positives were treated according to a protocol. Age at diagnosis was lower in the screening group (median age 7 weeks) compared with the no-screening group (median age 23 weeks). Nutritional status is being evaluated by anthropometric and biochemical methods in affected children in both groups and has been reported for the first 10 years of follow-up. It was found that children in the screening group were significantly heavier than their unscreened counterparts, both at time of diagnosis and during the follow-up period. However, although remaining better in the screened infants, these differences were less marked and of no statistical significance by 5–6 years of age. The authors concluded that 'neonatal screening provides the opportunity to prevent malnutrition in infants with cystic fibrosis'. Respiratory outcomes have not been reported from this trial but are proposed.

In an accompanying editorial, it was concluded that 'the results of this new study provide further evidence that the time has come for routine neonatal screening for cystic fibrosis'[67]. However, the issue of lead-time bias, a form of selection bias, has been raised in another editorial, which, it was suggested, may substantially alter the interpretation of the trial findings[68]. This arises because the probability of diagnosis in both arms of the trial is only equal after 4 years of age. Before this age, children diagnosed in the 'screening' group will include those with less severe disease which may not have presented clinically by this age, in contrast to those diagnosed by this age in the 'no screening' group, who are likely to have more severe disease[68]. Evidence for such a bias is suggested by the fact that the overall results presented in the original trial report were strongly influenced by the results in the first three years. The authors of this second editorial have proposed that further analyses comparing outcome in the screened and unscreened groups be restricted to outcomes measured after the age of four years. They concluded that 'the present evidence is not encouraging and does not warrant any change in policy from that suggested by the National Institutes of Health consensus statement'[1], which recommended that newborns should not be screened.

Results of (pilot) carrier screening programmes

Several pilot studies of CF carrier screening have been reported and these are summarised according to screening strategy (Tables 3 and 4). Uptake is highest for prenatal screening (either stepwise or couple) with a weighted average of 75%. The average uptake of preconceptional screening is 7–9% when individuals or couples are invited for screening, 38% and 76%, respectively, for opportunistically offered screening of individuals and couples. Uptake is influenced by the method of invitation to screening (opportunistic contact or written or other invitation) as well as the setting, with rates as low as 2% reported when the invitation is sent by post[82], compared with rates as high as 87% when screening is offered to visitors of a family clinic by committed researchers[83] (not shown in the table). Only two studies have been performed using a school setting: uptake was 42% in the Canadian study, and 42% and 75% in two high schools in Australia[45,46].

Table 3 Summary of studies reporting prenatal screening for CF carriers[69–79].

First author	Place	Population	Number of couples screened	Coverage (% of population screened)	Number of affected pregnancies detected	Number of affected pregnancies terminated	% of detected pregnancies terminated
Prenatal stepwise screening							
Harris[69]	Manchester	NA	127	NA	0	0	–
Schwartz[70]	Copenhagen	7,400	6,599	89%	1	1	100%
Jung[71]	Berlin	638	637	100%	1	1	100%
Cuckle[72]	Yorkshire	6,071	3,764	62%	NA	NA	NA
Miedzybrodzka[73]	Aberdeen	1,629	1,475	91%	0	0	–
Brock[74]	Edinburgh	6,030	4,978	83%	2	2	100%
Doherty[75]	Maine	NA	1,645	NA	1	1	100%
Loader[76]	Rochester	5,646	3,334	59%	0	0	–
Witt[77]	Northern California	6,617	5,161	78%	1	0	0%
Grody[78]	Los Angeles	4,739	3,192	67%	1	1	100%
All prenatal stepwise studies		38,770	29,140	75%	7	6	86%
Prenatal couple screening							
Harris[69]	Manchester	NA	117	NA	0	0	–
Miedzybrodzka[73]	Aberdeen	361	321	89%	0	0	–
Wald[79]	Oxford	810	543	67%	0	0	–
Brock[74]	Edinburgh	16,571	12,566	76%	6	6	100%
All prenatal couple studies		17,742	13,430	76%	6	6	100%

NA means that data are not available; these are omitted in the calculation of totals.

The most common reason for declining CF carrier screening was unwillingness to terminate an affected pregnancy[76,84,85]. This does not appear to be the case once a couple has consented to be screened. The results of published prenatal screening studies show that, of the 13 high risk couples with an affected fetus identified as a consequence of screening in early pregnancy, all but one chose to terminate that pregnancy. Data for preconceptional screening studies are not available.

Economic considerations

Previously, we have estimated the costs, effects and savings of prenatal, preconceptional, school and neonatal CF carrier screening for the Dutch situation where 1 in 30 persons is a carrier[86]. From this, we concluded that, in The Netherlands, savings of prenatal and single-entry two-step preconceptional screening have a favourable cost-savings balance (*i.e.* the savings of the programme are higher than the costs), but that double-entry two-step preconceptional screening and neonatal screening will only have

Table 4 Summary of studies reporting preconceptional screening for CF carriers[80–83].

First author	Place	Population	Number of couples screened	Coverage (% of population screened)	Method
Preconceptional stepwise screening					
Bekker[80]	London	3,951	234	6%	Invitation
Bekker[80]	London	1,208	556	46%	Opportunistic
Tambor[81]	Baltimore	2,713	101	4%	Invitation
Tambor[81]	Baltimore	608	143	24%	Opportunistic
Payne[82]	South Wales	739	166	22%	Invitation
Payne[82]	South Wales	802	303	38%	Opportunistic
All preconceptional stepwise studies		7,403	501	7%	Invitation
All preconceptional stepwise studies		2,618	1,002	38%	Opportunistic
Preconceptional couple screening					
Watson[83]	SW Hertfordshire	852	87	10%	Invitation
Watson[83]	SW Hertfordshire	944	714	76%	Opportunistic
Payne[82]	South Wales	135	2	2%	Invitation
Payne[82]	South Wales	NA	29	NA	Opportunistic
All preconceptional couple studies		987	89	9%	Invitation
All preconceptional couple studies		944	714	76%	Opportunistic

NA means that data are not available; these are omitted in the calculation of totals.

a favourable cost-savings balance if uptake of screening, prenatal diagnosis and induced abortion are high enough. The costs of school screening will be higher than the savings for all realistic assumptions.

In Table 5, we have applied the same methodology to the UK, where 1 in 25 persons is a carrier and 732,000 children were born in 1995[87]. Assuming that all couples will have exactly two children, 366,000 couples will then be screened yearly. As expected, the conclusions of this evaluation are comparable to those reached for The Netherlands, since the assumptions made are largely similar.

In the UK, we estimate the costs per carrier couple detected (not shown) to be lowest for neonatal carrier screening because it detects most carrier couples, as parents of detected carrier newborns are also tested, and they can use the test information for further reproduction. The costs per carrier couple detected through prenatal screening are approximately 10% lower than through preconceptional screening. Because the prevalence of CF carriers is higher in the UK than in The Netherlands, even the savings of double-entry two-step preconceptional screening and of neonatal screening (not shown) are greater than the screening costs. From this estimate, there would appear to be no economic objections to prenatal, preconceptional or neonatal screening in the UK. In contrast, the costs of carrier screening of school aged children are estimated to be higher than the savings (not shown). The

Table 5 Estimated costs, effects and savings of prenatal and preconceptional CF screening[†]

	Prenatal		Preconceptional	
	SETS	DETS	SETS	DETS
Costs of screening	£9,951,000	£14,450,000	£6,359,000	£8,900,000
Number of detected carrier couples	332	378	184	210
Number of couples with one detected carrier	9,624	19,249	6,367	12,734
Costs per detected carrier couple	£30,000	£38,000	£35,000	£42,000
Number of prenatal diagnoses	546	622	232	264
Number of terminations	109	124	46	53
Number of affected pregnancies averted*	113	128	59	68
Costs per affected pregnancy averted *	£88,000	£113,000	£107,000	£132,000
Net economic savings (savings – costs)	£16,492,000	£15,449,000	£7,298,000	£6,548,000

* The number of avoided patients is higher than the number of induced abortions since some detected carrier couples refrain from having children.
[†] Based on 366,000 couples screened. Costs and savings are converted to present values using a 3% discount rate.

most important assumption which might not hold is that the relative magnitude of the costs and savings in the UK is similar to that in The Netherlands. However, as reported in the original paper[86], the conclusions hold for a wide range of decision and cost assumptions.

We have compared our estimates of the cost per carrier couple detected through prenatal screening with those published for the UK by others. Our estimates are much higher than those reported by Cuckle *et al*[72], who calculated a cost per carrier couple detected of approximately £20,000. However, the latter analysis assumed 100% uptake of prenatal diagnosis and induced abortion and did not include costs of further diagnosis and treatment, in contrast to our study which assumed 85% uptake of prenatal diagnosis, 80% uptake of induced abortion, and included costs of further diagnosis and treatment. In contrast, the costs estimated by Morris and Oppenheimer[88] were similar to our estimates, being about £36,000 per carrier couple detected.

An assessment of CF screening

In The Netherlands, the Dutch Population Screening Act requires that central government approves certain screening programmes before they are implemented. Because genetic screening has some special implications, a committee of the Health Council of The Netherlands has issued a report on genetic screening[89]. In this report, the committee formulated criteria for the introduction of genetic screening programmes, taking the criteria of Wilson and Jungner[90] as a starting point. The committee divided these criteria into eleven absolute criteria that have to be complied with by every screening programme and ten weighing criteria that have to be provided to the review body so that the body can make an informed deliberation of the advantages and disadvantages of screening. Screening for cystic fibrosis is assessed in relation to these criteria in Table 6, which also identifies important gaps in the evidence required to support policy decisions. Although CF screening satisfies most of the criteria, some are not completely satisfied. These are discussed below.

Criterion 3 ('awareness of disease or carrier status') and **Criterion 5** ('voluntary participation and informed consent') are not met for school and neonatal screening, since minors are tested who legally can not give informed consent.

Criterion 4 ('practical courses of action') is also not completely met for school and neonatal screening, since the value of the information from screening for carriers detected as newborns or school aged children lies far in the future, by which time they may have forgotten their test results. Since preconceptional screening gives the carrier couple more options than prenatal screening (avoiding pregnancy, artificial insemination, pre-implantation diagnosis), preconceptional screening can be considered preferable with regard to this criterion.

With regard to **Criterion 6** ('accurate and comprehensible information'), there is a debate about the amount of information to be given to couples in the single-entry two-step version of carrier screening for cystic fibrosis where one partner is identified as a carrier and the other is not. Since the latter may have a mutation that is not detectable with currently available screening tests, these couples have a higher risk than the untested general population of an affected child but do not have the option of prenatal diagnosis. Understanding these and other implications of genetic testing for CF requires a high degree of genetic knowledge, including understanding of complex concepts such as test sensitivity, carrier status, patterns of inheritance, risk/probability and genotype-phenotype correlations[91]. Given the recognised gaps in genetic knowledge among the general public, it is essential that any genetic testing programme includes written informed consent as well as adequate resources for education and counselling[1].

Criterion 8 ('sufficient facilities for screening and diagnosis') is partially met. Approximately 350 carrier couples can be expected per year in the UK with prenatal screening and 200 couples with preconceptional screening (Table 5). For these carrier couples, there would be sufficient facilities for counselling in clinical genetic centres. This may not be the case for couples where one partner is identified as a carrier and the other is not, given that, each year, 19,249 such couples may be identified through prenatal couple screening and 12,734 through

Table 6 Criteria for assessing screening programmes proposed by the Health Council of The Netherlands, applied to CF carrier screening

		CF carrier screening strategy	
		Preconceptional or prenatal	School or neonatal
Absolute criteria			
1	The programme concerns a health problem or condition that can lead to a health problem	+	+
2	The target population is clearly defined	+	+
3	The programme enables participants to become aware of the disease or carrier status	+	+/–
4	Practical courses of action are open to the participants	+	+/–
5	Participation is voluntary and consent is based on good information	+	+/–
6	The target group is supplied with accurate and comprehensible information	+/–	+
7	A suitable test method is available	+	+
8	There are sufficient facilities for every step in screening and diagnosis	–	–
9	The personal privacy of the participants is protected	+	+
10	If scientific research is carried out, participants are properly informed about this	+	+
11	There is continuous quality assurance regarding tests, follow-up and participant information	+	+
Weighing criteria. There should be information about:			
12a	The prevalence of the disease or disorder	Y	Y
12b	The natural course of the disorder	Y	Y
12c	All possible target groups and the considerations which led to the selection of the target group and the time in life for testing	Y	Y
12d	The performance of the screening test, including the burden which testing imposes on the participants	Y	Y
12e	The available courses of action after a positive test result	Y	Y
12f	The time allowed for consideration and possible implementation of the courses of action	Y	Y
12g	The possible psychological, social and other repercussions of the offer, participation and non-participation to participants and other people	N	N
12h	The possibility and consequences of erroneous results	Y	Y
12i	The guarantees to prevent participants experiencing unjustified impediments from obtaining employment or private insurance cover as a result of (non-)participation in the screening and follow-up testing	Y	Y
12j	The costs which are linked to the screening and to the attainment of the requisite infrastructure	Y	Y

+   the criterion is or can be satisfied;
+/– the criterion is not completely satisfied;
–   the criterion is not satisfied or there are not enough data to enable a judgement;
Y   there is enough knowledge with regard to this criterion; and
N   there is not enough knowledge with regard to this criterion.

preconceptional couple screening. It has been suggested that these couples could be counselled by trained paramedics ('project-nurses'), who might also have a role in testing family members of detected carriers[92]. There are likely to be adequate facilities for an estimated maximum of 622 prenatal diagnoses and 124 induced abortions each year (Table 5).

Although **Criterion 11** ('continuous quality assurance') can in principle be satisfied in any CF screening programme, special attention has to be given to the quality control of CFTR typing. In a European Concerted Action on Cystic Fibrosis, Cuppens and Cassiman[93] found that only 25 of 40 participating laboratories throughout Europe (62.5%) were able to type correctly all nine samples with various CFTR alleles, and that 4 laboratories (10%) typed three or more alleles incorrectly. However, a significantly lower error rate was observed in laboratories from the UK, which is believed to be a direct consequence of their participation in a quality control scheme. This quality control testing has been operational for more than three years since the time of the study of Cuppens and Cassiman[93].

Insufficient knowledge is available regarding adverse psychological, social and other repercussions (**Criterion 12g**). Factors such as anticipated decision regret, perception of the severity of the condition as well as perception of risk influence the decisions to accept or decline screening[94]. The complexity of the concept of 'carrier status' and its implications for family members may also make the screening decision difficult[81]. Possible anxiety caused by the screening result appears to be short-lived, with most of those accepting the offer of screening expressing a preference for certainty over not knowing[95]. Furthermore, carriership could influence the self-perception and the perceptions of others who are not carriers, for example carriers view their future health with less optimism than people who are not carriers[96]. Most CF patients and their families appear to have a positive attitude to carrier screening and termination of affected pregnancies[97]. No adverse repercussions from a medical point of view have been reported.

Discussion

It is very important that the target group receives adequate and balanced information. It should include at least a description of the disease, inheritance patterns and relevant aspects of test performance. The offer of testing should be made to enable couples who wish to avoid the birth of a child with CF to do so, without influencing those who do not. Care should be taken to ensure that the decision to have testing is completely voluntary[1].

We agree with the National Institutes of Health consensus statement that CF testing be offered to couples seeking prenatal testing and couples currently planning a pregnancy, and should not be offered to other target groups[1]. Ideally, preconceptional screening should be provided because, with this strategy, all reproductive options remain open for carrier couples. Prenatal screening can be used as an alternative or as a 'safety net' for pregnant couples who have not been screened before conception. Particular emphasis should be given to the implementation of a routine quality control scheme in participating laboratories[93].

As for many diseases, advances in medical treatment for CF are and will be made. This progress in treatment will most likely have an impact on the length and quality of a CF patient's life[98]. As treatment improves the quality of life of CF patients, screening for CF gene carriers may in the future be a thing of the past.

References

1 Anonymous. Genetic testing for cystic fibrosis. *NIH Consensus Statement Online* 1997; **15**: 1–34

2 Fanconi G, Uehlinger E, Knauer C. Das Coeliakiesyndrom bei angeborener zysticher Pankreas-fibromatose und Bronchiektasien. *Wien Med Wochenschr* 1936; **86**: 753–6

3 Andersen DH. Cystic fibrosis of the pancreas and its relation to celiac disease: a clinical and pathologic study. *Am J Dis Child* 1938; **56**: 344–99

4 Welsh MJ, Tsui LC, Boat TF, Beaudet AL. Cystic fibrosis. In: Scriver CR, Beaudet AL, Sly WS, Valle D, eds. *The Metabolic and Molecular Basis of Inherited Disease*, vol 3: 7th edn. New York: McGraw-Hill, 1995; 3799–876

5 Rosenstein BJ, Zeitlin PL. Cystic fibrosis [review]. *Lancet* 1998; **351**: 277–82

6 Wildhagen MF, Verheij JBGM, Verzijl JG *et al*. Cost of care of patients with cystic fibrosis in The Netherlands in 1990–1. *Thorax* 1996; **51**: 298–301

7 Wildhagen MF, Verheij JBGM, Verzijl JG *et al*. The nonhospital costs of care of patients with CF in The Netherlands: results of a questionnaire. *Eur Respir J* 1996; **9**: 2215–9

8 Ornoy A, Arnon J, Katznelson D *et al*. Pathological confirmation of cystic fibrosis in the fetus following prenatal diagnosis. *Am J Med Genet* 1987; **28**: 935–47

9 Brugman SM, Taussig LM. The reproductive system. In: Taussig L. (ed) *Cystic fibrosis*. New York: Thieme Stratton, 1984: 323–37

10 Buchwald M. Cystic fibrosis: from the gene to the dream. *Clin Invest Med* 1996; **19**: 304–10

11 Aitken ML, Burke W, McDonald G *et al*. Recombinant human DNase inhalation in normal subjects and patients with cystic fibrosis. A phase 1 study. *JAMA* 1992; **267**: 1947–51

12 Mylett J, Johnson K, Knowles M. Alternate therapies for cystic fibrosis. *Semin Respir Crit Care Med* 1994; **15**: 426–33

13 Tamm M, Higenbottam T. Heart-lung and lung transplantation for cystic fibrosis: world experience. *Semin Respir Crit Care Med* 1994; **15**: 414–25

14 Wilson JM. Cystic fibrosis: strategies for gene therapy. *Semin Respir Crit Care Med* 1994; **15**: 439–45

15 Elborn JS, Shale DJ, Britton JR. Cystic fibrosis: current survival and population estimates to the year 2000. *Thorax* 1991; **46**: 881–5

16 Blythe SA, Farrell PM. Advances in the diagnosis and management of cystic fibrosis. *Clin Biochem* 1984; **17**: 277–83

17 Wright SW, Morton NE. Genetic studies on cystic fibrosis in Hawaii. *Am J Hum Genet* 1968; **20**: 157–68

18 Roberts G, Stanfield M, Black A, Redmond A. Screening for cystic fibrosis: a four year regional experience. *Arch Dis Child* 1988; **63**: 1438–43

19 Ten Kate LP. Cystic fibrosis in The Netherlands. *Int J Epidemiol* 1977; **6**: 23–34

20 De Vries HG, Collee JM, de Walle HE *et al*. Prevalence of delta F508 cystic fibrosis carriers in The Netherlands: logistic regression on sex, age, region of residence and number of offspring. *Hum Genet* 1997; **99**: 74–9

21 Turner G, Meagher W, Willis C, Colley P. Cascade testing for carrier status in cystic fibrosis in a large family. *Med J Aust* 1993; **159**: 163–5

22 Romeo G, Devoto M, Galietta LJV. Why is the cystic fibrosis gene so frequent? *Hum Genet* 1989; **84**: 1–5

23 Pier GB, Grout M, Zaidi T *et al*. *Salmonella typhi* uses CFTR to enter intestinal epithelial cells. *Nature* 1998; **393**: 79–82

24 Kerem BS, Rommens JM, Buchanan JA *et al*. Identification of the cystic fibrosis gene: genetic analysis. *Science* 1989; **245**: 1073–80

25 Riordan JR, Rommens JM, Kerem BS *et al*. Identification of the cystic fibrosis gene: cloning and characterization of complementary DNA. *Science* 1989; **245**: 1066–73

26 Rommens JM, Iannuzzi MC, Kerem BS *et al*. Identification of the cystic fibrosis gene: chromosome walking and jumping. *Science* 1989; **245**: 1059–65

27 Bear CE, Li CH, Kartner N *et al*. Purification and functional reconstitution of the cystic fibrosis transmembrane conductance regulator (CFTR). *Cell* 1992; **68**: 809–18

28 De Vries HG, Collee JM, van Veldhuizen MHR *et al*. Validation of the determination of deltaF508 mutations of the cystic fibrosis gene in over 11 000 mouthwashes. *Hum Genet* 1996; **97**: 334–6

29 Wilfond BS, Fost N. The cystic fibrosis gene: medical and social implications for heterozygote detection. *JAMA* 1990; **263**: 2777–83

30 Anonymous. Statement of the American Society of Human Genetics on cystic fibrosis carrier screening. *Am J Hum Genet* 1992; **51**: 1443–4

31 Ten Kate LP, Verheij JBGM, Wildhagen MF *et al*. Comparison of single-entry and double-entry two-step couple screening for cystic fibrosis carriers. *Hum Hered* 1996; **46**: 20–5

32 Brock DJH. Heterozygote screening for cystic fibrosis. *J Med Screen* 1994; **1**: 130–3

33 Dodge JA, Boulyjenkov V. New possibilities for population control of cystic fibrosis. *Bull World Health Organ* 1992; **70**: 561–6

34 Modell M. Screening for carriers of cystic fibrosis – a general practitioner's perspective. *BMJ* 1993; **307**: 849–52

35 Raeburn JA. Screening for carriers of cystic fibrosis. Screening before pregnancy is needed. *BMJ* 1994; **309**: 1428–9

36 Shapiro DA, Shapiro LR. Pitfalls in Tay-Sachs carrier detection: physician referral patterns and patient ignorance. *N Y State J Med* 1989; **89**: 317–9

37 Ten Kate LP, Tijmstra T. Screenen op dragerschap van het cystische-fibrose-gen [Screening for carrier state of the cystic fibrosis gene]. *Ned Tijdschr Geneeskd* 1989; **133**: 2402–4

38 Ten Kate LP. Genetische factoren [Genetic factors]. In: Van der Maas PJ, Hofman A, Dekker E. (eds) *Epidemiologie en gezondheidsbeleid*, vol 3. Alphen aan den Rijn: Samsom Stafleu, 1989; 133–44

39 Wald NJ. Couple screening for cystic fibrosis. *Lancet* 1991; **338**: 1318–9

40 Livingstone J, Axton RAA, Gilfillan A *et al*. Antenatal screening for cystic fibrosis: a trial of the couple model. *BMJ* 1994; **308**: 1459–62

41 Mennie ME, Gilfillan A, Compton M *et al*. Prenatal screening for cystic fibrosis. *Lancet* 1992; **340**: 214–6

42 Miedzybrodzka Z, Dean J, Haites N. Screening for cystic fibrosis [letter]. *Lancet* 1991; **338**: 1524–5

43 Bianco I, Graziani B, Lerone M *et al*. Prevention of thalassaemia major in Latium (Italy) [letter]. *Lancet* 1985; **2**: 888–9

44 Zeesman S, Clow CL, Cartier L, Scriver CR. A private view of heterozygosity: eight-year follow-up study on carriers of the Tay-Sachs gene detected by high school screening in Montreal. *Am J Med Genet* 1984; **18**: 769–78

45 Mitchell J, Scriver CR, Clow CL, Kaplan F. What young people think and do when the option for cystic fibrosis carrier testing is available. *J Med Genet* 1993; **30**: 538–42

46 Wake SA, Rogers CJ, Colley PW *et al.* Cystic fibrosis carrier screening in two New South Wales country towns. *Med J Aust* 1996; **164**: 471–4

47 Holtzman NA. Genetic screening: for better or for worse. *Pediatrics* 1977; **59**: 131–3

48 Kooij L, Tijmstra T, Verheij JBGM *et al.* Screening op gendragerschap van cystische fibrose: voor- en nadelen van verschillende scenario [Screening for cystic fibrosis gene carrier state: pros and cons of different scenarios]. *Ned Tijdschr Geneeskd* 1994; **138**: 818–23

49 Holloway S, Brock DJH. Cascade testing for the identification of carriers of cystic fibrosis. *J Med Screen* 1994; **1**: 159–64

50 Brock DJH. Heterozygote screening for cystic fibrosis [review]. *Eur J Hum Genet* 1995; **3**: 2–13

51 Schutt WH, Isles TE. Protein in meconium from meconium ileus. *Arch Dis Child* 1968; **43**: 178–81

52 Cain ARR, Deall AM, Noble TC. Screening for cystic fibrosis by testing meconium for albumin. *Arch Dis Child* 1972; **47**: 131–2

53 Ten Kate LP, Feenstra-de Gooyer I, Ploeg-de Groot G, Gouw WL, Anders GJPA. Should we screen all newborns for cystic fibrosis? *Int J Epidemiol* 1978; **7**: 323–30

54 Crossley JR, Elliott RB, Smith PA. Dried-blood spot screening for cystic fibrosis in the newborn. *Lancet* 1979; **1**: 472–4

55 Gregg RG, Simantel A, Farrell PM *et al.* Newborn screening for cystic fibrosis in Wisconsin: comparison of biochemical and molecular methods. *Pediatrics* 1997; **99**: 819–24

56 Gibson LE, Cooke RE. A test for concentration of electrolytes in sweat in cystic fibrosis of the pancreas utilizing pilocarpine by iontophoresis. *Pediatrics* 1959; **23**: 545–9

57 Doershuk CF, Matthews LW, Tucker AS, Spector S. Evaluation of a prophylactic and therapeutic program for patients with cystic fibrosis. *Pediatrics* 1965; **36**: 675–88

58 Huang NN, Macri CN, Girone J, Sproul A. Survival of patients with cystic fibrosis. *Am J Dis Child* 1970; **120**: 289–95

59 Shwachman H, Redmond A, Khaw KT. Studies in cystic fibrosis. Report of 130 patients diagnosed under 3 months of age over a 20-year period. *Pediatrics* 1970; **46**: 335–43

60 Stern RC, Boat TF, Doershuk CF *et al.* Course of cystic fibrosis in 95 patients. *J Pediatr* 1976; **89**: 406–11

61 Kraemer R, Hadorn B, Rossi E. Classification at time of diagnosis and subsequent survival in children with cystic fibrosis. *Helv Paediatr Acta* 1977; **32**: 107–14

62 Orenstein DM, Boat TF, Stern RC *et al.* The effect of early diagnosis and treatment in cystic fibrosis: a seven-year study of 16 sibling pairs. *Am J Dis Child* 1977; **131**: 973–5

63 Wilcken B, Chalmers G. Reduced morbidity in patients with cystic fibrosis detected by neonatal screening. *Lancet* 1985; **2**: 1319–21

64 Bowling F, Cleghorn G, Chester A *et al.* Neonatal screening for cystic fibrosis. *Arch Dis Child* 1988; **63**: 196–8

65 Dankert-Roelse JE, te Meerman GJ, Martijn A, Ten Kate LP, Knol K. Survival and clinical outcome in patients with cystic fibrosis, with or without neonatal screening. *J Pediatr* 1989; **114**: 362–7

66 Farrell PM, Kosorok MR, Laxova A *et al.* Nutritional benefits of neonatal screening for cystic fibrosis. Wisconsin Cystic Fibrosis Neonatal Screening Study Group. *N Engl J Med* 1997; **337**: 963–9

67 Dankert-Roelse JE, te Meerman GJ. Screening for cystic fibrosis – time to change our position? [editorial]. *N Engl J Med* 1997; **337**: 997–9

68 Wald NJ, Morris JK. Neonatal screening for cystic fibrosis. No evidence yet of any benefit [editorial]. *BMJ* 1998; **316**: 404–5

69 Harris H, Scotcher D, Hartley N *et al.* Cystic fibrosis carrier testing in early pregnancy by general practitioners. *BMJ* 1993; **306**: 1580–3

70 Schwartz M, Brandt NJ, Skovby F. Screening for carriers of cystic fibrosis among pregnant women: a pilot study. *Eur J Hum Genet* 1993; **1**: 239–44

71 Jung U, Urner U, Grade K, Coutelle C. Acceptability of carrier screening for cystic fibrosis during pregnancy in a German population. *Hum Genet* 1994; **94**: 19–24

72 Cuckle HS, Richardson GA, Sheldon TA, Quirke P. Cost effectiveness of antenatal screening for cystic fibrosis. *BMJ* 1995; **311**: 1460–3

73 Miedzybrodzka ZH, Hall MH, Mollison J *et al.* Antenatal screening for carriers of cystic fibrosis: randomised trial of stepwise v couple screening. *BMJ* 1995; **310**: 353–7

74 Brock DJH. Prenatal screening for cystic fibrosis: 5 years' experience reviewed. *Lancet* 1996; **347**: 148–50

75 Doherty RA, Palomaki GE, Kloza EM, Erickson JL, Haddow JE. Couple-based prenatal screening for cystic fibrosis in primary care settings. *Prenat Diagn* 1996; **16**: 397–404

76 Loader S, Caldwell P, Kozyra A *et al*. Cystic fibrosis carrier population screening in the primary care setting. *Am J Hum Genet* 1996; **59**: 234–47

77 Witt DR, Schaefer C, Hallam P *et al*. Cystic fibrosis heterozygote screening in 5,161 pregnant women. *Am J Hum Genet* 1996; **58**: 823–35

78 Grody WW, Dunkel-Schetter C, Tatsugawa ZH *et al*. PCR-based screening for cystic fibrosis carrier mutations in an ethnically diverse pregnant population. *Am J Hum Genet* 1997; **60**: 935–47

79 Wald NJ, George L, Wald N, MacKenzie IZ. Further observations in connection with couple screening for cystic fibrosis [letter]. *Prenat Diagn* 1995; **15**: 589–90

80 Bekker H, Modell M, Denniss G *et al*. Uptake of cystic fibrosis testing in primary care: supply push or demand pull? *BMJ* 1993; **306**: 1584–6

81 Tambor ES, Bernhardt BA, Chase GA *et al*. Offering cystic fibrosis carrier screening to an HMO population: factors associated with utilization. *Am J Hum Genet* 1994; **55**: 626–37

82 Payne Y, Williams M, Cheadle J *et al*. Carrier screening for cystic fibrosis in primary care: evaluation of a project in South Wales. The South Wales Cystic Fibrosis Carrier Screening Research Team. *Clin Genet* 1997; **51**: 153–63

83 Watson EK, Mayall E, Chapple J *et al*. Screening for carriers of cystic fibrosis through primary health care services. *BMJ* 1991; **303**: 504–7

84 Livingstone J, Axton RA, Mennie M, Gilfillan A, Brock DJH. A preliminary trial of couple screening for cystic fibrosis: designing an appropriate information leaflet. *Clin Genet* 1993; **43**: 57–62

85 Mennie ME, Gilfillan A, Compton ME, Liston WA, Brock DJH. Prenatal cystic fibrosis carrier screening: factors in a woman's decision to decline testing. *Prenat Diagn* 1993; **13**: 807–14

86 Wildhagen MF, Hilderink HBM, Verzijl JG *et al*. Costs, effects, and savings of screening for CF-gene carriers. *J Epidemiol Community Health* 1998; **52**: 45–67

87 Office for National Statistics. Birth statistics Series FM1, no 24. London: HMSO, 1995

88 Morris JK, Oppenheimer PM. Cost comparison of different methods of screening for cystic fibrosis. *J Med Screen* 1995; **2**: 22–7

89 Health Council of The Netherlands: Committee Genetic Screening. Genetic screening. The Hague: Health Council, 1994; publication no. 1994/22E

90 Wilson JMG, Jungner G. Principles and practice of screening for disease. *Public Health Papers 34*. Geneva: World Health Organization, 1968

91 Decruyenaere M, Evers-Kiebooms G, Denayer L, van den Berghe H. Cystic fibrosis: community knowledge and attitudes towards carrier screening and prenatal diagnosis. *Clin Genet* 1992; **41**: 189–96

92 Shickle D, Harvey I. 'Inside-out', back-to-front: a model for clinical population genetic screening. *J Med Genet* 1993; **30**: 580–2

93 Cuppens H, Cassiman JJ. A quality control study of CFTR mutation screening in 40 different European laboratories. The European Concerted Action on Cystic Fibrosis. *Eur J Hum Genet* 1995; **3**: 235–45

94 Tijmstra T. Het imperatieve karakter van medische technologie en de betekenis van 'geanticipeerde beslissingsspijt' [The imperative character of medical technology and the significance of 'anticipated decision regret']. *Ned Tijdschr Geneeskd* 1987; **131**: 1128–31

95 Mennie ME, Compton ME, Gilfillan A *et al*. Prenatal screening for cystic fibrosis: psychological effects on carriers and their partners. *J Med Genet* 1993; **30**: 543–8

96 Marteau TM, van Duijn M, Ellis I. Effects of genetic screening on perceptions of health: a pilot study. *J Med Genet* 1992; **29**: 24–6

97 Conway SP, Allenby K, Pond MN. Patient and parental attitudes toward genetic screening and its implications at an adult cystic fibrosis centre. *Clin Genet* 1994; **45**: 308–12

98 Rosenstein BJ. Cystic fibrosis in the year 2000. *Semin Respir Crit Care Med* 1994; **15**: 446–51

99 The Cystic Fibrosis Genetic Analysis Consortium. Population variation of common cystic fibrosis mutations. *Hum Mutat* 1994; **4**: 167–77

Evaluating newborn screening programmes based on dried blood spots: future challenges

Carol Dezateux

Department of Epidemiology and Public Health, Institute of Child Health, London, UK

A UK national programme to screen all newborn infants for phenylketonuria was introduced in 1969, followed in 1981 by a similar programme for congenital hypothyroidism. Decisions to start these national programmes were informed by evidence from observational studies rather than randomised controlled trials. Subsequently, outcome for affected children has been assessed through national disease registers, from which inferences about the effectiveness of screening have been made. Both programmes are based on a single blood specimen, collected from each infant at the end of the first week of life, and stored as dried spots on a filter paper or 'Guthrie' card. This infrastructure has made it relatively easy for routine screening for other conditions to be introduced at a district or regional level, resulting in inconsistent policies and inequitable access to effective screening services. This variation in screening practices reflects uncertainty and the lack of a national framework to guide the introduction and evaluation of new screening initiatives, rather than geographical variations in disease prevalence or severity. More recently, developments in tandem mass spectrometry have made it technically possible to screen for several inborn errors of metabolism in a single analytical step. However, for each of these conditions, evidence is required that the benefits of screening outweigh the harms. How should that evidence be obtained? Ideally policy decisions about new screening initiatives should be informed by evidence from randomised controlled trials but for most of the conditions for which newborn screening is proposed, large trials would be needed. Prioritising which conditions should be formally evaluated, and developing a framework to support their evaluation, poses an important challenge to the public health, clinical and scientific community. In this chapter, issues underlying the evaluation of newborn screening programmes will be discussed in relation to medium chain acyl CoA dehydrogenase deficiency, a recessively inherited disorder of fatty acid oxidation.

*Correspondence to:
Dr Carol Dezateux,
Senior Lecturer in
Epidemiology and Public
Health, Department of
Epidemiology and Public
Health, Institute of Child
Health, 30 Guilford St,
London WC1N 1EH, UK*

The UK national newborn screening programmes for phenylketonuria and congenital hypothyroidism are based on a single sample of capillary blood collected by heelprick from all infants between 6 and 14 days of age. These samples are usually stored dried on special filter papers,

---

previously referred to as Guthrie cards, after the originator of the main screening test for phenylketonuria[1]. These programmes are considered to be successful, achieving levels of population coverage, test performance and treatment effectiveness which compare favourably with other national screening programmes. A single blood sample is common to screening for both conditions and there is potential for the residual sample to be tested for other conditions. In 1995, Streetly *et al* estimated that about 16% of all infants born in the UK each year were routinely screened for cystic fibrosis, 12% for homocystinuria, 9% for haemoglobino-pathies, 9% for galactosaemia, and 3% for tyrosinaemia[2]. Such local variation is inequitable and emphasises the uncertainty that exists at the margins of screening policies and the susceptibility to local pressures. If national screening policy is to be based on evidence of effectiveness and cost-effectiveness[3], mechanisms are required to ensure that innovations in screening are introduced only within the context of an evaluative study, ideally a randomised controlled trial. In their absence, the opportunistic and piecemeal extension of the existing national newborn screening programmes is likely to continue. Prioritising which conditions should be formally evaluated and developing a national framework to support their evaluation poses an important challenge to the public health, clinical and scientific community.

In the UK, two commissioned systematic reviews of newborn screening for inborn errors of metabolism have been published[4,5]. Further commissioned reviews of cystic fibrosis and haemoglobinopathy screening are due to be reported (updated information can be obtained from the NHS R&D HTA website: http://www.soton.ac.uk/~hta/). Important issues for the organisation and delivery of newborn screening services have been identified through local audits[6–11] and, more recently, through a national audit of the screening programmes for phenyl-ketonuria and congenital hypothyroidism[12]. It is, therefore, timely to consider the future directions of newborn screening based on dried blood spots and the research required to inform and strengthen the scientific basis of these developments. In this chapter, some principles underlying the evaluation of proposed newborn screening programmes are discussed, using the example of screening for medium chain acyl CoA dehydrogenase deficiency.

Medium chain acyl CoA dehydrogenase deficiency

Over the last two decades, a number of disorders of fatty acid oxidation have been recognised, the most common of which is medium chain acyl CoA dehydrogenase (MCAD) deficiency. MCAD deficiency is a recessively inherited metabolic disorder that reduces the ability to maintain a normal blood sugar during episodes of metabolic stress[13]. During intercurrent infections and illnesses, affected children may develop profound hypoglycaemia, encephalopathy and hepatic dysfunction. Affected children are usually asymptomatic initially, although neonatal symptoms have been reported[14]. MCAD deficiency may not be suspected until late infancy or early childhood, when children present with an acute and frequently fatal episode of metabolic decompensation. These episodes are most frequent in the first 2 years of life and rare after 5 years of age. A spectrum of clinical severity is recognised and some affected individuals are not diagnosed until later childhood when they present with mild episodic hypoglycaemia or, in adult life, with symptoms of muscle weakness and fatigue[4,5].

Of those children presenting clinically, about one-quarter will die and about one-third of survivors will have irreversible neurological damage[4,5]. In the largest published case series based on 120 cases from the US, 19 of the 23 children who died had been previously well and had died during their first illness[15]. Failure to diagnose metabolic disease in those who die is a recognised problem, reflecting a low index of clinical suspicion for rare conditions as well as difficulties in making a biochemical diagnosis in an acutely sick child. It is estimated that 20–30% of cases may go undiagnosed clinically, either because they die without a diagnosis being considered or made, or because they remain asymptomatic and well throughout early childhood. However, this percentage, and the proportion at either extreme of the clinical spectrum, has not been directly measured.

A single point mutation of adenine to guanine at position 985 (termed A985G mutation) in the MCAD gene sequence has been identified which is thought to account for almost 90% of mutations[16,17]. Among those clinically diagnosed with MCAD deficiency, 81% are estimated to be homozygous and 18% heterozygous for this common mutation. Although this mutation is thought to have originated from the north-western European population[16], this genotype–phenotype relation has not been confirmed in Scotland[18]. Based on A985G mutation prevalence studies and assuming random mating, it has been suggested that the birth prevalence of MCAD deficiency in the UK may be as high as 10 per 100,000[19]. This is about twice the cumulative incidence to 16 years of age of clinically diagnosed MCAD deficiency reported from a national surveillance study[20]. This disparity suggests that cases are underdiagnosed clinically.

Once a diagnosis has been made, treatment during intercurrent illnesses or periods of anorexia consists of ensuring adequate calorie intake, either by mouth or intravenously. Clinical case series suggest that outcome is favourable following such treatment, although its effectiveness in preventing subsequent episodes has not been proven[15,21,22]. In the US, affected children are also given L-carnitine supplements. This is not currently used in the UK, but evidence to support either practice is lacking.

The rationale for screening

As major sequelae are often sustained during the presenting illness rather than at a later stage, the role of earlier diagnosis before symptoms have developed has received increasing attention. Although prenatal diagnosis has been reported, this is not considered an appropriate strategy, as affected children are believed to be normal provided severe metabolic decompensation can be avoided.

The screening test

The screening test for MCAD deficiency is based on detection and quantification of acyl carnitines using tandem mass spectrometry[23–25]. DNA analysis to detect A985G mutations can be undertaken on dried blood spots[19], but would not be suitable for primary screening. By linking two mass spectrometers together, tandem mass spectrometry allows the separation and analysis of complex samples such as dried blood spots to proceed simultaneously, so that a number of compounds can be identified in a single analytical step[25]. More than 20 inborn errors of metabolism can be detected with this technique, including phenylketonuria, tyrosinaemia type I, MCAD deficiency, other disorders of fatty acid oxidation and organic acidaemias[26]. However, at present, tandem mass spectrometry cannot be used to screen for congenital hypothyroidism and disorders such as cystic fibrosis, sickle cell disease and congenital adrenal hyperplasia, for which screening has been proposed or is currently undertaken.

A presumptive positive screening test for MCAD deficiency is based on the finding of raised concentrations of octanoyl (C8) carnitine. In one study from the US using isotope-dilution tandem mass spectrometry, octanoyl carnitine concentrations were raised (> 0.3 μM) in all ($n = 62$) cases of MCAD deficiency[23]. The authors reported that symptom status, carnitine supplementation or genotype (A985G homozygote or compound heterozygote) did not influence octanoyl carnitine concentrations but numbers were small. Octanoyl carnitine levels were > 0.3 μM in retrieved Guthrie card samples obtained for 8 clinically diagnosed subjects, and below this level among unaffected controls and normal neonates. In one UK report based on electrospray tandem mass spectrometry, octanoyl carnitine concentrations > 0.38 µM were reported in 35 children with proven MCAD deficiency and > 1.5 µM in the retrieved neonatal blood spots[21]. It has been suggested that all clinically ascertained cases may be identified with electrospray tandem mass spectrometry[26].

A presumptive positive screening test for MCAD deficiency may be confirmed by measuring blood spot *cis*-4-decenoic acid, white cell/fibroblast tritium release, or through a phenylproprionic acid load[21]. Plasma non-esterified fatty acid:3-hydroxy-butyrate ratios and urinary organic acids may be measured during an acute episode or after a provocative fast.

Current experience of screening for MCAD deficiency

Screening programmes have been established in the US and Saudi Arabia[4,5]. Published data from Pittsburgh suggest a birth prevalence for MCAD deficiency of 11 per 100,000, based on the identification of 9 affected infants among 80,371 newborns screened with tandem mass spectrometry[27]. In this report, quantitative thresholds were not specified but infants were identified through a 'characteristic pattern' of elevated octanoyl, hexanoyl and decanoyl carnitines. The ability to distinguish between simple heterozygotes (carriers of the A985G mutation who are not themselves at risk of metabolic decompensation) and compound heterozygotes (affected individuals who have two different MCAD mutations and are at risk) is clearly an important criterion for a screening test. In the Pittsburgh study, the methods used to confirm the presumptive positive screening result were not stated, although the results of DNA analyses were reported. Four were homozygous and five heterozygous for A985G, a higher proportion of heterozygotes than the authors predicted from clinical studies. One possible explanation for this is that A985G homozygotes may be relatively more common among clinically diagnosed cases than among those detected through screening. The authors considered it unlikely that these cases were simple heterozygotes, as raised octanoyl carnitine concentrations had not been reported previously among a small sample of obligate simple heterozygotes[23].

Although it is assumed that the true prevalence of MCAD deficiency is higher than that determined from clinically diagnosed cases, estimates of prevalence based on ascertainment through screening with tandem mass spectrometry are not yet available for the UK. Existing UK prevalence figures for MCAD deficiency are based on A985G carrier status determined in about 10,000 newborn blood spot specimens from Trent and three predominantly Caucasian English counties[19]. These suggest that MCAD deficiency may affect 10 out of every 100–200,000 children born in the UK.

Only limited information regarding outcome following screening is available from the Pittsburgh screening programme[27]. Two of the nine children identified through screening died subsequently: one (homozygote) developed a metabolic crisis after immunisation and one (heterozygote) during an intercurrent illness. The numbers involved are too small to allow any inferences to be drawn from these data. The effectiveness of treatment following early diagnosis through screening may also be reduced if clinical episodes occur before a screening test is performed or a result is available. Up to one-third of affected newborns may develop symptoms in the first 3 days of life, before a screening result would be available[14]. In the UK national surveillance study[20], 3 of 45 children without a family history of MCAD deficiency presented before 17 days of age (R Pollitt, personal communication).

What information is needed by decision makers?

What information is needed to determine whether screening for MCAD deficiency should be introduced in the UK? The objective of a screening programme for MCAD deficiency would be to prevent death and major neurological handicap through early diagnosis and treatment. Current experience of population-based screening for MCAD deficiency is very limited. What priority should be given to obtaining better information about effectiveness and what information is needed to determine policy? At a public health level, MCAD deficiency is a rare disorder. Clinically, it is a condition with potentially major consequences for affected children and their families. In health technology terms, MCAD deficiency is the tip of the tandem mass spectrometry iceberg, and technologies for other conditions, including congenital adrenal hyperplasia, have already emerged[28].

Some annual figures for a UK screening programme for MCAD deficiency can be estimated based on current data. If the birth prevalence of MCAD deficiency is assumed to be 10 per 100,000, this suggests that each year around 70 affected children are born in the UK, 49 (70%) of whom would be currently diagnosed clinically. Of the 49 clinically diagnosed cases, 12 (25%) would die while 12 of the 37 survivors would have irreversible neurological damage. Assuming a similar proportion of deaths among the 21 cases not diagnosed clinically, an additional 5 children would die, leaving 16 who are asymptomatic and presumed to be neurologically normal. If the true prevalence of MCAD deficiency were lower, say 5 per 100,000, these figures would be halved.

If screening combined with early treatment could reduce the proportion who die or sustain neurological damage by 50%, then, in the UK each year, screening might prevent 8–9 deaths and 6 children from becoming severely neurologically impaired. The benefits and harms to the 16 affected children who might never have developed symptoms have not been established. Potential consequences of diagnosis for this asymptomatic group include anxiety about the risk of hypoglycaemia during early childhood and genetic information for the parents which may have relevance for future children. The disbenefits to the false positives who are recalled for further testing include the potential anxiety and confusion caused to unaffected families, the risk of subsequent misdiagnosis among a truly unaffected child, and the health service resources required to recall, evaluate and diagnose all cases.

The magnitude of these outcomes depends on screening test performance and the prevalence of disease in the newborn population. If favourable assumptions about test performance are made (for example, a sensitivity of 99% and 0.5% false positive rate), 69 affected children would be correctly identified in the UK each year and 3500 unaffected children would require follow up for a presumptive positive screening result. This gives an odds of being affected given a positive result of 1:51 for a birth prevalence of 10 per 100,000. The number of children recalled for further investigation may be less than this: presumptive positive results can be investigated initially by using other dried spots from the same Guthrie card or by obtaining a second Guthrie card through the midwife or health visitor (currently a repeat sample is requested for about 1% of children in the UK). While DNA analysis could be used to select who should be recalled, at present this strategy would not allow the important question of phenotype–genotype associations within a screen-detected population to be assessed. The contribution of cis-4-decenoic acid and other in vitro assays suitable for dried blood spots to improving test specificity requires further investigation. It has been suggested[26] that the recall and retest rates for analyses carried out by tandem mass spectrometry are 'close to zero'. Further data are required from UK populations to confirm these views and to identify the determinants of the concentrations of individual acyl carnitine species in the neonatal period.

Distinct from the issue of recall policies is the issue of establishing or excluding a diagnosis of MCAD deficiency in a young baby who is well and without a family history. One recognised problem for families of newborn infants with a false positive screening diagnosis is residual anxiety despite re-assurance that the screening result has not been confirmed[29,30]. It is, therefore, extremely important that a definitive diagnosis can be provided as quickly and unequivocally as possible. The investigations and criteria that can be used to make a diagnosis of

MCAD deficiency in an asymptomatic presumptive positive infant are similar, but not identical, to those used to make a diagnosis in clinically symptomatic infants who are frequently investigated during an episode of metabolic decompensation. Diagnostic algorithms are required to avoid a potential risk of misdiagnosis and to ensure that a diagnosis may be confidently excluded in an asymptomatic presumptive positive infant. Without this there is a risk of misdiagnosis or of the screening result becoming a surrogate diagnostic result.

Current data are clearly insufficient for policy. This was effectively the conclusion of the teams responsible for both UK systematic reviews of screening for inborn errors of metabolism[4,5]. Both concluded that more UK based data were required to inform screening policies based on tandem mass spectrometry and identified a need for primary research on screening for MCAD deficiency and some other inborn errors of metabolism. The current debate relates to the nature of that primary research.

Information on likely benefits and possible harms is required to a precision that is meaningful in public health terms. In policy terms, this means identifying the level of benefit (in terms of mortality/disability) which would lead to a decision to introduce screening. An indication of the level of harm, and its relation to benefit, which would lead to a decision **not** to introduce screening is also required and is equally difficult to define. Given that a newborn infant will be screened for several conditions, the marginal disbenefits of each new screening programme may assume greater relevance. For most newborns screened, the probability of a false positive result will almost certainly exceed that of a true positive result. This issue has been discussed by Russell in relation to cervical screening, but applies equally to newborn screening where the probabilities of false positive diagnoses arising from each screening programme are likely to be additive[31].

Evaluating screening

The role of observational studies

Observational data can contribute to the assessment of potential screening, providing information about prevalence and test performance. Analysis of Guthrie specimens from large numbers of proven cases can be used to confirm current estimates of test sensitivity. However, these estimates will only apply to cases ascertained clinically. As the predictive value of a positive test will depend on pre-test probability of disease, geographically representative estimates of disease prevalence based on tandem mass spectrometry are required.

Observational study designs can also be used to determine the contribution of screen-detectable metabolic disorders such as MCAD deficiency to death in infancy and early childhood. This is currently being investigated through a UK collaborative case control study of death in the first 2 years of life. Finally, the role of further secondary data analyses designed to synthesise data from observational studies deserves mention. While the UK systematic reviews included some secondary economic analyses[4,5], further analyses based on decision trees and using existing observational data may be useful to assess cost-effectiveness and to identify key areas of uncertainty before a large and potentially expensive randomised controlled trial is undertaken[32,33].

The rationale for randomised controlled trials

More difficult is the issue of obtaining unbiased evidence that treatment is more effective following early detection than it is following clinical diagnosis, and that screening is not associated with significant risks to those screened. Is a randomised controlled trial of screening necessary or can observational studies of the outcomes of screening in 'pilot' regions provide this information? The rationale for a randomised controlled trial lies in its ability to overcome the biases inherent in observational studies of screening, whether they compare outcome before and after introduction of screening or outcome in different geographical areas with different screening strategies. Furthermore, because screening may be associated with unrecognised harms, which are difficult to assess within an observational study, a randomised trial is the best way to ensure that the potential risks of screening are minimised[34].

Bias due to differential methods used to ascertain cases is likely in an observational study of screening, as cases identified through screening will differ to those identified clinically. For example, an observational study of screening for MCAD deficiency may well show a reduction in mortality in screened periods or regions simply through identifying children with milder forms of the disease. To avoid ascertainment bias, the probability of ascertainment should be equal between the screened and an unscreened population at the time outcome is assessed. This approach was used in the Wisconsin trial of newborn screening for cystic fibrosis[35].

Outcome may be influenced by factors other than screening, such as variations in medical care over time or between different regions. The availability of tandem mass spectrometry as a diagnostic tool is likely to facilitate rapid diagnosis of a range of inborn errors of metabolism in symptomatic children or those with a relevant family history. The comparison of interest for a screening programme will be with a concurrent unscreened control group that has access to this technology. Geographically based comparisons will be difficult to interpret due to regional variation in disease prevalence as well as recognised variations within the UK in access to specialist paediatric metabolic services.

The key limitation of observational evaluative studies lies in their inability to quantify benefit and harm in an unbiased manner. Screening and early treatment may reduce mortality but result in survival of children with neurological impairment. It is difficult to see how this outcome could be satisfactorily measured within an observational study as a comparable control group would be lacking. Other outcomes are also important, notably the psychological effects of the information given to parents of true or false positive infants about their apparently well baby.

Despite an increasing commitment to requiring[3] 'evidence from high quality randomised controlled trials that a screening programme is effective in reducing mortality or morbidity', this kind of evidence is almost completely lacking for most newborn screening programmes. Neither congenital hypothyroidism nor phenylketonuria were assessed in this way before screening was introduced. For phenylketonuria, this was not because of lack of awareness about randomised controlled trials. Debates about how best to assess the effectiveness of early diagnosis and treatment for phenylketonuria when screening for this condition was first proposed bear an uncanny resemblance to the debates about screening for MCAD deficiency[36]. Birch and Tizard questioned the evidence for the effectiveness of dietary treatment of phenylketonuria which they regarded as 'not proven' on the basis of observational studies which they pointed out were subject to selection bias[36]. They proposed a randomised controlled trial of early treatment to assess the effectiveness of a low phenylalanine diet since 'it may not only be ineffective but harmful as a treatment'. In the end, screening policy was determined on the basis of observational data comparing outcome for cases diagnosed through screening in Scotland, where screening had already been introduced, and England, where it had not. Almost 30 years later, data from the UK national register confirm that outcome for classical severe phenylketonuria is much improved[37], but there remain some outstanding issues about the benefits and possible social and financial costs of treating milder forms of phenylketonuria.

Almost certainly screening has altered the concept of a 'case' of phenylketonuria. Genetic variation is increasingly recognised: phenylalanine levels are a continuous distribution determined largely by the specific mutations present[38]. The previous distinction between classical phenylketonuria (with little enzyme activity) and non phenylketonuria hyperphenylalaninaemia (with intermediate levels of enzyme activity) has become less meaningful as the genetic basis of phenylketonuria has been clarified and experience with screening has increased. Observational studies do not help assess the benefits or otherwise of treatment in individuals with borderline or mild phenotypes yet such information is highly relevant when determining screening policies.

The scientific case for trials of newborn screening is strong. There are also ethical reasons why such trials should be carried out[39]. Lumley[34] has suggested that evaluation through randomised controlled trials is an 'ethical imperative' and cites Silverman's[40] view of randomised trials as essentially 'risk minimising'. Objections to trials of screening usually arise because there are strongly held convictions that early treatment is effective and that the control group will be denied access to treatment, which will be beneficial. However screening, like most forms of medical treatment, is likely to produce marginal rather than dramatic benefits and the alternative possibility, that the intervention group may be offered something with unrecognised hazards, should also be considered. Potential hazards for MCAD deficiency include survival with neurological impairment, adverse effects of clinically-unwarranted treatment in asymptomatic individuals, the consequences of unwanted genetic information, misdiagnosis of false positives, anxiety among families of false positives.

How large a trial might be needed? Given the natural history of MCAD, mortality and/or neurological impairment as a combined measure and occurring in the first two years of life would be an appropriate primary outcome measure in a randomised trial. Provisional estimates of sample size based on this measure are summarised in Table 1, but cannot be considered definitive until more reliable data on birth prevalence are available. From this table, it can be seen that a trial would need to involve the entire UK population of births over a 5-year period in order to have sufficient power to detect a 50% reduction in the primary outcome of death and/or disability by 2 years of age. If a trial of this size and duration were to be undertaken, this would require that screening for MCAD deficiency using tandem mass spectrometry were only introduced into the UK as part of a randomised controlled trial.

There is no doubt that trials of newborn screening will pose a major challenge to the clinical, scientific and public health community and will

Table 1 Estimated number of live births required in each arm of a trial of screening for MCAD deficiency to detect specified reduction in death and/or neurological impairment*

% Reduction in outcome	Birth prevalence	
	5 per 100,000	10 per 100,000
25% reduction	15.1 million	7.5 million
50% reduction	3.2 million	1.6 million

*For 90% power and 5% significance.

require the informed participation of parents on a national scale. Parents will require better information and will need to give informed consent to screening and its evaluation, which is not currently requested. Clinical uncertainty will be made more publicly explicit than is currently the case[39]. The UK National Health Service and the existing infrastructure of the national newborn screening service could be developed to support such planned experiments and an investment in this aspect could increase the cost-effectiveness of newborn screening research. Lack of evidence for the effectiveness of early treatment for cystic fibrosis has been cited for over 15 years as the main reason for not introducing newborn screening[41]. Were neonatal screening for cystic fibrosis to be proved effective as the early results of the Wisconsin newborn screening trial[35] suggest, then affected children will have been denied an effective form of intervention for more than a decade because observational studies were not conclusive.

Conclusion

There are an increasing number of conditions for which neonatal screening is being proposed. Technological advances, such as tandem mass spectrometry, make it technically possible to test for several conditions in one analytical step. The priority given to evaluating these potential screening programmes will depend on the importance of the individual conditions, the performance of the proposed tests, as well as the anticipated benefits of screening. However, decisions to start new screening programmes should be informed by unbiased estimates of benefits and harms which cannot be derived from observational studies. These issues have been discussed in relation to screening for MCAD deficiency but apply to other proposed newborn screening programmes. The infrastructure established to support the current UK national newborn screening programmes for phenylketonuria and congenital hypothyroidism could be developed to allow new screening programmes to be introduced in the context of a formal trial. This would maximise the potential benefits of diagnostic and therapeutic advances to affected children and their families while minimising harm to the population being screened.

References

1 Guthrie R, Susi A. A simple phenylalanine method for detecting phenylketonuria in large populations of newborn infants. *Pediatrics* 1963; **32**: 338–43
2 Streetly A, Grant C, Pollitt RJ, Addison GM. Survey of scope of neonatal screening in the United Kingdom. *BMJ* 1995; **311**: 726
3 First report of the National Screening Committee. London: Department of Health, 1998

4   Pollitt RJ, Green A, McCabe CJ *et al.* Neonatal screening for inborn errors of metabolism: cost, yield and outcome. *Health Technol Assess* 1997; **1**: 1–203

5   Seymour CA, Thomason MJ, Chalmers RA *et al.* Newborn screening for inborn errors of metabolism: a systematic review. *Health Technol Assess* 1997; **1**: 1–97

6   Elliman D, Garner J. Review of neonatal screening programme for phenylketonuria. *BMJ* 1991; **303**: 471

7   Pharoah POD, Madden MP. Audit of screening for congenital hypothyroidism. *Arch Dis Child* 1992; **67**: 1073–6

8   Galloway A, Stevenson J. An audit of the organisation of neonatal screening for phenylketonuria and congenital hypothyroidism in the Northern Region. *Public Health* 1996; **110**: 119–21

9   Cappuccio FP, Hickman M, Barker M. Performance is hard to monitor. *BMJ* 1996; **312**: 182

10 Simpson N, Randall R, Lenton S, Walker S. Audit of neonatal screening programme for phenylketonuria and congenital hypothyroidism. *Arch Dis Child* 1997; **77**: F228–34

11 Ahmed SF, Barnes ND, Hughes IA. Initial evaluation of congenital hypothyroidism: a survey of general paediatricians in East Anglia. *Arch Dis Child* 1997; **77**: 339–41

12 Streetly A, Corbett V. An audit of phenylketonuria and congenital hypothyroidism screening in England and Wales. London: The Printed Word, 1998

13 Touma EH, Charpentier C. Medium chain acyl-CoA dehydrogenase deficiency. *Arch Dis Child* 1992; **67**: 142–5

14 Wilcken B, Carpenter KH, Hammond J. Neonatal symptoms in medium chain acyl coenzyme A dehydrogenase deficiency. *Arch Dis Child* 1993; **69**: 292–4

15 Iafolla AK, Thompson RJ, Roe CR. Medium-chain acyl-coenzyme A dehydrogenase deficiency: clinical course in 120 affected children. *J Pediatr* 1994; **124**: 409–15

16 Gregersen N, Winter V, Curtis D *et al.* Medium-chain acyl-CoA dehydrogenase (MCAD) deficiency: the prevalent mutation G985 (K304E) is subject to a strong founder effect from Northwestern Europe. *Hum Hered* 1993; **43**: 342–50

17 Andresen BS, Jensen TG, Bross P *et al.* Disease causing mutations in exon 11 of the medium-chain acyl-CoA dehydrogenase gene. *Am J Hum Genet* 1994; **54**: 975–88

18 Dundar M, Lanyon WG, Connor JM. Scottish frequency of the common G985 mutation in the medium-chain acyl-CoA dehydrogenase (MCAD) gene and the role of MCAD deficiency in sudden infant death syndrome (SIDS). *J Inher Metab Dis* 1993; **16**: 991–3

19 Seddon HR, Green A, Gray RGF, Leonard JV, Pollitt RJ. Regional variations in medium-chain acyl-CoA dehydrogenase deficiency. *Lancet* 1994; **345**: 135–6

20 Pollitt RJ, Leonard JV. Prospective surveillance study of medium chain acyl-CoA dehydrogenase deficiency in the UK. *Arch Dis Child* 1998; **79**: 116–9

21 Clayton PT, Doig M, Ghafari S *et al.* Screening for medium chain acyl-CoA dehydrogenase deficiency using electrospray ionisation tandem mass spectrometry. *Arch Dis Child* 1998; **79**: 109–15

22 Wilson CJ, Champion MP, Collins JE, Clayton PT, Leonard JV. Outcome of medium chain acyl-CoA dehydrogenase deficiency after diagnosis. Submitted

23 Van Hove JLK, Zhang W, Kahler SG *et al.* Medium-chain acyl-CoA dehydrogenase (MCAD) deficiency: diagnosis by acylcarnitine analysis in blood. *Am J Hum Genet* 1993; **52**: 958–66

24 Rashed MS, Ozand PT, Bucknall MP, Little D. Diagnosis of inborn errors of metabolism from blood spots by acylcarnitines and amino acids profiling using automated electrospray tandem mass spectrometry. *Pediatr Res* 1995; **38**: 324–31

25 Sweetman L. Newborn screening by tandem mass spectrometry (MS-MS). *Clin Chem* 1996; **42**: 345–6

26 Bartlett K, Eaton SJ, Pourfarzam M. New developments in neonatal screening. *Arch Dis Child* 1997; **77**: F151–4

27 Ziadeh R, Hoffman EP, Finegold DN *et al.* Medium chain acyl-CoA dehydrogenase deficiency in Pennsylvania: neonatal screening shows high incidence and unexpected mutation frequencies. *Pediatr Res* 1995; **37**: 675–8

28 Hughes IA. Congenital adrenal hyperplasia – a continuum of disorders. *Lancet* 1998; **352**: 752–4

29 Bodegard G, Fyro K, Larsson A. Psychological reactions in 102 families with a newborn who has a falsely positive screening test for congenital hypothyroidism. *Acta Paediatr Scand* 1983; **304** (Suppl): 1–21

30 Sorensen JR, Levy HL, Mangione TW, Sepe SJ. Parental response to repeat testing of infants with 'false positive' results in newborn screening program. *Pediatrics* 1984; **73**: 183–7

31 Russell LB. *Educated guesses*. Berkley: University of California Press, 1994

32 Parsonnet J, Harris RH, Hack HM, Owen DK. Modelling cost effectiveness of *Helicobacter pylori* screening to prevent gastric cancer: a mandate for clinical trials. *Lancet* 1996; **348**: 150–4

33 Torgerson DJ, Donaldson C. Economic evaluations before clinical trials. *Lancet* 1996; **348**: 687

34 Lumley J. Trials and evaluation of screening programs. In: Wilcken B, Webster D. (eds) *Neonatal screening in the nineties*. Sydney: 8th International Neonatal Screening Symposium, Australia, 1991; 11–17

35 Farrell PM, Kosorok MR, Laxova A *et al*. Nutritional benefits of neonatal screening for cystic fibrosis. *N Engl J Med* 1997; **337**: 963–9

36 Birch HG, Tizard J. The dietary treatment of phenylketonuria: not proven? *Dev Med Child Neurol* 1967; **9**: 9–12

37 Beasley MG, Costello PM, Smith I. Outcome of treatment in young adults with phenylketonuria detected by routine neonatal screening between 1964 and 1971. *Q J Med* 1994; **87**: 155–60

38 Walter JH. Neonatal screening for PKU and other metabolic disorders. *Semin Neonatol* 1998; **3**: 17–25

39 Fost N, Farrell PM. A prospective randomised trial of early diagnosis and treatment of cystic fibrosis: a unique ethical dilemma. *Clin Res* 1989; **37**: 495–500

40 Silverman WA. *Human experimentation: a guided step into the unknown*. Oxford: Oxford University Press, 1985

41 US Department of Health and Human Services. Newborn screening for cystic fibrosis: a paradigm for public health genetics policy development. *MMWR Suppl* 1997; **46**: 1–24

Screening for genital chlamydial infection

Judith M Stephenson

Department of Sexually Transmitted Diseases, University College London Medical School, London, UK

Genital chlamydial infection is a common, sexually transmitted infection that is often asymptomatic, but associated with long term morbidity in a sizeable proportion of women. Early infection can be diagnosed reliably using non-invasive methods and treated effectively with antibiotics. The case for screening in conventional high risk settings (*e.g.* genito-urinary medicine and termination of pregnancy clinics) is already clear. Screening in the wider community also needs evaluating if a significant impact on the problem is to be made since chlamydial infection is widely distributed among young, sexually active people who may have little contact with health services. Studies are in progress to assess the acceptability of different screening approaches to women and men in the community and to compare performance of newer diagnostic techniques. The cost-effectiveness of community-based screening in reducing morbidity needs to be evaluated empirically in randomised trials to encourage a coherent, evidence-based screening policy in this country.

In recent years, the control of genital chlamydial infection has emerged as an increasingly important public health problem. This chapter considers available evidence in support of screening, as well as some of the unresolved issues that need to be addressed before decisions can be made about the appropriateness of implementing a screening programme in the UK.

Why consider screening for chlamydial infection?

Chlamydia trachomatis is the most common sexually transmitted bacterial infection in the UK[1] and uncomplicated infection is easily treated with antibiotics. However, as it often causes no symptoms, most infected individuals are not diagnosed. As previous infection provides no immunity, re-infection occurs if infection in a sexual partner is not detected and treated. In about 30% of women[2], untreated infection leads to serious complications including pelvic inflammatory disease, tubal infertility and ectopic pregnancy. The risk of complications is high in women with recurrent infections[3] and the cost of treating complications has been conservatively estimated at £50 million per year in

*Correspondence to:
Dr Judith M Stephenson,
Department of Sexually
Transmitted Diseases,
University College
London Medical School,
Mortimer Market Centre,
off Capper Street,
London WC1E 6AU, UK*

the UK[4], although the true figure may be closer to £100 million. Vaccination against *C. trachomatis* may eventually be feasible, but is not currently an option for controlling either the acute infection or its complications[5]. The justification for screening is based on the premise that early detection and treatment of genital chlamydial infection effectively prevents the reproductive consequences of infection.

How strong is the case for screening?

Chlamydial infection fulfils several of the criteria for the implementation of a successful screening programme as outlined by Wilson and Junger[6]. Chlamydia is a common infection with important sequelae. Most of the burden of complications is borne by women, although infection in men may lead to epididymo-orchitis. Ascending infection of the genital tract in women may lead to pelvic inflammatory disease, which includes infection of the endometrium, fallopian tubes and their contiguous structures. The clinical features of pelvic inflammatory disease, which include pelvic pain, infertility and ectopic pregnancy, are thought to result from immune-mediated scarring in the presence of persistent upper genital tract infection. Intraluminal scarring of the fallopian tubes leads to ectopic pregnancy when occlusion is partial and to tubal-factor infertility when it is complete, while extraluminal scarring is associated with chronic pelvic pain. Ectopic pregnancy accounts for 1% of all conceptions and is the leading cause of maternal death during the first trimester of pregnancy in industrialised countries[7]. Because of its strong association with maternal age, the incidence of ectopic pregnancy has increased in recent years along with fertility rates in older women. There is a paucity of information on the epidemiology of pelvic inflammatory disease because of poor diagnostic precision[8]. Recent analysis of general practice morbidity data in England and Wales suggests a prevalence of 1.7% in women aged 16–46 years, or an annual number of 165,000 cases (I. Simms, personal communication). The incidence of tubal factor infertility, one of the most common causes of infertility[9], is unknown but demand for treatment is increasing. While the role of other infections, such as *Neisseria gonorrhoeae*, is well recognised in the aetiology of these complications, the incidence of gonococcal infection in women has declined. As a result, *C. trachomatis* has assumed greater importance, being responsible for an estimated 43% of ectopic pregnancies, 70% of cases of tubal infertility[10] and 50% of cases of pelvic inflammatory disease[11].

Simple and acceptable tests are now available for screening based on nucleic acid amplification tests using polymerase chain reaction (PCR) and ligase chain reaction (LCR). These tests can be used on urine samples making screening for chlamydia infection in both men and women feasible at a population level. Many of the earlier tests, such as enzyme immunoassays, were of lower sensitivity (60–75%) than these newer methods which have reported sensitivities of over 90%[12]. In addition, chlamydial infection in women was diagnosed previously from endocervix samples obtained with a swab or cytologic brush. The two main concerns about LCR testing are the increased cost, relative to previous methods, and the possible need for a 'cold chain' to be maintained from the collection of the urine specimen to laboratory testing[14]. If such a cold chain was necessary, this would clearly restrict the implementation of LCR urine testing for chlamydial infection in the community. However, current consensus seems to be that this is not a major issue, and that a loss of perhaps 5% sensitivity in the absence of a cold chain would be more than offset by a 30–50% improvement in sensitivity afforded by using urinary LCR instead of cervical or urinary enzyme immunoassay.

Effective treatment is available for people with uncomplicated chlamydial infection identified by screening. A tetracycline (*e.g.* 100 mg doxycycline by mouth, twice daily for 7 days) is the standard treatment[15]. Erythromycin (500 mg by mouth, twice daily for 7 days) is an effective alternative and is especially suitable for pregnant and lactating women. Azithromycin can be given as a single 1 g dose to guarantee compliance, and is as effective as doxycycline but nearly 4 times more expensive[16]. Effective treatment in this sense means negative chlamydia culture(s) or PCR testing a few weeks, or in one study up to 5 months, after appropriate antibiotic therapy[2,16,17]. However, only one randomised controlled trial has examined the impact of screening and treatment on the incidence of symptomatic complications[18,19]. In this trial, women from a Health Maintenance Organization in the US were selected on the basis of risk characteristics: 1009 were randomly assigned to screening, and 1598 to usual care. Only 645 (64%) women in the screening group were tested, of whom 44 tested positive and were treated. There was no mention of contact tracing of the sexual partners of the infected women. At the end of the 12 month follow-up period, there were 9 confirmed cases of pelvic inflammatory disease in the screening group and 33 among the women assigned to receive the usual care. The incidence of pelvic inflammatory disease in the screening group was significantly reduced (relative risk 0.44; 95% CI: 0.20, 0.90). However, 7 of the 9 cases in the screening group were women who had been tested for chlamydia infection. After adjusting for differences between the screening and comparison groups in baseline risk status, the relative risk was 0.42, (95% CI 0.20, 0.89), representing a 58% reduction in the risk of pelvic inflammatory disease associated with screening for chlamydia. Aspects of the trial design have been criticised[19]. Women were randomly assigned to screening or usual care before their eligibility to enter the trial was determined, and greater emphasis was then placed on recruiting those assigned to the screening group rather than those assigned to the control group. Consequently, the participation rate among controls was lower, which introduces the possibility of selection bias at the outset. Although the trial showed a marked reduction in pelvic inflammatory disease, with less than two-thirds of women assigned to screening actually being tested for chlamydia, these results need to be confirmed.

There is good information about who is most at risk of chlamydial infection. Prevalence surveys[20,21] and routine surveillance data[22] both show that the risk of infection is highly age-dependent, with the highest prevalence in teenage women. Other demographic and behavioural risk factors, which are markers for the probability of exposure to an infected sexual partner, include factors such as single status, number of sexual partners, previous history of a sexually transmitted infection and not using barrier contraceptive methods. Prevalence of infection in men is also strongly related to age, with peak levels in men aged 25–34 years[22], but less is known about other risk factors[23]. The target population for screening can, therefore, be defined loosely as sexually active young people.

Settings in which those at risk come into contact with health services include genito-urinary medicine, gynaecology, antenatal, general practice and family planning clinics. Best estimates of the prevalence of chlamydia range from about 7–12% in women seeking termination of pregnancy[24] to about 3–10% in women in general practice[20,25], although the use of different screening tests in different age groups hinders comparison between studies. These and other data sources show that *C. trachomatis* is much more widely distributed than, for example, gonorrhoea and not restricted to conventional 'high risk' groups. The case for routine screening of people attending genito-urinary medicine clinics or women seeking termination of pregnancy is strong, and already established or recommended by professional consensus[26,27]. The challenge is, therefore, to evaluate different strategies for screening young and sexually active people who have little or no contact with health services. The remainder of this chapter focuses on issues relating to population screening.

It is instructive to look at the achievements reported from Scandinavia since the introduction of a concerted approach to control chlamydial infection[28–30]. Swedish research groups reported high rates of chlamydia-associated acute pelvic inflammatory disease in young women during the late 1970s. This led to the introduction of liberal testing and treatment for chlamydial infection advocated by public health authorities in the early and mid-1980s. Diagnostic procedures were

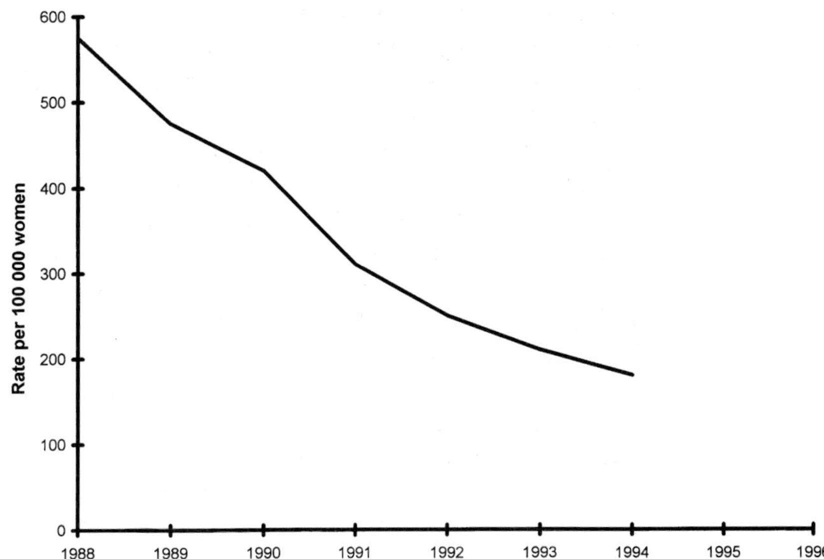

Fig. 1 New cases of chlamydial infection in Sweden, 1988–1994 (rate per 100,000 women). Adapted from Kamwendo et al[29].

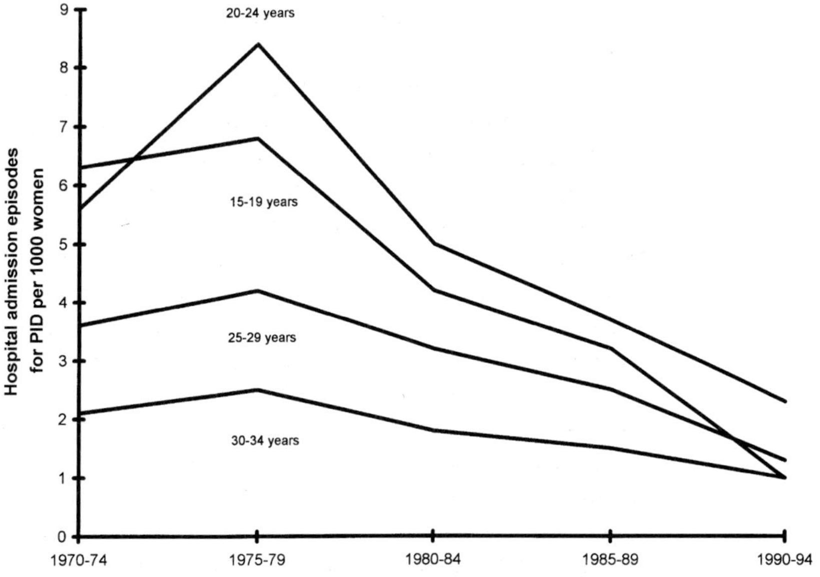

Fig. 2 Episodes of hospital admission for pelvic inflammatory disease per 1000 women in the catchment area for Orebro Medical Centre Hospital, Sweden, 1970–1994. Adapted from Kamwendo et al[29].

available free of charge in most areas of Sweden. Chlamydial prevalence rates were highest in teenage women and peaked in 1985–1987. Screening was directed at young, sexually active women in contact with health services, such as family planning and antenatal clinics, as well as those seeking termination of pregnancy or attending genito-urinary clinics. This approach was supported by a legal requirement to notify

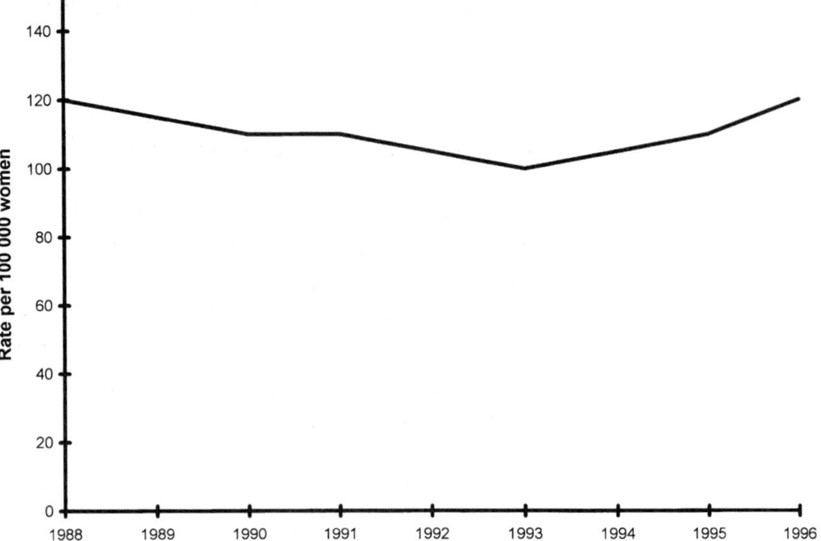

Fig. 3 New cases of infection with *C. trachomatis* seen in genito-urinary medicine clinics in England and Wales, 1988–1996 (rate per 100,000 women). Adapted from reference[1].

cases of chlamydial infection, active efforts to treat sexual partners, increased public awareness about chlamydial infection and compulsory education about sexually transmitted diseases in schools. Rates of reported chlamydial infection in women in Sweden have declined dramatically over the last couple of decades, as have rates of hospital admission for pelvic inflammatory disease (Figs 1 & 2). Data from genito-urinary medicine clinics in England and Wales have shown an increase in the prevalence of chlamydial infections over a similar period of time (Fig. 3).

Given the comprehensive package of public health measures undertaken in Sweden, it is uncertain how much of this decline can be attributed to screening *per se*, rather than, for example, more efficient contact tracing or changes in health-seeking behaviour and use of barrier contraceptive methods. Rates of chlamydia, gonorrhoea and pelvic inflammatory disease had all begun to fall before introduction of the public health measures described above (Fig. 1). Commenting on the decline in 1988, Westrom[30] suggested that 'the most important factor for the decrease in gonorrhoea and chlamydial infection, however, seems to be a more conservative attitude to sex and changes of partners in young people during the past decade'.

Although findings from other countries are important and instructive, they cannot readily be translated into a blueprint for a cost-effective community-based screening programme in the UK. It would be quite plausible for screening in this country to have little impact on desired outcomes if, for example, re-infection occurred during the screening interval or if men were not screened and contact tracing was inefficient.

Some of the issues that still need to be addressed are considered further below.

What are the important gaps in knowledge?

Areas of uncertainty that have an important bearing on the success or otherwise of screening include the natural history of chlamydial infection, the most appropriate approach(s) to screening and contact tracing in the community, whether to screen men as well as women, whether to select people on the basis of risk factors other than age, and the cost-effectiveness of screening. Raising awareness and understanding of chlamydial infection and its management among health care workers and the general public is another important issue.

The natural history of chlamydial infection in women has not been well documented, but it would be unethical now to attempt this prospectively. Scant data[31] from individuals with untreated chlamydial infection who were culture negative at follow-up suggest that infection clears spontaneously in perhaps 50% of women, although it is possible that these 'spontaneous cures' reflect the failure of cell culture to detect persistent infection because culture is relatively insensitive[12]. In a more recent, retrospective study using PCR testing, 21 (28%) of 74 patients with chlamydial infection who had not received treatment had apparent resolution of infection[32]. In this small study, resolution was inversely related to age, being greatest in those over 30 years of age, compared to teenagers aged 15–19 years.

A more important gap in understanding the natural history of chlamydial infection relates to the development of complications. It is often stated that 10–40% of women with chlamydial infection develop pelvic inflammatory disease, but the data on which these estimates are based are sparse. In one prospective study, 6 (30%) of 20 women with chlamydial infection developed pelvic inflammatory disease within 49 days[2]. Cross-sectional studies have reported the proportion of women with chlamydial infection who have co-incident pelvic inflammatory disease (8%)[33] or asymptomatic upper genital tract chlamydial infection (40%)[34], but these data are less useful because it is not clear whether the cervical infection was acquired before the onset of pelvic inflammatory disease or not. Without information from longitudinal studies about the temperal sequence of infection and onset of complications, appropriateness of screening and the screening interval cannot be reliably determined.

Although the new nucleic acid amplification tests represent an important advance in relation to those previously available, questions remain about their relative performance on different samples, *e.g.* urine, urethral, low vaginal or vulval, compared with endocervical[13]. Some samples are cheaper to process than others and these costs would need to be considered alongside the acceptability of different sampling methods and approaches to young people. It is now possible, for example, to invite people to produce their own urine sample at home and post it directly to a laboratory for testing. This approach has the advantage of reaching young, sexually active people, particularly men, who do not often come into contact with health services; it has been tried with promising results in women in Sweden[35]. Studies in the UK are underway to address the feasibility of home-based screening and its acceptability to women and men.

In view of the nature of this infection, contact tracing of an infected individual's sexual partners is key to the control of chlamydial infection[36]. However, this is often neglected in practice. Of a random sample of 374 general practitioners in England and Wales, 30% stated that they would refer a woman with chlamydia to a genito-urinary clinic for contact tracing, and 21% that they would treat or refer her partner[37]. In another study, 13% of 141 patients diagnosed in general practice in the Lothian region of Scotland were referred to a genito-urinary clinic[38]. A recent study from Denmark has suggested that home screening using urine samples might improve contact tracing of male partners of infected women, compared with the conventional approach of asking the partner to visit a doctor so that a urethral swab may be taken[39]. Further research into the most effective methods of contact tracing in this country is needed.

There has been much discussion about the most appropriate target population for screening. Clearly the target population needs to centre on sexually active young people, but should it include men? Should women (and men) be selected on the basis of age alone, or should other risk factors be taken into account? The cost-effectiveness of screening will depend on the prevalence of infection and distribution of risk factors in the local population. Some studies have considered the cost-effectiveness of different screening strategies[26,40–42], but others have only looked at increasing the yield of infection identified by screening, rather than the impact of screening on subsequent complications. The case for screening men, as well as women, is less clear. The consequences of chlamydia infection in men are minor compared with the complications in women. One of the main reasons for treating chlamydial infection in men is to reduce the risk of transmission to female sexual partners. This could be achieved by efficient male contact tracing or by screening men. The inefficiency of current contact tracing strengthens the rationale for screening men which is to reduce the pool of infection in the population. Further work is needed to address these issues adequately.

The success of any screening programme will also depend on the level of public awareness of chlamydial infection and its complications and an understanding of the benefits of screening. Current public awareness about sexually transmitted infections seems to be inversely related to their frequency. Awareness of HIV and gonorrhoea, which are uncommon outside certain risk groups in the UK, is much higher than public awareness of chlamydia[43]. However, it seems inevitable that knowledge about chlamydial infection will increase, with the accumulation of articles in women's magazines and the general press[44]. Training and education of doctors and other health care workers is key to the success of screening initiatives. Audit surveys have shown that the management of chlamydial infection and pelvic inflammatory disease in general practice is often inadequate[37,45]. In a recent survey in England and Wales, only 30% of general practitioners had prescribed appropriate antibiotic therapy to women with infection[37]. Issues about confidentiality and the sensitivities surrounding screening for sexually transmitted infections in general practice also need to be addressed.

How should the effectiveness of screening be evaluated?

Where possible, screening programmes should be rigorously evaluated through randomised controlled trials before being implemented[46]. Effectiveness needs to be shown by a decline in the prevalence of chlamydia and the incidence of complications in a screened population. In order to demonstrate that the decline is due to screening and not to unrelated factors, such as increased use of barrier contraceptives, a comparable non-screened group is required. No such trial has been conducted in the UK. A large, well designed trial, with communities or individuals randomised to screening or no screening, would enable several of the questions discussed above to be addressed. For example, information could be collected on the acceptability by men and women of screening methods, the efficiency of contact tracing, and the prevalence of infection in different areas or sub-groups.

Estimation of the cost-effectiveness of different screening programmes is important. There have been several economic analyses of the cost effectiveness of screening for chlamydia[26,40–42], most of which have ignored, or made dubious assumptions, about progression of infection to complications, re-infection rates, contact tracing and transmission dynamics. If an economic evaluation were built into the design of a screening trial, empirical data could then be used to provide more precise estimates of cost-effectiveness in terms of the number needed to screen to prevent one case of pelvic inflammatory disease, *etc.* Mathematical modelling techniques could also be applied to forecast the long term outcome of screening and clinical management policies in terms of their long term resource use and clinical effectiveness. The overall aim would be to provide an evidence-based picture of the likely outcome of community-based chlamydial screening that could contribute to health policy development. In practice, an effective screening programme might involve a combination of different strategies for different settings, but this should not be left to the hazards of encounters between individuals and health services. A screening programme needs to be centrally organised, with individual invitations to participate and adequate follow-up of infected persons, linked to routine monitoring of complications to allow evaluation of the impact of screening over time.

Much of the difficulty in assessing the benefits of screening relates to the difficulty of measuring chlamydial complications. Clinical diagnosis of pelvic inflammatory disease is notoriously imprecise[8]. Laparoscopic diagnosis is regarded as the diagnostic gold standard, but clearly this is inappropriate for ascertaining outcome in large studies[11]. Diagnosis of tubal infertility depends on a number of factors unrelated to chlamydial infection. Ectopic pregnancy is a life-threatening complication, but is uncommon, accounting for 1% of all conceptions. Despite these difficulties, trials are needed to examine the effect of screening on complications, as the goal of screening is to reduce the proportion of women developing PID, tubal infertility and ectopic pregnancy.

References

1 Anonymous. Sexually transmitted diseases quarterly report: genital infections with *Chlamydia trachomatis* in England and Wales. *Commun Dis Rep* 1996; 7: 394–5

2 Stamm WE, Guinan ME, Johnson C. Effect of treatment regimens for *Neisseria gonorrhoea* on simultaneous infection with *Chlamydia trachomatis*. *N Engl J Med* 1984; **310**: 545–9

3 Hillis SD, Owens LM, Marchbanks PA, Amsterdam LE, MacKenzie WR. Recurrent chlamydial infections increase the risks of hospitalisation for ectopic pregnancy and pelvic inflammatory disease. *Am J Obstet Gynecol* 1997; **176**: 103–7

4 Taylor-Robinson D. *Chlamydia trachomatis* and sexually transmitted disease. *BMJ* 1994; **308**: 150–1

5 Ward ME. The feasibility of preventing pelvic inflammatory disease by vaccinating against chlamydial and gonoccocal infection. In: Templeton A. (ed) *The Prevention of Pelvic Infection*. London: RCOG Press, 1996; 121–35

6 Wilson JMG, Junger G. Principles and practice of screening for disease. (*Public Health Papers* 34). Geneva:WHO, 1968

7 Simms I, Rogers PA, Nicoll A. The influence of demographic change and cumulative risk of pelvic inflammatory disease on the incidence of ectopic pregnancy. *Epidemiol Infect* 1997; **119**: 49–52

8 Kahn JG, Walker CK, Washington AE, Landers DV, Sweet RL. Diagnosing pelvic inflammatory disease. *JAMA* 1991; **266**: 2594–604

9 Healy DL, Trounson AO, Andersen AN. Female infertility: causes and treatment. *Lancet* 1994; **343**: 1539–44

10 World Health Organization Task Force on the Prevention and Management of Infertility. Tubal infertility: serologic relationship to past chlamydial and gonococcal infection. *Sex Transm Dis* 1995; **22**: 71–7

11 Bevan CD, Johal BJ, Mumtaz G, Ridgway GL, Siddle NC. Clinical, laparoscopic and microbiological findings in acute salpingitis: report on a United Kingdom cohort. *Br J Obstet Gynaecol* 1995; **102**: 407–14

12 Black CM. Current methods of laboratory diagnosis of *Chlamydia trachomatis* infection. *Clin Microbiol Rev* 1997; **10**: 160–84

13 Stary A. Chlamydia screening: which sample for which technique? *Genitourin Med* 1997; **73**: 99–102

14 Caul EO, Horner PJ, Leece J, Crowley T, Paul I, Davey Smith G. Population-based screening programmes for *Chlamydia trachomatis* [letter]. *Lancet* 1997; **439**: 1070–1

15 Management of genital *Chlamydia trachomatis* infections. *Drug Ther Bull* 1994; **32**: 87–8

16 Martin DH, Mroczkowski TF, Dalu ZA *et al.* A controlled trial of a single dose of azithromycin for the treatment of chlamydial urethritis and cervicitis. *N Engl J Med* 1992; **327**: 921–5

17 Workowski KA, Lampe MF, Wong KG, Watts MB, Stamm WE. Long-term eradication of *Chlamydia trachomatis* genital infection after antimicrobial therapy: evidence against persistent infection. *JAMA* 1993; **270**: 2071–5

18 Scholes D, Stergachs A, Heidrich FE, Andrilla H, Holmes KK, Stamm WE. Prevention of pelvic inflammatory disease by screening for cervical chlamydial infection. *N Engl J Med* 1996; **334**: 1362–6

19 Hillis SD, Wasserheit JN. Screening for chlamydia – a key to the prevention of pelvic inflammatory disease. *N Engl J Med* 1996; **334**: 1399–400

20 Stokes T. Screening for chlamydia in general practice: a literature review and summary of the evidence. *J Public Health Med* 1997; **19**: 222–32

21 Grun L, Tassano-Smith J, Carder C *et al.* Comparison of two methods of screening for genital chlamydial infection in women attending in general practice: cross sectional survey. *BMJ* 1997; **315**: 226–30

22 Simms I, Catchpole M, Brugha R, Rogers P, Mallinson H, Nicoll A. Epidemiology of genital *Chlamydia trachomatis* in England and Wales. *Genitourin Med* 1997; **73**: 122–6

23 US Department of Health and Human Services. Recommendations for the prevention and management of *Chlamydia trachomatis* infection, 1993. *MMWR* 1993; **42**: 1–37

24 Penney GC. Prophylactic antibiotic therapy for abortion. In: Templeton A. (ed) *The Prevention of Pelvic Infection*. London: RCOG Press, 1996; 211–22

25 Oakeshott P, Hay P. General practice update: chlamydia infection in women. *Br J Gen Pract* 1995; **45**: 615–20

26 Blackwell AL, Thomas PD, Wareham K, Emery SJ. Health gains from screening for infection of the lower genital tract in women attending for termination of pregnancy. *Lancet* 1993; **342**: 206–10

27 Recommendations arising from the 31st Study Group: the prevention of pelvic infection. In: Templeton A. (ed) *The Prevention of Pelvic Infection*. London: RCOG Press, 1996; 267–70

28 Ripa T. Epidemiologic control of genital *Chlamydia trachomatis* infections. *Scand J Infect Dis* 1990; **69**: 157–67

29 Kamwendo F, Forslin L, Bodin L, Danielsson D. Decreasing incidences of gonorrhoea and chlamydia associated acute pelvic inflammatory disease. *Sex Transm Dis* 1996; **23**: 384–91

30 Westrom L. Decrease in incidence of women treated in hospital for acute salpingitis in Sweden. *Genitourin Med* 1988; **64**: 59–63

31 McCormack WM, Alpert S, McComb DE, Nichols RL, Semine DZ, Zinner SH. Fifteen-month follow-up study of women infected with *Chlamydia trachomatis*. *N Engl J Med* 1979; **300**: 123–5

32 Parks KS, Dixon PB, Richey CM, Hook EW. Spontaneous clearance of *Chlamydia trachomatis* infection in untreated patients. *Sex Transm Dis* 1997; **24**: 229–35

33 Westrom L, Svensson L, Wolner-Hanssen P, Mardh P-A. Chlamydial and gonococcal infections in a defined population of women. *Scand J Infect Dis* 1982; **32 (Suppl)**: 157–62

34 Tait A, Duthrie SJ, Taylor-Robinson D. Silent upper genital tract chlamydial infection and disease in women. *Int J STD AIDS* 1997; **8**: 329–31

35 Ostergaard L, Moller JK, Andersen B, Olesen F. Diagnosis of urogenital *Chlamydia trachomatis* infection in women based on mailed samples obtained at home: multipractice comparative study. *BMJ* 1996; **313**: 1186–9

36　Johnson AM, Grun L, Haines A. Controlling genital chlamydial infection. *BMJ* 1996; **313**: 1160

37　Mason D, Kerry S, Oakshott P. Postal survey of management of cervical *Chlamydia trachomatis* infection in English and Welsh general practices. *BMJ* 1996; **313**: 1193–4

38　Ross JDC, Sutherland S, Coia J. Genital *Chlamydia trachomatis* infections in primary care. *BMJ* 1996; **313**: 1192–3

39　Andersen B, Ostergaard L, Moller JK, Olesen F. Home sampling versus conventional contact tracing for detecting *Chlamydia trachomatis* infection in male partners of infected women: randomised study. *BMJ* 1998; **316**: 350–1

40　Genc M, Mardh P-A. A cost-effectiveness analysis of screening and treatment for *Chlamydia trachomatis* infection in asymptomatic women. *Ann Intern Med* 1996; **124**: 1–7

41　Genc M, Ruusuvaara L, Mardh P-A. An economic evaluation of screening for *Chlamydia trachomatis* in adolescent males. *JAMA* 1993; **270**: 2057–64

42　Howell MR, Quinn TC, Gaydos CA. Screening for *Chlamydia trachomatis* in asymptomatic women attending family planning clinics. A cost effectiveness analysis of three strategies. *Ann Intern Med* 1998; **128**: 277–84

43　Goldsmith M. Health education to prevent pelvic infection. In: Templeton A. (ed) *The Prevention of Pelvic Infection*. London: RCOG Press, 1996; 229–4

44　Doyle C. Defusing a fertility timebomb. *The Daily Telegraph* 10 February 1998

45　Eynon-Lewis A. Audit of the management of pelvic inflammatory disease in general practice. *J R Coll Gen Pract* 1988; **38**: 492–3

46　Day NE. Screening for cancer of the cervix. *J Epidemiol Community Health* 1989; **43**: 103–6

Screening for abdominal aortic aneurysms

Malcolm Law

Department of Environmental and Preventive Medicine, Wolfson Institute of Preventive Medicine, St Bartholomew's and the Royal London Hospital, London, UK

Ruptured aneurysm of the abdominal aorta is a common preventable cause of death, accounting for 2% of all deaths in men over 60 years of age. Population screening could prevent such deaths. Aortic diameter (which can be measured accurately on ultrasound) is a strong predictor of the risk of rupture, which is about 17% per year with aortic diameter ≥ 6 cm, but below 0.5% per year with aortic diameter < 5 cm, with uncertainty regarding risk in the range 5.0–5.9 cm. Adopting an aortic diameter cut-off of 6.0 cm, the detection rate is estimated to be 86% (that is, 86% of all men who would rupture an aortic aneurysm could be identified and offered surgery) and the false positive rate only 0.6% (that is, 0.6% of men who would not rupture an aortic aneurysm would be so identified). In men with aortic diameter ≥ 6 cm, the risk of rupture of 17% per year greatly outweighs the peri-operative mortality of about 5%. A national screening programme for men over 60 years of age could prevent 2000 deaths per year and should commence. Uncertainty remains regarding the frequency with which men with smaller aneurysms should be re-examined and the value of intervention among those with an aortic diameter of 5.0–5.9 cm, but the screening programme itself would generate data to help resolve these issues.

Ruptured aneurysm of the abdominal aorta is a common preventable cause of death (Table 1), with 4940 deaths in men and 2062 in women in England and Wales in 1996 – 2% of all deaths in men aged 60 years and over[1]. The disorder is a candidate for a population screening programme and, in this paper, the effectiveness of screening is assessed.

Correspondence to:
Dr Malcolm Law,
Department of
Environmental and
Preventive Medicine,
Wolfson Institute of
Preventive Medicine,
St Bartholomew's and
the Royal London
Hospital, College of
Medicine and Dentistry,
Charterhouse Square,
London
EC1M 6BQ, UK

Natural history

For the abdominal aorta to rupture, an aneurysm must first form and grow to a critical size – the process has been compared to a blow out in an inner tube[2]. It is the section of the abdominal aorta below the renal arteries that is prone to aneurysmal enlargement, but the aneurysm may extend above the renal arteries or down into the common iliac arteries. The average rate of expansion of abdominal aortic aneurysms is relatively slow, but (like a balloon) the rate of expansion increases with

Table 1 The numbers and rates of deaths attributed to ruptured abdominal* aortic aneurysm by age and sex, England and Wales 1996[1]

Age (years)	Men			Women		
	No. of deaths (% total)		Rate/10,000	No. of deaths (% total)		Rate/10,000
< 50	9	–	–	2	–	–
50–54	27	(1)	0.2	3	–	–
55–59	97	(2)	0.7	14	–	–
60–64	272	(6)	2.3	35	(2)	0.3
65–69	598	(12)	5.4	127	(6)	1.0
70–74	1124	(23)	11.8	300	(15)	2.5
75–79	1099	(22)	16.7	427	(21)	4.4
80–84	1024	(21)	25.1	530	(26)	7.0
85–89	524	(11)	27.9	408	(20)	8.7
90+	166	(3)	29.0	216	(10)	8.6
	4940*	(100)		2062*	(100)	

*The totals include 1345 deaths in men and 724 in women with site not specified as thoracic or abdominal (with site specified, 8% of deaths in men and 26% of deaths in women were thoracic).

the diameter. From the available published data in 1994 the average rates of expansion were 0.14, 0.25, 0.36, 0.49 and 0.70 cm per year in patients whose aortic diameter was < 3, 3–3.9, 4–4.9, 5–5.9 and ≥ 6 cm respectively[2]. The extent of individual variation around these average rates is difficult to assess from the available data, as is the suggestion that growth may occur in 'spurts' rather than uniformly. Table 2 summarises the risk of rupture according to aortic diameter from the published prospective studies of patients who were observed without intervention (from older studies conducted before the availability of surgery or more recent studies in which surgery was not performed because the aneurysm was small, the patient declined or the risk was judged too high[3-14]). The risk of rupture, again like a balloon, increases with diameter; risk is relatively small when the aortic diameter is under 5 cm, but is large (about 17% per year) when aortic diameter is 6 cm or more. From the above average growth rates an aneurysm would take 7 years to expand from 2.0 cm (about the average infrarenal aortic diameter in men) to 3.0 cm (detectable as being above the normal range), and an additional 9 years to reach a diameter of 6 cm.

Table 3 shows the outcome when an abdominal aortic aneurysm ruptures, in 12 studies that attempted to identify all cases of ruptured abdominal aortic aneurysm in defined communities by combining data from hospital admissions, coroner's autopsies and death certificates[2,15]. About one-third of the patients die before reaching hospital and a further third reach hospital as emergencies but die before surgery can be arranged. Of the third who survive to surgery the operative mortality is about 50%, so only one patient in six survives a rupture.

Table 2 Prospective studies of the incidence of rupture (no. ruptured/total) according to aortic diameter

Study (first author)	Age (years) when reported range (mean)	Maximum aortic diameter (cm)				Duration of follow-up (years)
		3.0–3.9	4.0–4.9	5.0–5.9	≥ 6.0†	
Klippel[3]	41 – >80 (69)	–	–	–	2/10	2.8
Foster[4]	–	–	–	–	19/37	2.8
Bernstein[5]	49–87 (69)	1/26	1/18	1/14	3/6	2.4
Kremer[6]	62–92 (75)	0/20	0/12	0/3	3/7	3.1
Delin[7]	59–80	0/7	0/13	0/9	1/6	1.8
Nevitt[8]	–	0/85	0/45		9/46*	3.6
Collin[9]	65–74	0/52	0/10			2.7
Guirguis[10]	46–92 (70)	1/148	1/96		12/56*	2.8
Bengtsson[11]	54–84 (73)	0/30	0/12	0/2		2.7
Scott[12]	65–80	1/231	0/96			2.8
Lucarotti[13]	65 (65)	0/128	0/31			1.0
Smith[14]	65–75	0/140	0/23			1.1
Summary estimate of incidence per year† (95% confidence interval)		0.15% (0.10–0.46%)	0.24% (0.10–0.95%)	1.4% (0.22–10.2%)	17% (12–23%)	

*These were ≥ 5.0 cm; they are excluded from the summary estimate.
†Calculated from weighting the incidence in each study by its duration.

Table 3 Summary data from 12 studies (tabulated previously[2,15]) that identified all cases of ruptured aortic aneurysm in defined communities by combining data from hospital admissions and coroners' autopsies

Total number	2019 (100%)
Reached hospital	1253 (62%)
Operated on	720 (36%)
Survived surgery	318 (16%)

Aortic aneurysms are associated with smoking (the risk in smokers is about 4 times that in non-smokers), blood pressure (interquartile relative risk about 2-fold) and lipids[14–19]. The pathology of the disease is incompletely understood – aneurysms are generally associated with areas of the aorta affected by atheromatous disease, but destruction of elastin within the aortic wall is also important. However, the widely advocated means of preventing cardiovascular disease in general – not smoking and reducing lipids and blood pressure – would also be expected to reduce mortality from abdominal aortic aneurysm.

Deaths from ruptured abdominal aortic aneurysms must be undercertified, since sudden or unattended deaths are not invariably subject to autopsy. The well-recognised increase over time in the death rate from this cause in England and Wales (Fig. 1) may be due to a decline over time in under-certification. It may also be due to a true increase in incidence[20], though the decline over the same period in the

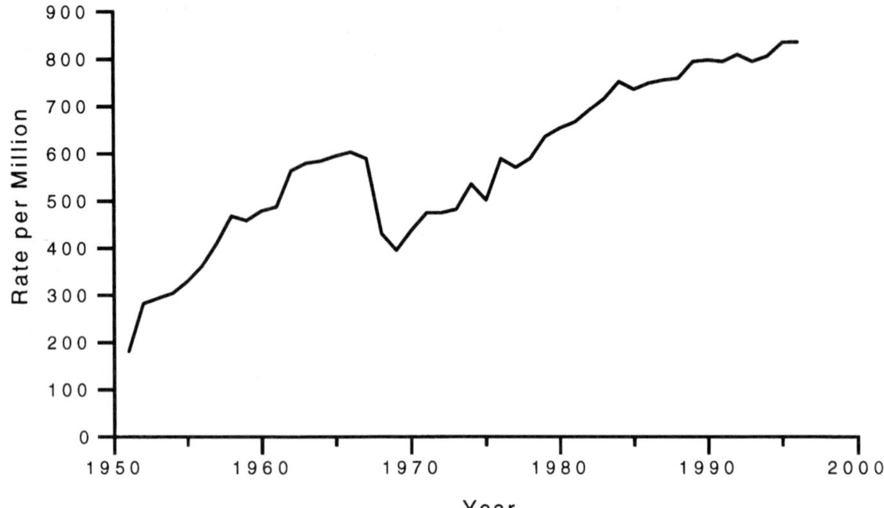

Fig. 1 Mortality ascribed to ruptured abdominal aortic aneurysms in men aged 65–74 years, England and Wales 1951–1996.

prevalence of smoking and the average blood pressure, two major causes of the disorder, weigh against this interpretation.

The screening procedure

As with many diseases, age and sex are important as an initial screening enquiry. The disorder is predominantly one of men: age specific death rates in men correspond to those in women 20 or more years younger (Table 1). Of the 4940 deaths in men, 97% occurred in men aged 60 years and over. Screening might, therefore, be limited to men, and to men aged 60 years and over.

Age and sex apart, maximum aortic diameter is the principal screening variable. This is the greater of the antero-posterior and transverse diameters, measured by ultrasound scanning of the abdominal aorta. This test is safe, free of discomfort, repeatable to 0.5 cm, and requires equipment which is portable[21–24]. It does not usually identify aneurysms as bulges, but a maximal external infrarenal diameter in the antero-posterior or transverse planes of ≥ 3.5 cm in men indicates aneurysmal enlargement with certainty and 3.0–3.4 cm with high probability; uncertainty occurs in the range 2.5–2.9 cm[25]. Patients with aortic diameters ≥ 3.0 cm are, therefore, followed as further expansion can be expected. Screening programmes have operated successfully in various localities in England. Table 4 summarises published data on these programmes. The rate of acceptance of the invitation is high – generally above 75%, and the aorta can be visualised on ultrasound scanning (allowing a measurement of the aortic diameter) in 97–100% of men.

Table 4 Population screening programmes in five localities in England

Locality	Age (years)	No invited	Attended*	Aorta visualised on scanning	Aortic diameter > 3.0cm	
					men	women
Gloucester[13]	65	5,337	4,232 (79%)	4,229 (100%)	167 (3.9%)	–
Oxford[25]	65–74	843	426 (51%)	426 (100%)	20 (4.7%)	–
Birmingham[14,18]	60–75	13,000	10,061 (76%)	9,771 (97%)	706 (7.2%)†	–
Northumberland[26]	65–79	800	628 (79%)	612 (97%)	40 (6.5%)	–
Chichester[12,27]	65–80	14,057	8,944 (64%)†	8,806 (98%)	294 (7.5%)	62 (1.3%)

*Letters sent to wrong address, illness and known aortic aneurysm account for some instances of failure to attend.

†Increasing over time; recent proportions are (men/women) 81%/73% at age 65 years, declining with age to 66%/58% at age 76–80 years[29].

In men judged at sufficiently high risk of rupture of the aorta, the remedy is an elective surgical insertion of a prosthetic aorta. The peri-operative mortality of this operation is about 5% on average[5,21,28]. It varies according to centre, being between 1–3% in the most experienced centres[12,14,26,27,29,30]. The most representative study is one of all surgical cases in The Netherlands in 1990, in which the overall peri-operative mortality was 6.7%, increasing markedly with age (2%, 4%, 10% and 17% in persons in their 50s, 60s, 70s and 80s)[28]. Peri-operative mortality will be lower in a screening programme than in clinical practice because sick individuals are less likely to attend for screening. During a 5 year screening study[29], mortality from all causes was almost twice as high in those who did not accept screening as in those who did (19.0% *versus* 10.4%), indicating that sick people tend to decline screening.

Conceptually, the aim of screening is not to identify all aneurysms but only those that will rupture. The prevalence in men of aortic diameter ≥ 3.0 cm diameter is about 5% at age 65 years and 9% at age 75–80 years[12–14,27,29], but screening would be inefficient if it directed all these men to medical attention when only a minority will rupture (2% of men die from this cause). Growth rates are slow (see preceding section) and most men die from other causes before their aneurysm is sufficiently large to be at significant risk of rupture. If the remedy was simple and safe it might be offered to all men with detectable aneurysms, even the smallest. In view of the 5% peri-operative mortality intervention must be limited to men in whom the risk of imminent rupture is judged sufficiently high to warrant this risk. The objective of screening is to select a 'cut-off' value of aortic diameter that identifies a large proportion of persons who will rupture the aorta (high detection rate) while intervening in a small proportion who will not (low false positive rate).

Estimating detection rates and false-positive rates

Data such as those in Table 2 are insufficient to assess the value of a screening programme. It is necessary to estimate the detection rate and the false-positive rate associated with a specific cut-off value of aortic diameter. This requires knowledge of the distribution of aortic diameter in subjects with (affected) and without (unaffected) a ruptured aortic aneurysm.

In affected subjects, estimates of the distribution of maximum aortic diameter in cases of ruptured aortic aneurysm are available from two sources – patients presenting for emergency surgery for acute rupture (measuring aortic diameter with callipers), and studies reporting the distribution from measurements taken at autopsy in patients who died of acute rupture. Data are available from three surgical studies and two autopsy studies; their results (similar in the two types of study) have been summarised[2] (the average aortic diameter at rupture is about 8.5 cm). From this distribution, it is simple to calculate the cumulative distribution of the percentage of affected subjects with aortic diameter greater than or equal to specified values. This is shown in Table 5 as the detection rate.

The distribution of maximum aortic diameter in unaffected subjects can be determined from ultrasound surveys in men of similar age distribution to that of the affected subjects in the studies used to determine the detection rate[2]. From this, the percentage of unaffected subjects with aortic diameter greater than or equal to specified values is shown in Table 5 as the false-positive rate. The distributions of aortic diameter may underestimate (by 2–3 mm) the true measurement in both affected and the unaffected individuals – in the affected because the measurements were made at zero blood pressure when aneurysms collapse slightly[8], and in the unaffected because measurements on ultrasound are slightly lower than on computed tomography or at operation[23,24]. The estimates of detection rate and false positive rate are based on the difference between the two distributions, so the similar measurement error in both will not affect the estimate of screening performance.

Table 5 shows that, given a policy of offering surgery to all men with aortic aneurysms of diameter of 6 cm or greater, about 86% of all men who would rupture an aortic aneurysm could be identified and offered surgery (detection rate 86%). Only 0.6% of the men who would not have ruptured an aortic aneurysm would be offered surgery (false-positive rate 0.6%). The ratio of the two, 143, is the likelihood ratio – that is, the 'concentrating power' of the screening test or the risk in screen positive men relative to that in the general population. Multiplying this likelihood ratio by the mortality rate provides an estimate of the risk of rupture over the next year in screen positive men. This is 18% – remarkably close to the estimate of 17% from prospective

Table 5 Estimated screening parameters, and risk of rupture calculated from them[2]

Diameter of 'screen-positive' aorta (cm)	Detection rate* (i)	False positive rate† (ii)	Likelihood ratio (i)/(ii)	Risk of rupture in 1 year‡
≥ 3.0	100%	7.4%	14	1.7%
≥ 4.0	100%	2.7%	37	4.6%
≥ 5.0	97%	1.1%	88	11%
≥ 6.0	86%	0.6%	143	18%
≥ 7.0	68%	0.2%	340	42%

*Proportion of all subjects with a ruptured abdominal aortic aneurysm who are identified by the cut-off.
†Proportion of all subjects without a ruptured abdominal aortic aneurysms who are identified by the cut-off.
‡From the likelihood ratio multiplied by the annual mortality in men aged 65–79 years, increased to take account that 16% of ruptures are not fatal (Table 3).

studies shown in Table 2. There is uncertainty, however, about the relative value of intervention when aortic diameter is in the range 5.0–5.9 cm.

The most rational screening policy, therefore, would use a conservative intervention policy initially – say aortic diameter ≥ 6.0 cm (this may later be revised). The risk of rupture is about 17% in the next year or 50% in the next three years – an order of magnitude greater than the peri-operative mortality after elective surgery of about 5%[5,21,28]. The prevalence of large aneurysms increases with age, but no major influence of age on the risk of rupture for a given aortic diameter is recognised. A randomised trial has confirmed fewer deaths from, or emergency operations for, ruptured aortic aneurysm in 3205 men offered screening than in 3228 men not offered screening (9 *versus* 20; $P = 0.06$)[29]. In women, the number of events was too small to allow a conclusion (3 *versus* 2). The trial confirms net benefit from early detection in men, but trials necessarily underestimate the size of the benefit. Events in those who declined the screening test must be included in the intention-to-treat analysis. Also, deaths from acute rupture may have been undernumerated in the unscreened group if sudden or unattended deaths were wrongly ascribed to heart disease or other causes; this will not have occurred in the screened group as the presence of an aneurysm was known.

Screening policy

A national screening programme should be established. It could save 2000 lives per year (from the number of deaths in England and Wales in men aged 60–79 years; Table 1) if the detection rate was 86% (Table 5) and 75% of all men accepted screening (Table 4)). Screening might commence at age 60 years and be repeated at age 70 years; alternatively, the number of deaths prevented by scanning each man only once may not be much fewer[27]. Invitations to attend for an ultrasound scan would be sent to men using a population age-sex register. Those with aortic diameter ≥ 3 cm would be scanned again at appropriate intervals. There is uncertainty over where to set the cut-off value of aortic diameter for surgery, but this is not a reason to defer the initiation of screening. Screening can be introduced using a high cut-off (6.0 cm) which could be lowered later in the light of data generated by the screening programme and other studies. The co-ordinators of the screening programme would be notified of all deaths and emergency hospital admissions due to ruptured aortic aneurysm so that risk in men with smaller aneurysms could be determined. The appropriate intervals at which aortic diameter should be remeasured in men with small aneurysms is also not known: there are sufficient data to estimate **average** rate of expansion but insufficient to estimate the **fastest** rate (say, the 95th centile). This too is not a reason to defer screening; frequent (say 6–12 monthly) ultrasound examinations would be performed until sufficient data were obtained, and then the interval between examinations would be lengthened. Detecting men with smaller aneurysms may also be worthwhile in itself. Patients should be encouraged to stop smoking as this slows the rate of expansion[31]. Treatment with beta-blockers also slows expansion[32,33], but it is uncertain whether the benefit justifies the cost and side effects of treatment.

There is concern that screening for abdominal aortic aneurysm may not be worthwhile because of the associated risk of atherosclerotic disease: even after successful elective surgery, susceptibility to heart disease, stroke and other circulatory diseases must shorten life expectancy. This excess risk has been quantified: life expectancy is reduced by only 2 years[2]. The average number of years of life lost by men who die from ruptured abdominal aortic aneurysms between the ages of 60 and 79 years is 9.1 years; the population average life expectancy in the same age range in England and Wales is 11 years[2].

Screening to prevent deaths in people over 60 years of age may be perceived as not worthwhile. Routine invitations for breast and cervical screening are discontinued at age 65 years in Britain; it would be inconsistent to terminate two screening programmes at an age when another is commenced. Resolving the issue by value judgements on the quality of life at different ages is invidious; the pragmatic solution is to allow individuals themselves to decide whether the quality of their life justifies a screening test which may extend it. The high uptake of invitations for abdominal aneurysm screening (about 75%, Table 4) confirms that most older people judge that it is.

Financial costs

Some studies have indicated that the costs associated with screening for abdominal aortic aneurysm are prohibitively high. These high costs have been based largely on inappropriate calculations – screening younger men (in whom the death rate is too low to warrant screening), using a lower cut-off of aortic diameter (and thereby a high false-positive rate), screening that included physical examination by a doctor (which is expensive and adds nothing to the ultrasound measurement), or using American data with relatively high health care costs. Based on British costs of screening and of elective surgery in 1994, and taking into account the savings on hospital resuscitation and emergency surgery for acute aneurysms prevented, the cost per life saved was an estimated £6787, or £746 per year of life saved[2].

Endovascular prostheses

Use of an endovascular prosthesis (inserted through the femoral artery) has potential advantages over open abdominal surgery[22,34–36], including lower peri-operative mortality and morbidity and lower cost. The procedure might permit a less conservative policy on surgery, though at present the proportion of patients in whom conversion to an open abdominal procedure is necessary is too high for this to be considered. The ultimate success of the procedure remains to be determined.

Conclusions

A national screening programme for abdominal aortic aneurysms should commence for men over 60 years of age. The benefits outweigh the costs and 2000 deaths in men in England and Wales could be prevented each year. Life expectancy after surgery in these patients is equivalent to that of an average man 2 years younger.

References

1   Office for National Statistics. *Mortality Statistics, cause: England and Wales 1996*. London: The Stationery Office, 1998
2   Law MR, Morris J, Wald NJ. Screening for abdominal aortic aneurysms. *J Med Screen* 1994; **1**: 110–5
3   Klippel AP, Butcher HR. The unoperated abdominal aortic aneurysm. *Am J Surg* 1966; **111**: 629–31

4   Foster JH, Bolasny BL, Gobbel WG, Scott HW. Comparative study of elective resection and expectant treatment of abdominal aortic aneurysm. *Surg Gynecol Obstet* 1969; **129**: 1–9

5   Bernstein EF, Chan EL. Abdominal aortic aneurysm in high-risk patients. *Ann Surg* 1984; **200**: 255–63

6   Kremer H, Weigold B, Dobrinski W, Schreiber MA, Zöllner N. Sonographische Verlaufsbeobachtungen von Bauchaortenaneurysmen. *Klin Wochenschr* 1984; **62**: 1120–5

7   Delin A, Ohlsen H, Swedenborg J. Growth rate of abdominal aortic aneurysms as measured by computed tomography. *Br J Surg* 1985; **72**: 530–2

8   Nevitt MP, Ballard DJ, Hallett JW. Prognosis of abdominal aortic aneurysms. *N Engl J Med* 1989; **321**: 1009–14

9   Collin J, Heather B, Walton J. Growth rates of subclinical abdominal aortic aneurysms – implications for review and rescreening programmes. *Eur J Vasc Surg* 1991; **5**: 141–4

10   Guirguis EM, Barber GG. The natural history of abdominal aortic aneurysms. *Am J Surg* 1991; **162**: 481–3

11   Bengtsson H, Bergqvist D, Ekberg O, Janzon L. A population based screening of abdominal aortic aneurysms. *Eur J Vasc Surg* 1991; **5**: 53–7

12   Scott RAP, Wilson NM, Ashton HA, Kay DN. Is surgery necessary for abdominal aortic aneurysm less than 6 cm in diameter? *Lancet* 1993; **342**: 1395–6

13   Lucarotti M, Shaw E, Poskitt K, Heather B. The Gloucestershire Aneurysm Screening Programme: the first 2 years' experience. *Eur J Vasc Surg* 1993; **7**: 397–401

14   Smith FCT, Grimshaw GM, Paterson IS, Shearman CP, Hamer JD. Ultrasonographic screening for abdominal aortic aneurysm in an urban community. *Br J Surg* 1993; **80**: 1406–9

15   Bengtsson H, Bergqvist D. Ruptured abdominal aortic aneurysm: a population-based study. *J Vasc Surg* 1993; **18**: 74–80

16   Reed D, Reed C, Stemmermann G, Hayashi T. Are aortic aneurysms caused by atherosclerosis? *Circulation* 1992; **85**: 205–11

17   Strachan DP. Predictors of death from aortic aneurysm among middle-aged men: the Whitehall study. *Br J Surg* 1991; **78**: 401–4

18   Grimshaw GM, Thompson JM, Hamer JD. Prevalence of abdominal aortic aneurysm associated with hypertension in an urban population. *J Med Screen* 1994; **1**: 226–8

19   Doll R, Peto R, Wheatley K, Gray R, Sutherland I. Mortality in relation to smoking: 40 years' observations on male British doctors. *BMJ* 1994; **309**: 901–11

20   Fowkes FGR, Macintyre CCA, Ruckley CV. Increasing incidence of aortic aneurysms in England and Wales. *BMJ* 1989; **298**: 33–5

21   Ernst CB. Abdominal aortic aneurysm. *N Engl J Med* 1993; **328**: 1167–72

22   Harris PL. Reducing the mortality from abdominal aortic aneurysms: need for a national screening programme. *BMJ* 1992; **305**: 697–9

23   Lederle FA, Wilson SE, Johnson GR *et al*. Variability in measurement of abdominal aortic aneurysms. *J Vasc Surg* 1995; **21**: 945–52

24   McGregor JC, Pollock JG, Anton HC. The value of ultrasonography in the diagnosis of abdominal aortic aneurysm. *Scot Med J* 1975; **20**: 133–7

25   Collin J, Araujo L, Walton J, Lindsell D. Oxford screening programme for abdominal aortic aneurysms in men aged 65 to 74 years. *Lancet* 1988; **2**: 613–5

26   Holdsworth JD. Screening for abdominal aortic aneurysm in Northumberland. *Br J Surg* 1994; **81**: 710–2

27   Khoo DE, Ashton H, Scott RAP. Is screening once at age 65 an effective method for detection of abdominal aortic aneurysms? *J Med Screen* 1994; **1**: 223–5

28   Akkersdijk GJM, van der Graaf Y, van Bockel JH, de Vries AC, Eikelboom BC. Mortality rates associated with operative treatment of infrarenal abdominal aortic aneurysm in The Netherlands. *Br J Surg* 1994; **81**: 706–9

29   Scott RAP, Wilson NM, Ashton HA, Kay DN. Influence of screening on the incidence of ruptured abdominal aortic aneurysm: 5-year results of a randomized controlled study. *Br J Surg* 1995; **82**: 1066–70

30 Mutirangura P, Stonebridge PA, Clason AE *et al*. Ten-year review of non-ruptured aortic aneurysms. *Br J Surg* 1989; **76**: 1251–4

31 MacSweeney STR, Ellis M, Worrell PC, Greenhalgh RM, Powell JT. Smoking and growth rate of small abdominal aortic aneurysms. *Lancet* 1994; **344**: 651-2

32 Gadowski GR, Pilcher DB, Ricci MA. Abdominal aortic aneurysm expansion rate: effect of size and beta-adrenergic blockade. *J Vasc Surg* 1994; **19**: 727–31

33 Leach SD, Toole AL, Stern H, DeNatale RW, Tilson D. Effect of β-adrenergic blockade on the growth rate of abdominal aortic aneurysms. *Arch Surg* 1988; **123**: 606–9

34 Marin ML, Veith FJ. Transfemoral repair of abdominal aortic aneurysm. *N Engl J Med* 1994; **331**: 26

35 Paaski WP, Laustsen J. Early results of 132 aortic-iliac arterial reconstructions with the new stretch ePTFE vascular prosthesis. *Int Angiol* 1994; **13**: 296–9

36 Chiesa R, Melissano G, Castellano R *et al*. A new ePTFE stretch graft for aorto-iliac reconstructions. Surgical evaluation and one year follow-up with magnetic resonance imaging. *J Cardiovasc Surg* 1995; **36**: 134–41

Is screening for osteoporosis worthwhile?

Karen Walker-Bone, David M Reid* and Cyrus Cooper

*MRC Environmental Epidemiology Unit, Southampton General Hospital, Southampton, UK and *Department of Medicine and Therapeutics, Medical School Buildings, Aberdeen, UK*

Osteoporosis is a common condition, which is recognised by the occurrence of fragility fractures and leads to considerable mortality and morbidity with huge financial implications world-wide. Based on predicted demographic changes, the implications of this disease are set to increasingly affect the healthcare budgets of all nations.

The determinants of fracture are skeletal factors, such as peak bone mass, the rate of bone loss and extra-skeletal factors, which include trauma and the response to that trauma. Some of these factors are genetically determined, but several have environmental origins, which could, theoretically, be manipulated.

There are two potential means whereby osteoporotic fractures might be prevented. Measures could be targeted at the entire population, with the aim of shifting the distribution of bone mass in a beneficial direction, through modifying the behaviour of all individuals. The alternative is a high risk approach, whereby intervention is targeted only at those considered to have the greatest risk of future fracture. Mass bone density screening falls into the second approach. Bone density is a good predictor of future fracture risk, and cost-effectiveness analyses of the high risk approach suggest economic benefits of policies targeting pharmacological treatment to those individuals at highest risk.

However, there are important concerns about the levels of compliance achievable with such therapeutic interventions, the balance of risks and benefits for some of these interventions (for example, hormone replacement therapy), and the outcome when treatment is discontinued. On current evidence, it is certainly not appropriate to target hormone replacement therapy for women at the menopause on the basis of a bone density screening programme. However, newer bone-specific agents are being developed which might be administered at later ages, closer to the time when fracture incidence rates rise steeply. Bone densitometry has been shown to predict fractures even in the elderly, and high risk strategies for the targeting of such agents (for example, the bisphosphonates or selective oestrogen receptor modulators) will remain important research issues for the future.

Correspondence to: Prof. C. Cooper, MRC Environmental Epidemiology Unit, Southampton General Hospital, Southampton SO16 6YD, UK

Osteoporosis is defined as[1]: 'a systemic skeletal disorder characterised by low bone mass and micro-architectural deterioration of bone tissue, with a consequent increase in bone fragility and susceptibility to fracture'. Clinically, osteoporosis is recognised by the occurrence of characteristic fragility fractures. These fractures share the following features: incidence rates which are greater in women; rates which rise steeply with age; and occurrence predominantly at sites with high trabecular bone content[2]. The most important sites for these fractures are the hip, distal forearm and spine. Osteoporotic fractures result in pain, disability and death and have profound socio-economic implications for all healthcare providers, particularly those who serve an ageing population.

The burden of fracture

Frequency of fragility fractures

In the UK, it is estimated that approximately 60,000 hip, 50,000 wrist and 40,000 clinically diagnosed vertebral fractures occur each year as a consequence of osteoporosis[3]. Beyond 50 years, the remaining lifetime risk of an osteoporotic fracture for a British white woman has been estimated at 14% for the hip, 11% for the spine and 13% for the radius[4,5]. These figures are estimated to be 25% higher in the US (17.5%, 15.6% and 16%, respectively), giving an overall remaining lifetime risk for a 50 year old woman in the US approximating to 40% in white women for any fragility fracture[6]. Fracture incidence is lower in men: the lifetime risk of hip fracture at age 50 years is 6%, of vertebral fracture 5% and of wrist fracture 2.5%, giving an overall remaining lifetime risk of 13% in white men for any fragility fracture[6]. However, fragility fractures occur at sites other than the spine, hip and distal forearm, and, if these were also included, the lifetime risk might be as high as 70% for an American woman aged 50 years[7].

Mortality associated with fragility fractures

A survey of men and women after osteoporotic fractures in Rochester, MN, USA, demonstrated no adverse effect on mortality after Colles' fractures, but the survival rate 5 years after hip and vertebral fractures was only 80% of that expected for age-matched individuals without fracture[8].

Hip fractures are the most serious of all fragility fractures, and are associated with an overall reduction in survival of 10–20%[9], with most of the excess deaths occurring in the first 6 months. These mortality rates differ, however, by age and sex, with older, male patients having the lowest survival. Mortality is also greater in patients with poorer function prefracture or with co-existent diseases. Postoperative confusion and co-existing disease are both independent predictors of an increased risk of death after hip fracture, suggesting that the high mortality results from an interaction between acute trauma and comorbid pathology[10].

Population-based data have shown that osteoporotic vertebral fractures also carry an excess mortality which increases progressively after a fracture has been diagnosed[8]. This is more pronounced if the fracture is secondary to mild or moderate, rather than severe, trauma and is more apparent in men than in women. However, only 8% of the excess deaths are directly attributable to the fracture itself. It appears that the clinical presentation of a vertebral fracture is associated with underlying poor health, because the observed survival curve in these patients diverges from the expected curve with time after the point of diagnosis.

Morbidity associated with fragility fractures

It is difficult to quantify precisely the morbidity caused by osteoporotic fractures, because both the prevalence of disability and osteoporosis correlate strongly with age. It has been estimated that osteoporotic fractures of the hip, distal forearm and spine cause 7.6% of women to become dependent in activities of daily living and another 7.8% to require nursing home care for an average of 7.6 years. Overall, a 50 year old white American woman will have a 13% chance of having functional impairment after any type of fragility fracture[11].

Most of the morbidity is caused by hip fractures, which lead to hospitalisation. Many hip fracture patients (20%) cannot walk independently prefracture, making them a group at high risk of acute complications, but the most significant long-term disability is further impairment of mobility. Up to one-third of hip fracture patients may become totally dependent and require long-term institutionalisation. Inevitably, the long-term morbidity is skewed towards the older age range, such that 55% of the patients over 90 years were discharged to nursing homes in the US in 1990[12]. One year after a hip fracture, 40% of people could not walk independently, 60% required assistance with at least one essential activity of daily living, and 80% could not perform at least one other activity of daily living, such as shopping[7].

The morbidity attributable to vertebral fracture is more difficult to quantify, since the presentation of these fractures is frequently subclinical. The clinical outcomes of vertebral fractures are back pain, kyphosis and loss of height[13]. An acute compression fracture of the spine typically causes considerable local pain and tenderness, which gradually settles over weeks or months. However, a more chronic pattern is observed in some patients, lasting up to 6 months. This leads to adverse effects on physical function, self-esteem and increased depressive illness. The pain and loss of confidence caused by the fracture leads to reduced physical exercise, with an inevitable exacerbation of osteoporosis and further increased risk of fracture[14]. The European Vertebral Osteoporosis Study, which is a large population-based study of vertebral fractures, also showed that the presence of radiographically evident vertebral fracture was associated with a 40–70% increase in risk of limb fractures[15].

Distal forearm fractures rarely require hospital admission, except in the older age groups, but they account for 400,000 hospital outpatient consultations in the US each year[16]. Wrist fractures do, however, carry a high morbidity, with only 50% reporting a good functional recovery at 6 months[17].

Costs of fragility fractures

It is difficult to estimate the financial burden of osteoporosis, because the costs are incurred at many different levels of healthcare. Minor fractures are dealt with in an outpatient or primary care setting, whilst more serious fractures necessitate acute hospital assessment and treatment. Furthermore, the long-term disability caused by fractures has financial implications in terms of institutionalisation and burdens on informal carers. It is particularly difficult to estimate the cost in this last group. Cost estimates are also confounded by the fact that it is difficult to dissociate those fractures caused by osteoporosis from those which would have occurred without osteoporosis.

Despite these difficulties, the total costs of osteoporotic fracture in England and Wales in 1994 were estimated to be £742 million. Of this total, £237 million was accounted for by acute inpatient services[18], the majority of which were incurred through hip fractures. For example, in England and Wales in 1985, 3,500 beds were used daily, with an average length of stay of 30 days. The estimate for 1998 has risen to £942 million. The costs in the US may be as high as $20 billion annually, with hip fractures accounting for one-third of this total[19].

The pathophysiology of fracture

There are two ultimate determinants of osteoporotic fracture: bone strength and propensity to trauma. Bone mineral density is a key correlate of bone strength, but other characteristics of the skeleton (geometry and architecture) may contribute to strength independently of bone density. The bone density of an adult in later life is dependent upon the peak bone mass gained during growth and its subsequent loss rate.

Peak bone mass

Skeletal mass increases progressively during growth with an accelerated phase at the time of the prepubertal growth spurt[20]. The determinants of peak bone mass are not completely understood. Twin studies confirm a genetic influence[21], but the genotype of an individual interacts with several environmental influences during intra-uterine life, infancy and childhood. The importance of prenatal and infant environment is supported by observations that weight in infancy predicts adult skeletal size and bone mineral content[22-25]. These environmental influences are thought to programme endocrine and metabolic systems during critical periods of early life, thereby establishing the skeletal growth trajectory. During later childhood, lifestyle factors such as calcium nutrition and physical activity are also important[26,27]. Finally, skeletal development is closely linked with normal sexual maturation from the prepubertal growth spurt onwards. Primary or secondary amenorrhoea from any cause may be associated with reduced peak bone mass.

Determinants of bone loss

Bone loss commences during the fourth decade of life in both men and women. Although cross-sectional studies suggested an accelerated phase of bone loss among women during the decade following the menopause, prospective studies suggest a more linear progression of bone loss in both sexes (around 1% each year), which continues throughout life[28-30]. Non-hormonal factors which influence bone loss include thin body build, cigarette smoking, heavy alcohol consumption, poor dietary calcium and vitamin D intake, and physical inactivity. In addition, several diseases and medications (most notably corticosteroids) are also associated with accelerated bone loss.

Propensity to trauma

Falls are a common occurrence in elderly individuals. The prevalence of falls is greater among women than men at all ages above 65 years. Around 6% of falls culminate in a limb fracture and 1% in a hip fracture, among elderly women. Comparisons between elderly fallers who fracture and those who do not, suggest that the nature of the fall is an important risk factor. Elderly people who suffer a direct injury to the greater trochanter of the hip have a marked increase in risk of hip fracture, while those falling onto the outstretched arm have a marked increase in the risk of wrist fracture. The risk factors for falls include a host of intrinsic and extrinsic problems. Chronic illness, impaired mental function, defective vision or hearing acuity, chronic disease, and use of sedative/hypnotic agents are all important intrinsic risk factors. Poor lighting and environmental hazards around the home are important extrinsic risk factors. Although trauma modification is an attractive means of preventing hip fractures, strategies to reduce the risk of falling among the institutionalised elderly, even when intensive, have not yielded large reductions in the incidence of falls and have not shown a commensurate reduction in the rate of fracture. The use of devices which modify the effects of low trauma to the hip appears a more promising avenue. Small controlled trials of protective hip pads which may be fitted into the undergarments of elderly people have reported reductions in hip fracture among subjects who are compliant.

Strategies to prevent osteoporotic fracture

Two approaches may be adopted in the prevention of osteoporotic fractures in the community: the population strategy and the high-risk strategy[31].

Population strategy

An example of the population strategy would be to move the entire population bone density distribution in a beneficial direction. It is often argued that lifestyle modification, for example avoidance of tobacco and heavy alcohol consumption; maintenance of weight-bearing physical activity; and encouragement of a high dietary calcium intake, might reduce the overall incidence of fracture in the general population.

A recent meta-analysis examined the relationship between cigarette smoking, bone mineral density and the risk of hip fracture[32]. Postmenopausal bone loss was greater in current smokers than non-smokers, and was associated with an increased risk of hip fracture beyond the age of 50 years. The relative risk of fracture increased with the number of cigarettes smoked and with age, and risk seemed to be lower in former smokers than current smokers. This evidence implies that a large anti-smoking campaign might reduce hip fractures, above the general health benefits to the population. Cost-effectiveness data are required to support such an approach, as well as supporting evidence to suggest that it would be effective.

Similarly, epidemiological data consistently suggest a link between physical inactivity and fracture, most notably hip fracture[33]. Most of the data come from case-control studies, with a small proportion from follow-up studies. The current evidence points to a protective effect of physical activity against hip fracture in a strong and consistent association, which may well be dose-related. However, these data have not clarified what type of activity is most beneficial. It seems that weight-bearing activity increases bone mineral density but low intensity activity also prevents fractures, perhaps by improving co-ordination and balance, and, thereby, reducing falls. At the present time, there are no large case-controlled studies, using fractures as the outcome, which can demonstrate the efficacy of any type of physical activity programme, such that a large population-based strategy could be advocated.

An increased calcium intake has been proposed as one population-based strategy for the prevention of fractures. The evidence for this has been recently reviewed[34]. Whilst there have been several studies, few have been randomised trials with fracture as the endpoint. It is encouraging that the small number of such trials which have been performed with calcium supplementation have shown a reduction in fracture risk, but these studies were not all directly comparable, and the largest also involved vitamin D supplementation[35], leaving no clear conclusion as to the effect of calcium alone. There have not been any randomised trials of dietary calcium and fracture risk and the observational and case-control data are inconsistent, although meta-analysis suggests a reduction in hip fractures, and possibly fractures at other sites. Thus, the current evidence is promising that a policy of improved calcium intake may prove to be effective, but there are still questions to be answered in a randomised controlled setting before such a programme could be extrapolated to a population-based strategy.

The current evidence to support a population-based approach to the prevention of osteoporosis is far from conclusive in view of the lack of large controlled studies with fractures as an outcome, demonstrating the effectiveness of lifestyle modifications. Until such evidence is available, it seems sensible to broadly recommend safe lifestyles, but the confidence that these will achieve a real reduction in the fracture burden remains limited[36].

The high-risk strategy

This approach involves an assessment of an individual's future fracture risk, with an intervention targeted at those at greatest risk. Among the various possible means of assessing future fracture risk, bone densitometry has been the most exhaustively studied. Initial observations that bone density measurements predicted future fractures led to an enthusiastic call for widespread bone density measurement to target hormone replacement therapy at the time of the menopause.

Evaluation of a bone density screening programme requires consideration of: (i) the characteristics of the disease; (ii) the characteristics of the test; (iii) the intervention; and (iv) the programme. These aspects of bone density screening will be discussed with particular reference to the targeting of hormone replacement therapy at the menopause. When taken together, the evidence argues strongly that such a strategy would not be appropriate. However, recent innovations in the prevention of bone loss using other pharmacological agents will lead to a re-appraisal of the high risk strategy in different guises. These newer developments will be highlighted in the conclusion.

Evaluation of screening for osteoporosis

The disease

Screening for any disease cannot be justified simply on the basis that more individuals will be diagnosed at an earlier time. It is an essential requirement that the natural history of the disease in question is well-characterised, with evidence that earlier interventions will successfully alter the long-term prognosis. Osteoporosis fulfils these criteria, as described above. There is now unequivocal evidence that fractures can be prevented by several different interventions[37]. Osteoporosis is an important public health problem, and predictions based on future demographic changes suggest that the costs are likely to increase. One model suggests that there may be 6.26 million hip fractures world-wide per annum by the year 2050[38]. The costs of a population screening programme may well be justifiable, offset against the financial burden which these fractures are likely to cause, but there are not yet sufficient data to support this approach.

The test

Bone mineral measurement is currently the primary tool used to identify women at high risk of osteoporosis and fracture. Several different techniques have been developed for the assessment of bone mineral density[39]. Dual energy X-ray absorptiometry is widely used because of its ability to assess bone mass at both axial and appendicular sites, its high reproducibility, and the very low doses of radiation associated with measurement (less than the daily natural background levels). Recently, devices have been developed which perform dual X-ray measurements exclusively at appendicular sites such as the forearm; these are portable and relatively inexpensive. Quantitative computed tomography enables differential measurement of cortical and cancellous bone in the spine or peripheral skeleton, but the equipment required is expensive and the radiation dose relatively high. Finally, ultrasound velocity and attenuation at the os calcis, tibia or patella may also be used to predict future fractures. Ultrasound devices are radiation free and, like the absorptiometric instruments which measure appendicular sites, the machines are portable and relatively cheap. To date, evidence supports the use of ultrasound techniques for the assessment of fracture risk in elderly women but there is currently insufficient knowledge of reference ranges, a lack of data in younger women and men, and limited standardisation of calibration, for which reasons, its use in the diagnosis and monitoring of osteoporosis is not yet clear[40].

Several limitations of absorptiometric techniques should be recognised. First, the absolute bone mineral density for a given bone mass varies with different systems, and there are also differences in reference data provided by the manufacturers, so that the same measured value may lie within different parts of the reference range depending on the system used. Second, measurement of bone mineral density in the spine may be affected by the presence of extraskeletal calcification, osteophytes, scoliosis and vertebral deformity[41]. Third, the distribution of osteoporosis within the spine may be heterogeneous, with differential involvement of the dorsal spine. Finally, osteomalacia also results in low bone mineral density measured by absorptiometric techniques.

Despite these limitations, bone densitometry is our best available predictor of future fracture risk[42] and a recent meta-analysis suggests a 2.6-fold increase in the risk of hip fracture for each standard deviation drop in bone density at the femoral neck[43]. The strength of this relationship is similar to that between blood pressure and stroke, and is substantially greater than that between serum cholesterol and myocardial infarction, particularly if the site of biological interest is being measured. If one assumes a relative risk increase of 2.5 for each SD drop in bone density and a threshold for the definition of high risk at the 30th centile, estimates suggest a sensitivity of 74% and a specificity of 80% for the prediction of lifetime fracture risk[44]. There are few data on the acceptability of bone densitometry in the context of a screening programme. One study achieved uptake rates of 54–75%, depending on the way in which patients were contacted[45]. People who did not take up the offer gave reasons such as inconvenience and fear of irradiation.

The extent to which risk factor profiles, ultrasonic assessments of bone, and biochemical markers of bone turnover might improve the predictive capacity of bone densitometry, remains uncertain. In epidemiological studies, these additional investigations have been shown to predict fracture independently of bone density. However, clear algorithms for their use and the establishment of decision thresholds for intervention remain major obstacles to their utilisation. The single most useful historical risk factor is the presence of a previous fragility fracture. In a recent population-based randomised controlled trial of a new bisphosphonate (alendronate), women selected on the basis of low bone density and a prevalent vertebral deformity, were randomised to receive alendronate or placebo[46]. Over a 3 year period, there was an approximately 50% reduction in the incidence of new vertebral, hip and all limb fractures in the alendronate treated women. However, the recruits to the study were healthy volunteers, and only comprised a small proportion of all potential subjects. Translation of these findings to a screening programme for prevalent vertebral deformities would require the evaluation of compliance with such radiographic measurements on a large scale in the general population.

The intervention

Clinical trials have demonstrated that postmenopausal hormone replacement therapy effectively prevents bone loss. However, only two controlled trials have studied the effect of hormone replacement on the incidence of osteoporotic fractures[47]. Most of the evidence for fracture prevention arises from case-control and cohort studies, which are limited by their susceptibility to selection bias. A synthesis of epidemiological information suggests that the long-term use of hormone replacement therapy has major extraskeletal effects. In terms of benefit, cardiovascular disease incidence rates will be reduced in addition to the benefits stemming from fracture reduction. Important risks are associated, most notably that of breast cancer[48]. Given this complex balance of risks and benefits, it does not seem sensible to target hormone replacement therapy simply on the basis of bone density measurement. Furthermore, compliance with long-term oestrogen use is known to be poor and the pattern of bone loss when such therapy is discontinued remains controversial[49]. Some studies suggest that an accelerated phase of bone loss follows cessation of therapy, with the consequence that fracture protection wears off rapidly after this time-point. Should this be the case, lifelong hormone replacement therapy would be required to have a substantial effect on fracture incidence. This would add further to the burden of non-compliance with postmenopausal oestrogens. For all these reasons, a national screening programme to target hormone replacement therapy at the time of the menopause cannot be justified.

Other interventions are now available which have been shown to retard bone loss in later life and reduce fracture rates. The most important class of compounds is the bisphosphonates (alendronate and cyclical etidronate). These agents may be used at older ages, and their cost utility is enhanced as a consequence[50]. The inclusion of these agents into high risk strategies to prevent fracture forms the basis of several current randomised controlled trials, for example the Fracture Intervention Trials[46].

The programme

At present, no screening programme for osteoporosis has been validated by randomised controlled trials. The availability of bone densitometry is patchy throughout the country, the reference ranges against which measurements in individuals are compared have not been widely agreed, and no policy of treatment is established.

Conclusions

This review has demonstrated that screening for osteoporosis is not justified at the present time. However, several developments might lead to a re-appraisal of screening programmes in this disease area. It is now clear that bone loss continues even beyond the age of 80 years and that therapeutic interventions can have a positive impact on bone mass and fracture risk at these ages. Bone densitometry continues to predict future fracture with comparable sensitivity and specificity at age 75 years as at age 65 years. The incidence of fractures in the general population rises steeply between 65 and 75 years. Compliance with therapy is likely to be greater among those whose baseline fracture incidence is highest. Therapeutic agents are now available which act on the skeleton to reduce bone loss and fracture incidence and these have been demonstrated to be effective in later life (age 65–80 years). The identification through screening of late postmenopausal and elderly women for the targeting of effective antiresorptive agents (for example, the bisphosphonates and selective oestrogen receptor modulators) provides a potentially cost-effective strategy against osteoporotic fracture. Over the next decade, further evaluation of such strategies will provide a sounder evidence base for policy makers who have to choose between competing health demands with ever scarcer resources.

References

1   Consensus development conference: diagnosis, prophylaxis and treatment of osteoporosis. *Am J Med* 1993; **94**: 646–50

2   Cooper C, Melton LJ III. Magnitude and impact of osteoporosis and fractures. In: Marcus R, Felman D, Kelsey J. (eds)*Osteoporosis*. San Diego: Academic Press, 1996; 419–34

3   Cooper C. Epidemiology and public health impact of osteoporosis. *Clin Rheumatol* 1993; **7**: 459–77

4   Donaldson LJ, Cook A, Thompson RG. Incidence of fractures in a geographically defined population. *J Epidemiol Community Health* 1990; **44**: 241–5

5   Cooper C, Melton LJ III. Vertebral fractures. How large is the silent epidemic? *BMJ* 1992; **304**: 793–4

6   Melton LJ III, Chrischilles EA, Cooper C, Lane AW, Riggs BL. Perspective. How many women have osteoporosis? *J Bone Miner Res* 1992; **7**: 1005–10

7   Cooper C. The crippling consequences of fractures and their impact on quality of life. *Am J Med* 1997; **103**: 12S–19S

8   Cooper C, Atkinson EJ, Jacobsen SJ *et al*. Population-based study of survival after osteoporotic fractures. *Am J Epidemiol* 1993; **137**: 1001–5

9   Melton LJ III, Epidemiology of fractures. In: Riggs BL, Melton LJ III. (eds) *Osteoporosis: Etiology, Diagnosis and Management*. New York: Raven Press, 1988; 133–54

10   Poor G, Atkinson EJ, O'Fallon WM, Melton LJ III. Determinants of reduced survival following hip fractures in men. *Clin Orthop* 1995; **319**: 260–5

11   Chrischilles EA, Butler CD, Davis CS, Wallace RB. A model of lifetime osteoporosis impact. *Arch Intern Med* 1991; **151**: 2026–32

12   Office of Technology Assessment, Congress of the United States. Hip fracture outcomes in people aged 50 and over: mortality, service use, expenditures, and long-term functional impairment. Washington DC, 1993. In: US Department of Commerce publication NTIS PB94107653

13   Ettinger B, Black DM, Nevitt MC *et al*. Contribution of vertebral deformities to chronic back pain and disability. *J Bone Miner Res* 1992; **7**: 449–56

14   Ross PD, Ettinger B, Davis JW, Melton LJ III, Wasnich RD. Evaluation of adverse health outcomes associated with vertebral fractures. *Osteoporos Int* 1991: **1**; 134–40

15   Cooper C, O'Neill TW, Egger P *et al*. Vertebral deformities: clinical impact and relation to fractures at other sites [Abstract]. *J Bone Miner Res* 1995; **10**: S145

16   Holbrook TL, Grazier K, Kelsey JL, Stauffer RN. Frequency of occurrence, impact and cost of selected musculoskeletal conditions in the United States. *American Academy of Orthopaedic Surgeons, Chicago*, 1984

17   Kaukonen JP, Karaharju EO, Porras M, Luthje P, Jakobssen A. Functional recovery after fractures of the distal forearm. *Ann Chir Gynaecol* 1988; **77**: 27–31

18   Department of Health Advisory Group on Osteoporosis. Chairman D. Barlow. November 1994: 34

19   Praemer A, Furner S, Rice DP, Musculoskeletal conditions in the United States. *American Academy of Orthopaedic Surgeons Park Ridge*, 1992

20   Bonjour JP, Theintz G, Buchs B, Losamn D, Rizzoli R. Critical years and stages of puberty for bone and femoral bone mass accumulation during adolescence. *J Endocrinol Metab* 1991; **73**: 555–63

21   Ralston S. Osteoporosis. *BMJ* 1997; **315**: 469–72

22   Johnston FE. Somatic growth of the infant and pre-school child. In :Faulkner F, Tanner DIM. (eds) *Human growth: A Comprehensive Treatise, vol 2*. New York: Polonium Press, 1986; 3–24

23   Widows EM, McCance RA. The effect of finite periods of undernutrition at different stages on the composition and subsequent development of the rat. *Proc R Soc Lond B Biol Sci* 1963; **158**: 329–42

24   Cooper C, Cawley M, Bhalla A *et al*. Childhood growth, physical activity and peak bone mass in women. *J Bone Miner Res* 1995; **10**: 940–7

25   Cooper C, Fall C, Egger P, Hobbs R, Eastell R, Barker D. Growth in infancy and bone mass in later life. *Ann Rheum Dis* 1997; **56**: 17–21

26 Johnston CC, Miller JZ, Slemenda CW *et al*. Calcium supplementation and increase in the development of skeletal mass in children. *N Engl J Med* 1992; **327**: 82–7

27 Slemenda CW, Miller JZ, Hui SL *et al*. Role of physical activity in the development of skeletal mass in children. *J Bone Miner Res* 1993; **306**: 1357–8

28 Falch JA, Sandvik L. Perimenopausal appendicular bone loss: a 10-year prospective study. *Bone* 1990; **11**: 425–8

29 Aitken DIM *et al*. Osteoporosis after oophorectomy for non-malignant disease in premenopausal women. *BMJ* 1973; **ii**: 325–8

30 Richelson LS, Wahner HW, Melton LJ III, Riggs BL. Relative contributions of ageing and oestrogen deficiency to postmenopausal bone loss. *N Engl J Med* 1984; **311**: 1273–5

31 Cooper C, Melton LJ III. Epidemiology of osteoporosis. *Trends Endocrinol Metab* 1992; **3**: 224–9

32 Law M, Hackshaw A. A meta-analysis of cigarette smoking, bone mineral density and risk of hip fracture: recognition of a major effect. *BMJ* 1997; **315**: 841–6

33 Joakimsen R, Magnus J, Fonnebo V. Physical activity and predisposition for hip fractures: a review. *Osteoporos Int* 1997; **7**: 503–13

34 Cumming R, Nevitt M. Calcium for prevention of osteoporotic fractures in postmenopausal women. *J Bone Miner Res* 1997; **12**: 1321–9

35 Chapuy MC, Arlot ME, Delmas PD, Meunier PJ. Effect of calcium and cholecalciferol treatment for three years on hip fractures in elderly women. *BMJ* 1994; **308**: 1081-2

36 World Health Organization. Assessment of fracture risk and its application to screening for postmenopausal osteoporosis. *World Health Organ Tech Rep Ser* 1994; No 843

37 Reid IR. The management of osteoporosis. *Baillières Clin Endocrinol Metab* 1997; **11**: 63–81

38 Cooper C, Campion G, Melton LJ III. Hip fractures in the elderly: a worldwide projection. *Osteoporos Int* 1992; **2**: 285–9

39 Compston JE, Cooper C, Kanis JA. Bone densitometry in clinical practice. *BMJ* 1995; **310**: 1507–10

40 Gluer C. Quantitative ultrasound techniques for the assessment of osteoporosis: expert agreement on current status. *J Bone Miner Res* 1997; **12**:1280-8

41 Reid IR, Evans MC, Ames R, Wattie DJ. The influence of osteophytes and aortic calcification on spinal bone mineral density in postmenopausal women. *J Clin Endocrinol Metab* 1991; **72**: 1372–4

42 Cooper C. Femoral neck bone density and fracture risk. *Osteoporos Int* 1996; **3**(Suppl **2**): S6–8

43 Cummings SR, Black DM, Nevitt MC *et al*. Bone density at various sites for the prediction of hip fractures. *Lancet* 1993; **341**: 72–5

44 Barlow D, Cooper C, Reeve J, Reid D. Department of Health is fair to patients with osteoporosis. *BMJ* 1996; **312**: 297–8

45 Garton MJ *et al*. Recruitment methods for screening programmes: trial of a new method within a regional osteoporosis study. *BMJ* 1992; **305**: 82–4

46 Black DM, Cummings SR, Thompson D. Alendronate reduces risk of vertebral and clinical fractures in women with existing vertebral fractures: results of the fracture intervention trial. *Lancet* 1996; **348**: 1535–41

47 Compston JE. HRT and osteoporosis. *Br Med Bull* 1992; **48**: 309–44

48 Daly. Hormone replacement therapy: a cost-effective analysis. *Report for the Department of Health by the Oxford HRT study group* 1992

49 Felsen DT, Zhang Y, Hannan MT, Kiel DP, Wilson PW, Anderson JJ. The effect of postmenopausal estrogen therapy on bone density in elderly women. *N Engl J Med* 1993; **3**: 1141–6

50 Black DM. Why elderly women should be screened and treated to prevent osteoporosis. *Am J Med* 1995; **98** (Suppl 2A): 67S–75S

Screening in child health

David M B Hall and ***Sarah Stewart-Brown**

*The Children's Hospital, Sheffield, UK and *Health Services Research Unit, Institute of Health Sciences, Oxford, UK*

Screening programmes in child health have evolved on the basis of individual enthusiasm and professional consensus, rather than being based on objective evidence of benefit. Three reviews have been carried out in the UK over the past 10 years. The only programmes which show robust evidence of effectiveness are those for PKU and hypothyroidism. The value of screening for hearing loss and vision defects is widely accepted, but there are many unresolved issues. Programmes for detection of congenital dislocation of the hip, congenital heart disease and growth disturbances are of doubtful value. Early identification of developmental problems is stressed by parents, but screening may not be the best way to achieve this. The UK programme of well-child care places increasing emphasis on promotion of physical and emotional health; screening tests should either be subjected to quality monitoring, or removed from the programme if they cannot fulfil the classic criteria of Wilson and Jungner.

The routine checking of apparently healthy children is a popular activity throughout the western world, but does it offer value for money? Screening in childhood is rarely carried out in isolation; rather, it is packaged with other tasks such as immunization, advice and support in a programme commonly known in the UK as child health surveillance (CHS). Three working parties have reported on the role of CHS in the past 10 years[1] and many systematic reviews and much research have been commissioned. The evidence is not, and probably never will be, complete; nevertheless, pragmatic guidelines and decisions about screening policy have to be made. This evidence-based approach has produced a programme of preventive child care that is probably the leanest in the western world and the one with the most clearly articulated aims[2]. It remains to be shown how the benefits will compare with more intensive packages such as the Bright Futures programme in the US[3].

Four types of child health screening programme can be identified (Table 1). The screening tests with the most robust evidence of effectiveness are those for PKU and hypothyroidism. There are many other procedures for which the evidence is scanty and many have been discontinued because they did not fulfil the classic criteria and may even

Correspondence to:
Prof. David M B Hall, The Children's Hospital, Sheffield S10 2TH, UK

Table 1 Four types of screening programmes currently available

1	**Biochemical**: PKU, hypothyroidism; additional screening possible for other inherited metabolic disorders by tandem mass spectrometry; screening for cystic fibrosis, Duchenne muscular dystrophy, neuroblastoma, haemoglobinopathies, fragile-X, maternal HIV, lead intoxication.
2	**Screening involving objective measurements**: vision screening; hearing screening; blood pressure; growth monitoring – height, weight and head circumference.
3	**Screening involving physical examination procedures**: congenital dislocation of the hip; spinal defects; congenital heart disease; genitalia and undescended testes; adolescent scoliosis. It is also possible to consider the complete physical examination as a single screening entity.
4	**Screening involving an understanding of child development**: recognition of cerebral palsy and other motor disorders; speech, language and communication disorders, including autism; behavioural and emotional disorders; screening for parental mental health problems which may affect the child.

do harm, or because they were unlikely to improve on what parents could achieve by identifying problems in their children[4]. For example, vision screening in infancy has been discontinued in the UK[5], while the emphasis on developmental screening has been much reduced in the US[6] where professionals are learning to use parents' knowledge of their own children more effectively.

In this article, we will discuss hearing and vision screening, which have been the subject of much recent research and debate. Then we will briefly consider the context in which these screening programmes are offered.

Screening for hearing and vision deficits

Fifty years ago it was not uncommon for deaf, blind or partially sighted children to be misdiagnosed as mentally retarded or behaviour disordered. A screening method for hearing loss was developed by the Ewings[7] and introduced in 1957. Sheridan was the first to seek simple methods of testing for visual deficits – the STYCAR tests[5,8] (Sheridan Tests for Young Children and Retardates). The emerging concept of the critical or sensitive period in biological research suggested that early deprivation of input, via the special sense organs to the brain, would result in irreparable limitation of neural development, lending a sense of urgency to the detection and remediation of defects.

To most parents and professionals it seemed self-evident that early detection of sensory deficits must be desirable. By the end of the 1960s these procedures had become a cherished part of routine well-child care and were not questioned for another 10 years. The difficulties that now arise in evaluating and changing, or discontinuing these long-established activities exemplify the hazards of launching screening programmes before they have been fully assessed.

Hearing screening

Justification.   Approximately 840 children each year are born in the UK with a hearing impairment that substantially affects quality of life for them and their family[9]. The vast majority of these children have sensorineural hearing loss. Children with even a modest permanent congenital hearing impairment (PCHI) have increased difficulty in language acquisition and those with a hearing loss of 55 dB or greater rarely learn to talk without intervention. Provision of amplification and expert teaching ensure that most children will acquire at least some spoken language and comprehension of speech.

Middle ear disease – an added complication.   The following discussion focuses on PCHI, but the difficulties of evaluating screening for PCHI are compounded by the explosion of interest in screening for conductive deafness due to secretory otitis media, or otitis media with effusion (OME), over the past two decades. This arose from concern that mild hearing loss due to OME might have subtle but potentially serious and long-lasting effects on behaviour, language acquisition, reading and general health. Screening tests which had been introduced to identify PCHI of moderate degree or worse, were now asked to take on the job of identifying OME, a task for which they were quite unsuitable. Recent evidence suggests that these supposed adverse outcomes from OME are of less concern than originally predicted and screening is no longer thought appropriate for a condition which is in a state of constant change and has a highly variable natural history[10]. Parent and professional vigilance is the key to detecting those cases of OME which are of real significance to the child (Table 2).

The justification for screening is 2-fold: first, that early diagnosis improves outcome; second, that PCHI is not obvious to the parents. Evidence as to whether age of diagnosis and of intervention is important to outcome is very difficult to gather. In the absence of any screening programme, the age of diagnosis is affected by parents' attitudes and education and by the severity of the hearing loss, factors which also affect the prognosis[9]. Outcome can be measured in terms of early progress in language development, but arguably the most important outcomes are to do with quality of life as an adult, in terms of mental and emotional health, employment and relationships. Furthermore, if

Table 2 Epidemiology of hearing loss

Estimated birth prevalence of congenital sensorineural hearing loss (SNHL) defined as > 40 db in the better ear averaged over the frequencies 0.5, 1, 2, and 4 kHz is 1.16 per 1000.

1.3 children per 1000 have this degree of hearing loss and need a hearing aid. The difference between this and the birth prevalence is accounted for by acquired hearing loss and conductive hearing loss.

The incidence of SNHL is at least 10 times higher in babies admitted to neonatal intensive care units.

At least half of all children have at least one episode of otitis media with effusion (OME). Around 7% have OME for at least half the time between 2 and 4 years.

parents are pressured into compliance with intensive early intervention before they are emotionally prepared to handle the diagnosis of deafness, they may become alienated from the whole process. Some parents who are themselves deaf and reliant on sign language resent the implication that their language is somehow second best to spoken language and prefer to teach their child signing as his first language[11].

Notwithstanding all these difficulties, however, a recent review[9] concluded that early diagnosis is beneficial – early, in this context, means in the first few months of life. There remains some uncertainty about the magnitude of the benefit, but the need to identify cases and give a trial of conventional amplification before cochlear implantation have added impetus to the arguments for early detection. Although much remains to be learned about long-term prognosis for cochlear implants, the excellent results now being obtained when this procedure is undertaken at a young age have transformed the outlook for many severely and profoundly deaf children

Screening would only be justified if parents could not identify PCHI themselves. Hearing impaired children look normal and apparently behave like other children, though there are subtle changes in their pattern of babble and communication. Parents do identify a proportion of cases, but a combination of uncertainty about what is normal and, perhaps, an element of denial, result in many children being diagnosed as late as 3 years of age. Modest improvements in this situation can be obtained by parent education and increased professional sensitivity to parents' worries, but on their own these are not sufficient to deliver the very early diagnosis now thought desirable.

What screening tests are available? In the UK, the mainstay of screening in infancy is the Ewing distraction test, though it was never widely adopted overseas and indeed screening for PCHI in infancy was included in the child care programmes of few other countries. The screening test, traditionally performed by two health visitors working together, is known as the health visitor distraction test (HVDT). It relies on the fact that there is a narrow window in development, between 6 or 7 months when a baby learns to sit and balance, and 12 or 13 months when he has acquired a sense of object and person permanence, during which he will repeatedly turn his head in search of an unfamiliar sound. By presenting a series of quiet sounds of known frequency and intensity, the hearing levels can be assessed.

In expert hands, and for diagnostic purposes, this apparently crude test provides surprisingly accurate results. As a screening test, its performance has consistently been poor due to inadequate training, lack of commitment, poor feedback, inclusion of other screening and health promotion tasks in the same appointment, high background noise levels, and the exceptional visual alertness and searching behaviour characteristic of deaf babies. As a result, the test has low sensitivity, sometimes as low as 20%, and poor specificity, with some screeners referring 10 or even 15% of all babies for further investigation[9]. Notwithstanding this damning evidence, there has until very recently been great reluctance to abandon the HVDT.

The concept of high risk infants.   The incidence of PCHI is much higher in certain groups of infants[12]. The risk factors are: history of more than 48 h care in neonatal intensive care (whatever the reason); family history of permanent childhood deafness; craniofacial anomalies; congenital infections due to rubella or cytomegalovirus. Around 60% of children with PCHI have one or more of these risk factors, and could, in theory, be identified by testing 10% of the population. In practice, it is difficult to identify all at risk babies so that the 60% target is unlikely to be achieved and 40–50% is a more realistic figure. In addition, it is considered good practice to test the hearing of any infant or child with other neurological problems, such as cerebral palsy, though the yield is small. The most important cause of acquired hearing loss in childhood is meningitis[13] and failure to check the hearing promptly after recovery in these children is negligent.

Neonatal screening,   Identification of PCHI in the new-born offers an alternative to the HVDT and can be applied either to high risk infants (targeted neonatal screening, TNS) or to all infants (universal neonatal screening, UNS). It is attractive for two reasons. First, it permits very early diagnosis and intervention; second, there is a captive population, which simplifies the logistics of screening.

Three methods are available to test newborns. The auditory response cradle (ARC) is a behavioural test, relying on automated analysis of sudden head movements and changes in respiratory pattern in response to loud sounds[14]. It is easy to use, acceptable to parents and effective at identifying severe and profound PCHI in otherwise normal babies. Doubts about its sensitivity for moderate PCHI, coupled with repeated technical problems, are largely responsible for the current low profile of this method[15].

The two methods that now dominate debate about neonatal screening are oto-acoustic emissions (OAE) evoked by clicks, and brainstem evoked response audiometry (BSER). The method of OAE is based on an observation by Kemp that when the cochlea is stimulated by sound input, it emits sound energy in response by an active physiological mechanism[16]. This has been variously called an echo or regarded as a form of resonance, though neither is strictly a true description of the physiology. The sound output can be collected via a microphone placed in the ear canal and the pattern analysed and displayed graphically, with automatic pass-fail criteria built into the algorithm. In principle, the method is quick and easy to use, but it is very sensitive to correct placement of the probe in the ear canal and the emission is abolished by even minor hearing deficits or by middle ear fluid. As a result, its use in the first few days of life produces a significant number of false positive results, but most of these are eliminated by a second OAE test[17]. Since hearing in one ear is sufficient for language acquisition, for screening purposes it is enough to show normal responses in one ear and this reduces the number of re-tests and referrals required.

Those infants in whom no emission can be detected in either ear after two tests are then tested using BSER. This measures the changes in EEG activity in response to sound stimuli using computer averaging techniques. It requires electrode placement and is more demanding and time-consuming than OAE, so it is used as a second filter after OAE for most infants. For those newborns designated high risk, particularly graduates of neonatal intensive care, BSER may be a better primary screening test.

Does the programme work? There is extensive experience of targeted neonatal screening in the UK. Only three centres have operated universal neonatal screening programmes; one used the auditory response cradle[18] and two used OAE backed up by BSER[17]. In the US, similar programmes now operate in many centres. High coverage of over 90%, yields of confirmed cases in the predicted range and generally high parent acceptability are being reported. However, implementation and quality assurance of UNS will test the managerial and technical skills of both health and education professionals in districts where there is no previous experience of TNS.

Unresolved issues. Since coverage of neonatal screening will never be 100%, because of refusals, early hospital discharges and home deliveries, and some forms of PCHI are progressive, the ideal programme would need to include a safety net to test children missed in the neonatal screen and identify those with progressive hearing loss. This could be achieved by retaining the HVDT for those children, as suggested in the recent systematic review. However, no such scheme has yet been implemented, so any economic assessment must be based on theoretical projections from existing data. It would present considerable logistic problems and would probably be costly in terms of incremental yield. The practical implications of the proposal need to be tested in pilot trials before it could be adopted as policy.

Costs of hearing screening. If the HVDT is performed according to standards set out in 1981 and endorsed many times since, it is labour intensive and, therefore, expensive[19]. The estimated programme cost is £15–25,000 per 1000 children born, with the variability being due primarily to differing grades of staff doing the test. The test is considerably cheaper if done as part of a health promotion review but, given the evidence of poor performance even when carried out in protected time, without other intrusions on the health visitors' attention, there seems little value in doing it in obviously sub-optimal conditions. The cost per case detected is probably around £75,000 and this figure is rising as TNS becomes more effective, reducing the pool of children still waiting to be diagnosed after the first month of life. If UNS is introduced, the cost per case detected by the HVDT, even if working at maximum effectiveness, will possibly exceed £100,000. In contrast, the programme cost for UNS is around £12–13,000 per 1000 births and the cost per case detected is around £18–20,000.

Cost and policy issues. These costs are high for a condition that is not life threatening and where the magnitude of benefit from early intervention is not yet certain. If a proposal were now made to introduce UNS *de novo*, it would probably be rejected pending better evidence on the value of early diagnosis. However, it is ethically and politically difficult to withdraw the existing HVDT screening programme and abandon the goal of early detection, when a much more effective approach is available at considerably less cost. The logical course of action is to withdraw resources from the HVDT and re-invest them in a UNS programme, but this too will present difficult management challenges.

Screening after infancy. If most PCHI can be detected in the first year of life, and children recovering from meningitis are screened, there will be very few seriously hearing impaired children undetected in the community after the first year of life. The incremental yield of any further screening will be very low and the cost per case detected will be high. The main argument regarding any further screening in early childhood (age 2–4 years) and at school entry now centres on the issue of OME, as discussed above. However, in some communities high coverage of screening may be difficult to achieve even with a neonatal programme and a steady arrival of children in the UK from overseas may mean that some hearing impaired children might still be undetected when they start school. The extent of this problem has yet to be fully assessed and, until further data are available, most authorities will continue to advise a universal screen for hearing loss at school entry.

Vision screening

The debate on hearing screening has focused on the imperative to identify children with serious PCHI and screening for mild hearing impairment due to OME is not widely supported. In contrast, serious visual defects are not the subject of any current screening debate and the controversy centres around screening for mild defects. This is because infants with serious visual impairment are usually identified by the obviously abnormal appearance of the eyes or their visual behaviour with diminished response to visual stimuli, failure to establish eye contact or inability to develop fixation and tracking. Screening is not needed for such problems[5] and the crucial issue is the quality of service response to parental worries about their baby's vision, which often leaves much to be desired. The only screening initiatives for severe vision defects are examination of the eyes with an ophthalmoscope to detect congenital cataract (a procedure which is not as easy as it sounds and is of uncertain effectiveness in the hands of non-specialists) and expert examination of infants at risk of retinopathy of prematurity[20]. Occasionally, visual impairment develops later in childhood (for example, optic atrophy due to intracranial tumour) but the incidence of new cases is too low for screening to be justified on these grounds alone, though a visual acuity check is part of good practice in any child with neurological complaints or school problems.

The conditions to be sought by screening. Minor defects of vision include squint, refractive error and amblyopia. These are collectively very common, with 5–10% of children being affected, and there is much debate about whether they merit a screening programme (Table 3).

Justification for vision screening

Squint. This is usually cosmetically obvious and is considered unattractive in our society. Failure to refer and receive treatment is usually due not to lack of identification but to parental or professional

Table 3 Terminology for vision screening

Visual acuity is a measure of how well a person can separate adjacent visual stimuli.

Refractive error is a disturbance of the optical system of the eye so that a sharp image is not formed precisely on the retina.

Myopia or short sight is a condition in which the image falls in front of the retina. It is correctable by concave spectacles. Distant vision is affected but close work is not impaired.

Hypermetropia or long sight is a condition in which the image falls behind the retina. It is correctable by convex spectacles. Distant vision is not impaired; close vision may be. The child can accommodate to overcome this but this may be associated with squint.

Astigmatism means that the degree of refractive error is different between the axes of the eye.

Anisometropia means that the degree of refractive error is different between the two eyes; the resulting difference in image size may predispose to amblyopia.

Amblyopia is a condition of reduced vision in which the eye is healthy but the brain has either suppressed or failed to develop the ability to perceive a clear image from that eye.

ignorance about its possible significance. Micro-squint or small angle squint is not visible to simple inspection. It can be detected by expert orthoptic examination, but usually presents with amblyopia. Identification of micro-squint is not sufficiently important to justify vision screening, nor would screening be feasible by anyone other than an orthoptist, because of the level of skill involved.

Refractive error. This is a commonly used term but is difficult to define. Few eyes are perfect optical systems. Measurements of the refraction of healthy eyes in childhood form an approximately normal distribution curve but there is no exact correlation between the optical properties of the eye as measured by refraction and the visual acuity. Mild degrees of myopia (short sight) or hypermetropia (long sight) are common and are probably of little significance. More severe hypermetropia in the first year of life is thought to be a pre-disposing factor to squint and amblyopia.

There is no precise definition of what constitutes refractive error, nor is there any evidence as to whether or how much hypermetropia or myopia cause any disability. Reduced visual acuity may adversely affect sporting and academic achievement. In early childhood, however, the common refractive error is hypermetropia which is more likely to present with a squint than to seriously reduce visual acuity. Severe astigmatism is uncommon but significantly reduces visual acuity.

Detection of myopia is the main goal of vision screening in older children and teenagers. It is uncommon in young children and is more prevalent in the teens and early twenties. It is associated with better educational performance, though possibly has an opposite effect on sporting skill. While screening is still widespread, the benefits are modest at best. Many mild cases of myopia are identified and glasses are prescribed, but few children with mild myopia wear their glasses regularly. Myopia becomes important when it impacts on quality of life; in these circumstances individuals become aware of their impaired visual acuity because of difficulties with sports, cinema screens or reading bus numbers. Vision screening may well be superfluous in later childhood and adolescence, provided that children have easy access to diagnostic testing whenever there is doubt about their visual acuity; and in many places vision screening after the first year at school is being reduced or even phased out altogether[21].

Amblyopia. The detection of refractive error and squint are not the primary motivation for screening for vision defects in young children. The main argument in favour of vision screening in young children is the identification of amblyopia[1,6]. This is usually associated either with either a squint (which may be the presenting feature) or with refractive error (hypermetropia or astigmatism). A difference in the degree of refractive error between the two eyes (anisometropia) may be found. Amblyopia reduces the visual acuity in the affected eye to a variable degree, with the worst cases being effectively blind in that eye.

The disability associated with amblyopia is not easy to define[22]. Some impairment of stereopsis is inevitable and this might interfere with, for example, ball games and some careers, though many people seem to compensate well by using other cues to gain depth perception. Loss of the good eye through disease or trauma might leave the individual functionally blind or partially sighted, though this appears to be a very uncommon event and little is known about how much recovery in the amblyopic eye can be expected at various ages under these circumstances. Amblyopia also may bar an individual from certain career choices where sudden temporary loss of vision in the one good eye, due for instance to a foreign body, is judged to be unduly hazardous.

Does treatment for amblyopia work? In addition to doubts about the extent of the disability caused by amblyopia, little is known about the effectiveness of treatment[23], which usually involves correction of any refractive error and occlusion of the normal eye. Animal experiments some 20 years ago suggested that there may be a critical period for development of the visual pathways and connections. These findings not only created an enthusiasm for detection of vision defects as young as possible, but also generated a belief that any trials of the benefits of such an approach would be unethical.

Occlusion therapy has been in use for at least 50 years but there are still no satisfactory trials to show the magnitude or permanence of the benefits obtained from this treatment[24,25]. Furthermore, although it is generally agreed that improvement in amblyopia is less likely to occur after the age of 7 years, there is no evidence that treatment at age three or four is more beneficial than at age five or six. It is often said that children will experience less distress if treated before they start school and that occlusion therapy after starting school will lead to teasing or bullying. There is no evidence to confirm or refute this opinion.

Minimum age for screening.   Primary prevention of amblyopia by early identification and treatment is an attractive goal. As refractive errors may predispose to amblyopia, spectacle correction of refractive errors in the first two years of life might reduce the incidence of squint and amblyopia in childhood[26]. There is some evidence that this is so, but it does not eliminate them; many cases with amblyopia and squint are found among those who did not have significant refractive error in the first year of life. Automated refraction methods allow screening for vision defects in infancy, but much remains to be done before this could either be justified or considered as a practical proposition.

Most children younger than 3.5 years cannot reliably co-operate with a visual acuity test and their vision can only be assessed indirectly by refraction, which in young children needs considerable skill. Screening for vision defects currently is only a practical proposition at around the age of 3–3.5 years onwards. At this age, the issue is the detection and treatment of established amblyopia rather than its primary prevention. Since amblyopia is generally a unilateral condition, each eye must be tested separately, and children find this more difficult than tests with both eyes open. If screening is attempted with children who lack the maturity to give reliable unilateral visual acuity measures, there will be many incorrect results and a high re-test rate.

Policy issues.   As with hearing screening, decision making is much more difficult with the existing programme than would be the case with a new proposal. Since the evidence suggests that vision defects, though common, are of only modest importance to the individual, and the effectiveness of treatment for the most potentially important condition, amblyopia, is in doubt, it is difficult to justify substantial expenditure on a vision screening programme and it could be argued that the programme should be discontinued altogether. However, it is counter-intuitive to suggest that there is no value in checking a child's eyesight. A small number of children do have severe refractive errors which are worth correcting, and ophthalmologists remain convinced that occlusion therapy is indeed effective. For these reasons, it is probably necessary to continue with some form of vision screening, at least until more evidence is available, and the aim, therefore, is to devise the most cost-effective programme possible[27].

If the aim of screening is primarily to identify amblyopia, then the *sine qua non* is a visual acuity check of each eye separately, *i.e.* with one eye closed. Visual acuity testing is difficult for young children and acceptable results without a high re-test rate can probably only be achieved at 3.5 or even 4 years of age. In this age group, some children have started school; many attend playgroups or nurseries, and a large proportion of parents are at work. As a result, few screening programmes in this age group achieve a coverage of over 70% and often the figure is lower. Several studies have shown that acceptable sensitivity and specificity for vision screening in this age group are achieved only by orthoptists, who are trained specifically for the assessment of vision in children. Health visitors, who see many healthy children for routine checks, and doctors, are not cost-effective vision screeners.

The simplest and cheapest solution is to test the visual acuity when each child starts school at the age of 4 or 5 years. A captive population is then available and the quality of, and conditions for, testing can be monitored. As there is no evidence that a slightly later start of treatment for amblyopia is a disadvantage, this is an acceptable approach[28].

An orthoptic service to community clinics can greatly streamline the process of deciding who needs a full ophthalmic examination whenever a parent or professional suspects a squint or impaired vision. This service is cost-effective and is said to reduce inequity between prosperous and poor neighbourhoods in the age at which vision disorders are diagnosed[29], but it does not seek to see every child and is not, therefore, a screening programme.

If the goal is achieved of ensuring that every child has a competent visual acuity test by or soon after the age of 5 years, essentially all cases of amblyopia will be detected. New cases of amblyopia, thereafter, are exceedingly uncommon and certainly do not merit screening. Indeed, there is probably no justification for further visual acuity screening after the age of 5 years and this can be replaced by written information to parents regarding optometrist services for any child about whom there is concern.

What next? Uncertainty about the benefits of occlusion therapy for amblyopia could be resolved by a large randomised trial, but the complexities of such a trial are such that it will be expensive and protracted. More work on assessing the true disability caused by amblyopia is needed. The literature is virtually silent on the prevalence of varying degrees of impaired visual acuity due only to refractive error or colour vision defects[30] or on the disability associated with these impairments.

Meanwhile, pragmatic decision making will continue. Even the minimal programme set out above is probably more than can be justified on purely evidence based grounds but equally it is probably the slimmest programme that would be acceptable to parents and professionals.

Other aspects of screening in childhood – the policy context

Changing the policy regarding one aspect of child health screening has knock-on effects for many other parts of routine well-child care. For example, if universal neonatal hearing screening is introduced successfully, the number of children with serious hearing loss still to be detected in the 2–5 year-old group will be very small indeed. Some projections suggest that over 90% of cases would be found within the first year. This means that there may be only one or two cases per 10,000 preschool children with undetected permanent hearing impairment.

It is considered good clinical practice to exclude hearing loss as the cause of delay in speech and language acquisition. This is an extremely common problem; although the exact prevalence depends on how it is defined, figures quoted range between 3–7%. Conventional audiological assessment of these children is quite time-consuming and there is often a long waiting list, which, when combined with the waiting list for assessment by a speech therapist, can result in considerable delays in diagnosis and intervention. The yield is small and is largely confined to otitis media with effusion, which is disabling to a few children but an incidental or trivial finding in most. Universal neonatal screening will mean that the probability of permanent hearing loss being the cause of delayed speech and language development will decline further. Although this will still be an important condition to consider, the rarity of permanent hearing loss coupled with changing perceptions of the importance of middle ear disease suggest that detailed audiological testing may not be an efficient first-line procedure in these children and that we need more efficient ways of identifying or excluding hearing problems in this group of children.

The arguments about vision screening in preschool children provide another example of how decision making must be integrated with other children's services. It is national policy to offer a child health surveillance review to all children at around 3.5 years of age and this is usually undertaken by the family's health visitor. The coverage varies widely, from as low as 40% to over 80%. It has become clear in the last few years that health visitors are good at prioritising their workload if permitted to do so; for example a review of a healthy 3.5 year old in a stable competent family might take second place to working with families who have problems. This policy has been officially endorsed by many community managers and as a result, the coverage of the 3.5 year assessment is falling. Even if it were thought desirable for health visitors to carry out a vision screening examination in this age group, it would be increasingly difficult to deliver without substantial new resources.

In contrast, the assessment of all 5 year old children starting school is widely accepted by parents and professionals. It is easy to achieve high coverage. It fulfils a statutory duty laid on the Secretary of State to provide for the health of school children to be assessed. It is possible to carry out several screening procedures at the same time, so that the cost of any one test is low and the savings to be made by discontinuing any procedure are marginal. No screening test should be undertaken if it produces more harm than good. However, currently the school nursing service has the opportunity to screen for vision and hearing defects, to measure height and weight, and to identify children who have missed out on preschool health care, and this is thought to offer reasonable value for money. Health care must be based on evidence as far as possible, but decision making must take account of the political climate, legislation, public perceptions and demands, and professional opinion.

References

1   Hall DMB. *Health For All Children*. Oxford: OUP, 1996
2   Butler J. *Child Health Surveillance in Primary Care – a critical review*. London: HMSO, 1989
3   Green M. *Bright Futures: guidelines for the health supervision of infants, children and adolescents*. Arlington, VA: National Centre for Education in Maternal and Child Health, 1994
4   Glascoe FP, Dworkin PH. The role of parents in the detection of developmental and behavioral problems. *Pediatrics* 1995; **95**: 829–36
5   Hall SM, Hall DMB, Pugh A. Vision screening in the under-fives. *BMJ* 1982; **285**: 1096–9
6   Dworkin PH. British and American recommendations for developmental monitoring: the role of surveillance. *Pediatrics* 1989; **84**: 1000–10
7   Ewing IR, Ewing AWC. Ascertainment of deafness in infancy and early childhood. *J Laryngol Otol* 1944; **59**: 309–33
8   Sheridan M. *Manual for the Stycar vision tests*. Windsor: NFER, 1976
9   Davis A, Bamford J, Wilson I, Ramkalawan T, Forshaw M, Wright S. A critical review of the role of neonatal hearing screening in the detection of congenital hearing impairment. *Health Technol Assess* 1997; **1**: 23–32
10 Haggard MP, Hughes E. *Screening Children's Hearing*. London: HMSO, 1991
11 Lane H. *When the Mind Hears: a history of the deaf*. New York: Random House, 1984
12 Arnold B, Schorn K, Stecker M. Screening program for selection of hearing loss in newborn infants instituted by the European Community. *Laryngorhinootologie* 1995; **74**: 172–8
13 Fortnum HM, Davis AC. Epidemiology of bacterial meningitis. *Arch Dis Child* 1993; **68**: 763–7
14 Bhattacharya J, Bennett MJ, Tucker SM. Long term follow up of newborns tested with the auditory response cradle. *Arch Dis Child* 1984; **59**: 504–11
15 Davis AC, Wharrad HJ, Sancho J, Marshall DH. Early detection of hearing impairment: what role is there for behavioural methods in the neonatal period? *Acta Oto-Laryngol Suppl* 1991; **482**: 103–9
16 Stevens JC, Webb HD, Hutchinson J, Connell J, Smith MF, Buffin JT. Click evoked otoacoustic emissions in neonatal screening. *Ear Hear* 1990; **11**: 128–33
17 Watkin PM, Baldwin M, McEnery G. Neonatal at risk screening and the identification of deafness. *Arch Dis Child* 1991; **66**: 1130–5

18 Tucker SM, Bhattacharya J. Screening of hearing impairment in the newborn using the auditory response cradle. *Arch Dis Child* 1992; **67**: 911–9

19 Stevens JC, Hall DM, Davis A, Davies CM, Dixon S. The costs of early hearing screening in England and Wales. *Arch Dis Child* 1998; **78**: 14–9

20 Anonymous. Screening examination of premature infants for retinopathy of prematurity. A joint statement of the American Academy of Pediatrics, the American Association for Pediatric Ophthalmology and Strabismus, and the American Academy of Ophthalmology. *Ophthalmology* 1997; **104**: 888–9

21 Cummings GE. Vision screening in junior schools. *Public Health* 1996; **110**: 369–72

22 Snowdon SK, Stewart-Brown SL. *Amblyopia and Disability: a qualitative study*. Oxford: Health Services Research Unit, 1997

23 Snowdon SK, Stewart-Brown SL. *Pre-school Vision Screening: a systematic review*. Oxford: Health Services Research Unit, 1997

24 Newman DK, Hitchcock A, McCarthy H, Keast-Butler J, Moore AT. Preschool vision screening: outcome of children referred to the hospital eye service. *Br J Ophthalmol* 1996; **80**: 1077–82

25 Bray LC, Clarke MP, Jarvis SN, Francis PM, Colver A. Preschool vision screening: a prospective comparative evaluation. *Eye* 1996; **10**: 714–8

26 Atkinson J, Braddick O, Robier B *et al*. Two infant vision screening programmes: prediction and prevention of strabismus and amblyopia from photo- and videorefractive screening. *Eye* 1996; **10**: 189–98

27 Wright MC, Colville DJ, Oberklaid F. Is community screening for amblyopia possible, or appropriate? *Arch Dis Child* 1995; **73**: 192–5

28 Williamson TH, Andrews R, Dutton GN, Murray G, Graham N. Assessment of an inner city visual screening programme for preschool children. *Br J Ophthalmol* 1995; **79**: 1068–73

29 Smith LK, Thompson JR, Woodruff G. Children's vision screening: impact on inequalities in central England. *J Epidemiol Community Health* 1995; **49**: 606–9

30 Holroyd E, Hall DMB. Re-appraisal of screening for colour vision defects. *Child Care Health Dev* 1997; **23**: 391–8

Multidimensional assessment of elderly people in the community

Astrid Fletcher

Department of Epidemiology and Population Health, London School of Hygiene and Tropical Medicine, London, UK

Multidimensional assessment has been advocated as the most appropriate type of screening activity for elderly people. The emphasis has traditionally been on screening for problems with function, disability and dependency in order to identify service and treatment needs. Several randomised trials of multidimensional assessment have been conducted. The UK trials have been conducted in the setting of general practice, while trials in other European countries as well as the US have targeted elderly people living in the community. Although there appear to be possible benefits from multidimensional assessment, for example in reduced mortality, disability and hospital inpatient admissions, these trials have not been consistent in their findings, nor have they been large enough to produce results of sufficient precision and certainty to inform policy. There is stronger evidence that multidimensional assessment can prevent falls but the size of the benefit for serious falls is quite small. The UK health policy of regular assessment of people aged 75 years and above to be carried out in general practice has been implemented haphazardly with little guidance on appropriate methods and levels of assessment. A large randomised trial is currently underway in the UK which will provide evidence on the cost effectiveness of a range of different strategies for assessment.

Correspondence to:
Dr Astrid Fletcher,
Department of
Epidemiology and
Population Health,
London School of
Hygiene and Tropical
Medicine, Keppel Street,
London WC1E 7HT, UK

Screening, in its classic definition, as the identification of precursors of disease in asymptomatic people is not, for the most part, an appropriate description of the activities that have been undertaken among elderly people. The exception to this is screening for some cancers, such as colorectal and prostatic cancer, which occur mainly in elderly people and are reviewed elsewhere in this issue. In general, screening activities among elderly people have focused on the identification of disability in order to identify service and treatment needs. The term **assessment** has tended to be used, in preference to screening, to describe this mixture of case-finding and needs assessment. Several historical strands in the development of these activities can be traced.

Table 1 UK Department of Health contract of service with general practitioners 1990

Annual invitation to each patient aged 75 and over to 'participate in consultation'

Assessment should include ***where appropriate***

sensory function
mobility
mental condition
physical condition including continence
use of medicines
social environment

Indications for possible benefit from regular assessment of elderly people came from early studies several decades ago in the UK, which found high levels of undetected problems in elderly people[1-3]. These included asymptomatic problems (such as a high blood pressure or glucose level), and problems that were symptomatic but unknown to the primary care team. GP consultation rates are high among elderly people, suggesting that undetected problems could not be attributed to lack of contact but were unreported or unrecognized, either by the patient or the doctor. These studies highlighted the need for a systematic approach to problem detection. Around the same time, an approach emerged which emphasized function and disability in the medical care of elderly people and questionnaires were developed to assist in the assessment of a range of physical, mental and social dimensions[4]. Doubts about the feasibility of routine assessment of elderly people[5] led to the notion of two stage targeted screening to identify those at greatest risk or greatest need[6-8].

In the 1980s, results from three randomised controlled trials were published[9-12], which examined the benefit of socio-medical assessment. Two of these trials took place in the UK[9,10] in the setting of general practice and one in Denmark among elderly people living in the community[11,12]. These trials (described in detail below) suggested some possible benefits on mortality and hospital admissions (mainly the Danish trial) but neither of the UK trials provided convincing evidence for regular assessment of elderly people.

UK policy: the 1990 contract of service

Despite these equivocal results, the UK Health Departments introduced an annual health check for people aged 75 years and above[13]. The offering of this health check became a requirement of the 1990 contract of service for general practitioners. The contract specified the broad area for the health check (Table 1) but also added the words 'as appropriate'. By leaving it to the doctor's discretion about which areas to cover (if any), the likelihood of a systematic health check being carried out was reduced. A paragraph in the contract allowed GPs to delegate the health check to an authorised and competent person.

Since the introduction of the 1990 contract, several randomised trials have reported their results. Below is a review of the evidence to date on the benefits of multidimensional assessments in elderly people.

Randomised controlled trials of multidimensional assessment of elderly people in the community

Randomised controlled trials in the UK

Randomised controlled trials in the UK have been conducted in the setting of general practice, mostly using an intervention carried out by a health visitor or equivalent (Table 2). Most studies have taken place in a single general practice[9,14,16] and two studies[10,15] took place in two general practices. The first randomised controlled trial was carried out by Tulloch and Moore and published in 1979. The intervention group were interviewed by a nurse in their homes about social, economic and functional problems, and this was followed by a medical screen by the GPs. Study patients attended a surveillance 'geriatric' clinic run by the primary care team. After 2 years, hospital out-patient referrals and admissions tended to be increased in the intervention group (30% and 25%, respectively, in the intervention group compared with 17% and 19% in the control group) but duration of stay was reduced (median of 12 days compared with 16 days). None of these differences were statistically significant. Use of other agencies, such as social services and chiropody, was also higher in the intervention group (20%) compared to the control group (5%). There was no difference in the prevalence of 'socio-economic and medical problems' but a tendency to less dependency in the intervention group (84% fully dependent compared with 73% of controls). Cost effectiveness was not formally measured, but the intensive involvement of the primary care team and extra service use in the intervention group together with relatively small benefits in terms of hospital admissions and dependency make it unlikely that the intervention would be cost effective. Mortality was almost identical in both groups.

Vetter *et al* used a simple intervention of a health visitor making an extra unsolicited visit[10]. No formal screening protocol was used. Very mixed results were obtained, with the rural practice showing no effects of the intervention on measures of disability, quality of life and use of services, while the urban practice found a significant reduction in mortality (12% in the intervention group compared to 21% in the control

Table 2 Randomised controlled trials of multidimensional assessment in the UK

Study (ref)	Setting	Sample size	Age (years)	Intervention	Follow-up	Results	Intervention *versus* control
Tulloch & Moore 1979[9]	One general practice	C = 150 I = 145 P = 99%	70+	Socio-medical assessment by nurse Follow-up by primary care team	2 years	Mortality OP referrals Hospital admissions Median stay Other services No differences in disability or dependency	20% *versus* 20% 30% *versus* 17% 25% *versus* 19% 12 days *versus* 16 days, *P* < 0.01 20% *versus* 5%
Vetter *et al* 1984[10]	Two general practices (urban,rural)	Rural C = 273 I = 281 Urban C = 298 I = 296 *P* = 96% both	70+	Health visitor made one extra unsolicited visit annually Semi-structured questionnaire on physical, mental and social function	2 years	Rural Mortality Physical disability Quality of life Urban Mortality Physical disability Quality of life	16% *versus* 17% 24% *versus* 31% 23% *versus* 24% 12% *versus* 21%, *P* < 0.001 37% *versus* 28% 32% *versus* 39%, *P* = 0.09
McEwan *et al* 1990[14]	One general practice	C = 145 I = 151 P = 89%	75+	Detailed protocol for nurse assessment Full physical, mental and social assessment	20 months	Mortality Quality of life No differences in medical problems or ADLs	11% *versus* 16% Significantly improved effect size not calculated
Carpenter & Demopolous 1990[15]	Two general practices	C = 267 I = 272 P = 90%	75+	Visits by unskilled volunteers with frequency determined by ADL questionnaire	2 years	Mortality Hospital admissions Median stay Residential Median stay No differences in ADLs	24% *versus* 20% 34% *versus* 25% 16 days *versus* 12 days, *P* < 0.05 7% *versus* 9% 125 days *versus* 168 days
Pathy *et al* 1992[16]	One general practice	C = 356 I = 369 P = not given	65+	2 stage screening Postal questionnaire with home visits on triggered responses	3 years	Mortality Hospital admissions Average stay	18% *versus* 24%, *P* = 0.05 70% *versus* 80% 12.5 days *versus* 14.6 days

ADL = activities of daily living, C = control, I = intervention, OP = outpatient, P = participation rate.

group), and a tendency to improved quality of life. There was some suggestion that the lower death rate in the intervention group resulted in more people surviving with greater levels of disability. The health visitor in the urban group made considerably more referrals to other agencies, especially to social services, compared to the health visitor in the rural area. A difficulty in generalising the results of this study is that the health visitors did not follow a protocol for screening and referral.

In contrast, a structured protocol for screening and referral was followed in the study by McEwan and colleagues[14]. A comprehensive screening approach was employed which included assessment of basic self care (activities of daily living: ADLs), sensory functions, social, mental, emotional and medical problems, as well as urine analysis and measurement of blood pressure and haemoglobin levels. After 20 months of follow-up, no significant differences were observed in the death rate (11% in the intervention group compared with 16% in the control group), or in the prevalence of medical problems or ADLs, but the intervention group had improved morale and emotional well-being scores. This study also collected data on the direct costs of delivering the intervention although extra referral and services were not costed.

Carpenter and Demopolous[15] used unskilled volunteers to screen elderly people for problems with ADLs with regular follow-up of those with higher disability scores. It was unclear how referral to services were made by the volunteers. The intervention group tended to have more acute hospital admissions and a significantly longer duration of stay. There was a tendency for control patients to spend more days in institutional care.

The trial by Pathy and Harding[16] recruited patients at a lower age range (> 65 years) than the trials reviewed above, with 60% being in the age range 65–74 years The trial used targeted screening by a postal questionnaire with follow-up nurse visits for the 60% identified as being in need. At the end of 3 year follow-up, there was a significant difference in mortality in favour of the intervention group (18% compared with 24%). There were no differences in hospital admissions, but the duration of stay was 5 days shorter for younger patients in the intervention group, but not for the group as a whole. There was some improvement in self-rated health status, but not in quality of life. Use of services increased in the intervention group, for example for chiropody, home helps and the proportion receiving attendance allowance.

Randomised controlled trials in other European countries

Two randomised controlled trials have been conducted in other European countries (Table 3). Hendriksen *et al* randomly selected subjects aged 75 years or more living in a Copenhagen suburb[11,12]. The intervention

Table 3 Randomised controlled trials of multidimensional assessment in other European countries and the US

Study (ref)	Setting	Sample size	Age (years)	Intervention	Follow-up	Results	Intervention *versus* control
Hendriksen et al 1984[11], 1989[12]	Randomly selected residents of Copenhagen suburb	C = 300 I = 300 P = 96%	75+	Structured interview assessing health and social problems conducted by nurses or medical practitioner	3 years	Mortality Hospital admissions Hospital days Nursing homes	20% *versus* 26%, $P < 0.05$ 10% *versus* 12% 4884 *versus* 6442, $P = 0.01$ 1.3% *versus* 1.9%
van Rossum et al 1993[17]	Elderly people in defined area of southern Netherlands	C = 288 I = 292 P = 78%	75+	Structured checklist by nurse on functional state, social contacts and housing	3 years	Mortality Hospital admissions Average bed days OP referrals No differences in self rated health or ADLs	14% *versus* 17% 41% *versus* 46% 13 *versus* 17 55% *versus* 66%
Fabacher et al 1994[18]	Volunteers recruited by mailing voters lists in Los Angeles suburb, CA, USA	C = 123 I = 131 P = 12%	70+	HAPSA programme intensive assessment including physical exam and health promotion	1 year	Mortality and hospital and institutional admissions not reported Small changes (effect size 0.3) for improved high grade ADLs and fewer OTC drugs in favour of intervention	
Stuck et al 1995[19]	Volunteers recruited from voter list in Santa Monica, CA, USA	C = 199 I = 215 P = 37%	75+	HAPSA programme	3 years	Mortality Hospital admissions Hospital days Nursing homes Days ADL dependent	11% *versus* 13% 46% *versus* 47% 197 *versus* 160 4% *versus* 10%, $P = 0.02$ 128 *versus* 820 12% *versus* 22%
Wagner et al 1994[20]	Randomly sampled health maintenance enrollees in Seattle, WA, USA	C = 607 I1 = 635 I2 = 317 P = 46%	65+	Intervention group 1 received multidimensional assessment, intervention group 2 health promotion only	2 years	Mortality No results for hospital or nursing home admissions No differences in physical function or proportion with restricted activity days Total number of restricted days less in intervention group difference of 3 days, $P < 0.05$ Fewer falls after one year of follow-up	2.6% *versus* 4.1% and 3.7%

ADL = activities of daily living, C = control, HAPSA = Home Assessment Program for Successful Ageing, I = intervention, OP = outpatient,

OTC = over the counter, P = participation rate,

consisted of a structured interview in the patient's home assessing social and health problems. No physical or clinical examinations were carried out. If indicated, arrangements for medical and social services were initiated and co-ordinated by the interviewers. Two of the interviewers were nurses and one was a medical practitioner. Intervention subjects were visited every 3 months and extra visits could be arranged if requested. After 3 years of follow-up, there was a significant difference in mortality in favour of the intervention group (20% compared to 26% in the control group) and length of hospital stay, but not in the cumulative proportion admitted to hospital. There was a small reduction in nursing home admissions, and a favourable trend to fewer nursing home and hospital admissions in the intervention group. The intervention group received significantly more social services, in particular home helps, aids and equipment for the home. Thus, this trial suggested some considerable benefits from a simple questionnaire based intervention. Details of the questionnaire contents were not published and it is difficult to assess to what extent the questionnaire, or the fact that the interviewers were professionally trained nurses and a doctor, contributed to the better outcome.

In contrast, a randomised controlled trial in The Netherlands[17], using a similar design to the Danish study, did not find similar benefits for mortality, measures of well-being, functional state, hospital or nursing home admissions. Outpatient referrals were significantly reduced but this was analysed with a one-sided significance test. The intervention of home visits by public health nurses focused mainly on broad health topics using a structured checklist of functional state, medication, social contacts and housing conditions and included no physical examinations. Four visits per year were conducted with extra visits if necessary. Use of social and medical services was increased in the control group particularly for home help and home nursing care while meals on wheels, physiotherapy and contacts with general practitioners were similar in both groups. There was a tendency to reduced hospital stay but the magnitude of the difference was small (less than 3 bed days per person assessed). There was some suggestion of a larger benefit in favour of intervention in a small subgroup of patients with initially poor health. These patients showed greater improvements in self-rated health and performance of household activities, and possible large benefits for reduced mortality and hospital admissions. This led the authors to recommend that targeted screening might offer more potential.

Randomised controlled trials in the US

Studies have also been conducted in the US but their generalisability to the UK is uncertain due to differences in the health care setting in which the intervention was delivered[18–20]. The studies which are most comparable have evaluated home geriatric assessments (usually delivered by nurses with specialist training in geriatric assessment) which, in some studies, also involved case management with geriatricians (Table 3).

Fabacher *et al* targeted community dwelling elderly people who were not currently enrolled in a Veterans Administration outpatient clinic[18]. The participation rate was very low (12%). The intervention comprised an initial in-home assessment by a physician's assistant or research nurse trained in geriatrics. The intervention was intensive – the Home Assessment Program for Successful Ageing (HAPSA) – which included a physical examination (blood pressure, audiometry and acuity, height and weight, gait and balance and an oral inspection), blood sample, faecal occult blood test, functional status, mental health, social support, and inspection of the home for safety hazards. Each case was discussed with the study geriatricians and recommendations developed. In-home follow up visits were conducted every 4 months to monitor implementation, facilitate compliance and to administer a brief screen to detect new problems. These follow-up visits were conducted by trained volunteer nurses and social workers. Subjects without regular health care were referred to the Veterans Administration geriatric clinic. The most common new problems or suboptimally treated problems detected were impotence, gait/balance disorders, dental problems, hearing and vision deficits, obesity (each occurring in around 20%). 58% of those participating were referred to physicians, of whom half were treated and a third evaluated but not treated. Outcomes were measured only up to one year. Controls consumed significantly more over the counter medications and showed more decline in high grade activities of daily living (although this was of a very small order). Mortality and use of health services was not reported.

In a study using a similar intervention including the HAPSA methods, Stuck *et al* invited people aged over 75 years from the voter lists[19]. 37% agreed to participate and a further 15% were excluded (mainly due to cognitive impairment or language problems). After 3 years, mortality was similar in both groups (11% intervention and 13% control) as were hospital admissions and length of stay. The proportion admitted to nursing homes was significantly lower in the intervention group (4% compared with 10%). Dependency in basic activities of daily living was also reduced in the intervention group (12% *versus* 22%). There was no difference in hospital admissions or use of in-home support services but the intervention group made more use of services promoting socialisation and made more physician visits. It was estimated that each disability free year of life gained by the intervention cost $6000 and each day of prevented nursing home stay $35.

Both US trials included some health promotion interventions, including recommendations on nutrition and exercise, and use of preventive services such as influenza vaccination, mammographic and cervical screening, as well as advice to stop smoking and reduce alcohol consumption. Only Fabacher *et al* reported any results for the health promotion component. These were based on self-reported compliance with recommendations which was high for vaccine uptake but low for physical activity, stopping smoking advice and reducing alcohol intake. It is unlikely that any benefits observed in the trials were due to the health promotion component.

A stronger emphasis was given to health promotion in addition to assessment in a randomised trial of a younger age group (aged 65 years and over) of Health Maintenance enrollees conducted by Wagner and colleagues[20]. Of those eligible, 54% did not reply or refused the invitation, while a further 16% with any baseline disability were excluded. Participants were randomised to one of three groups: intervention, visit only or usual care. The intervention assessed risk factors for falls and disability including exercise, alcohol, home safety, drugs use and also screened for problems with hearing and vision. The 'visits only' group received health promotion only, focusing on lifestyle factors for cardiovascular disease prevention, breast and cervical cancer detection, influenza vaccine and seat belt use. Very small effects were observed at one year with differences between usual care and intervention of 3 fewer restricted activity days, 1.3 fewer bed days, less deterioration in physical function score (15% in intervention compared to 20% in usual care) and fewer injurious falls (10% compared to 14.5% respectively). Disability outcomes in the 'visit only' group tended to be intermediate between the intervention group and the usual care group. For example, a deterioration in physical function score was observed in 17% of the 'visit only' group which was not significantly different from either of the two comparator groups. None of the differences between intervention and usual care persisted at 2 years. Many other outcomes, such as problems with vision or hearing, showed no differences between any of the groups at the 1 or 2 year follow-up.

The results of trials of multidimensional assessment have tended to focus on major outcomes such as mortality, hospital and institutional admission, use of services and overall measures of disability. A few trials have also reported their results for other outcomes, most commonly risk of falls.

Multidimensional assessment to reduce risk of falls

Four of the randomised trials discussed above provided data on falls or fractures. In addition several trials whose primary outcome was falls or fractures used a multifactorial approach to screen for risk of falls[21–24]. In Hendriksen's study[12], the distribution of falls by randomised group was

Table 4 Odds of a fall among elderly people assigned to specified intervention *versus* controls

Intervention	Outcome	Odds ratio (95% confidence interval)
Multidimensional assessment	Any fall	0.79 (0.65–0.96)
	Fall requiring medical care	0.70 (0.47–1.04)
	Fall resulting in injury	0.73 (0.51–1.04)
Exercise alone	Any fall	1.05 (0.74–1.48)
	Fall requiring medical care	1.85 (0.85–4.03)
	Fall resulting in injury	1.31 (0.60–2.84)

From Gillespie *et al*[25].

not reported, although falls were the most common reason for hospital admissions and hospital admissions were reduced in the intervention group. Carpenter and Demopolous[15] reported fewer falls in the intervention group based on data in the month before the final interview, but the cumulative rate of falls in both groups was not described.

The efficacy of multidimensional assessment in the prevention of falls has recently been reviewed by Gillespie and colleagues for the Cochrane Database[25] (Table 4). Results obtained by pooling data from five studies show a significant 20% reduction in risk of falls. The UK study by Vetter and colleagues[22] found no benefit, and possibly an adverse effect, on falls and differed significantly in its results from the other trials. In the meta-analysis, there was also a tendency for the intervention group to have fewer serious falls, that is those resulting in injury or requiring medical care, but, as these benefits were quite small, prior economic modelling was recommended before implementing multifactorial programmes. The Cochrane team also found that trials using exercise alone, or in conjunction with health education, were not effective.

Multidimensional assessment to improve socialization

There is an extensive literature which suggests that low social support among elderly people is predictive of poor health outcomes. This is a complex area, both in the construct and measurement of social support and in elucidating the key components. A few of the multidimensional assessment trials also included strategies to enhance social support, or have reported results for some measure of socialization even though this was not specifically described as part of the assessment procedure. The trial by Stuck *et al*[19], which included an assessment of the extensiveness of social networks and quality of social support found significantly greater use by the intervention group of services promoting socialization (college courses for seniors, visitor schemes and community transport). However it is not known whether this in turn resulted in improvements in quality of life or health outcomes. In McEwan's study[14], which showed a benefit of multidimensional assessment on measures of quality of life, this was in part due to benefits on the subscale of loneliness. No improvement in measures of social isolation or reported contacts with friends and relatives or feelings of loneliness were observed in the trial of Pathy *et al*[16] or Vetter *et al*[10]. Hendriksen and colleagues[12] attributed the benefits observed in their study to an improved social network because of the home help service and the regular visits by the intervention team, but there was no suggestion that these visits in turn stimulated an increase in non-professional social networks.

Only one randomised controlled trial has focussed entirely on an intervention to promote social contacts and social support[26]. This trial took place in the setting of a single general practice in the UK in 523 people aged 75 years and over. The level of intervention varied according to the subject's baseline social contact score and included social, nursing, and medical referrals. Only 39% of study participants accepted offers of assistance and those who refused were found to be fitter, and to have higher morale and social contact scores. At the 3 year follow-up, there were no differences in mortality, physical status, use of health and social services, or measures of morale and loneliness. The intervention group showed significantly more improvement in self-reported health status than the control group.

Value of screening for specific problems

The essential feature of multidimensional assessment is that it is an overall package of different assessments with the objective of reducing disability and dependency and hence improving quality of life. However, a drawback of studies of multidimensional assessment is that it is difficult to attribute the benefits (if any) to a particular component of the package, or to examine the benefit of specific components of the package. Most studies have not provided sufficient data to examine separately different types of assessment. The benefits of screening for visual impairment in elderly people have recently been reviewed by Smeeth and colleagues[27] as part of a Cochrane effectiveness review. There has been no randomised trial assessing the effectiveness of vision screening alone in elderly people. Five multidimensional assessment trials provided the reviewers with data on visual outcomes at least 6 months after the intervention. No trial measured visual acuity and all used self-reported problems, such as difficulty in seeing even when

Table 5 Odds of improved vision outcomes after vision screening in multidimensional studies versus control

Study	Odds ratio (95% confidence interval)
Vetter *et al*[10]	1.10 (0.83–1.44)
McEwan *et al*[14]	1.05 (0.53–2.08)
Vetter *et al*[22]	0.93 (0.62–1.38)
van Rossum *et al*[17]	1.16 (0.79–1.68)
Wagner *et al*[20]	1.04 (0.71–1.32)
Total*	1.04 (0.89–1.22)

*Pooled weighted odds ratio; from Smeeth *et al*[27].

wearing glasses, or difficulty in reading newsprint, even with glasses. All outcome data were also self-reported usually with the same assessment questionnaire. None of the studies found improvements in vision function as a result of screening (Table 5) and the reviewers concluded that screening elderly people for vision impairment was not justified. Several reasons may be suggested why the trials failed to find a benefit. All the studies used self-reported vision problems which have low sensitivity. None of the studies provided more detailed data on process, such as the medical reasons for poor vision, referral recommendations, uptake and barriers to uptake.

Conclusions

Although there appear to be possible benefits from multidimensional assessment of elderly people, for example in mortality, reduced hospital bed days, and measures of disability, the trials have not been consistent in their findings, nor have they been large enough to produce results of sufficient precision and certainty to inform policy decisions. There is stronger evidence that multidimensional assessment can prevent falls but the size of the benefit for serious falls is quite small.

Existing trials of multidimensional assessment demonstrate a range of methodological problems. The studies conducted in general practice used within-practice individual randomisation and this may have resulted in 'contamination' of the control group, with dilution of benefits. Most of the European trials suffered from 'black box' effects: the intervention was described in such general terms that it was not clear exactly what it comprised. This was particularly problematic for the trial by Hendriksen and colleagues which showed the greatest benefit. A detailed description of the assessment protocol and follow-up was given in only one European trial[14]. The US trials of geriatric screening were conducted in randomly sampled volunteers in the community. A striking feature of these trials is the low participation rates, compared with rates in excess of 90% in the European studies, as well as the over-representation of high-income fit elderly. The intervention in the US studies was usually well described.

In none of these trials was there adequate information regarding the cost-effectiveness of multidimensional assessment. If properly implemented, multidimensional assessment should lead to significant extra health and social service costs as a result of identifying unknown or untreated morbidity and disability. It is essential, therefore, that a comprehensive evaluation of the resource implications, as well as of the benefits of multidimensional assessments, be included.

A meta-analysis published in 1993[28] and including a range of diverse studies using some form of comprehensive geriatric assessment found no significant benefits from home assessment on mortality at 12 months and 24 months and a 14% reduction at 36 months (95% CI, 1–25%). The result was heavily weighted by the Danish study. Hospital admissions were reduced by 16% (OR = 0.84; 95% CI, 0.73–0.96). The study by Tulloch and Moore, which showed no effect on mortality and a trend to increased hospital admissions in the intervention group was incorrectly assigned to the geriatric out-patient group of studies and therefore not included in the results for community based assessment.

The UK policy of health checks for elderly people was introduced prematurely, in the absence of convincing evidence of the benefit of multidimensional assessment. Not surprisingly, most GPs view the policy unfavourably while nurses and elderly people are enthusiastic about the health checks and consider them to be of value[29–31]. Evaluations of the contract have shown variable implementation with few examples of good practice[32–34].

The policy has many of the characteristics of a screening programme. It is doctor rather than patient led; implies to the patient a benefit from the health check; requires resources (personnel, laboratory facilities, questionnaires/tests, *etc.*) to carry out the check; requires adequate tests/instruments for detection of health problems; requires that appropriate services be in place to meet the problems identified as a result of the check; requires identification of optimal frequency of assessment (currently required annually). Unfortunately there is little evidence that any of these requirements have been systematically considered. A recent evaluation of the policy concluded that the NHS has not given priority to the development of the assessment programme for elderly people[34].

The current situation is unsatisfactory but simply abandoning the health checks is not a sensible option. As Illiffe and colleagues point out, this would undermine the work that has been done to promote the health of older people[32]. There are some models of good practice and ongoing research. Within the UK, a large randomised trial is currently in progress, which has two major objectives: first, to evaluate different methods of assessing elderly people within primary care as required by the 1990 contract and, secondly, to evaluate two models for the management of elderly people with problems identified from the assessment process, namely a multidisciplinary geriatric team versus a primary care team. The trial is comparing targeted versus universal screening, as well as three methods of delivering the screen – postal, lay person or nurse. The methods that are being tested in the study are, to some extent, already being used in general practice albeit in an unsystematic fashion. They represent a range of strategies from the minimal approach (postal questionnaire) to a fully comprehensive nurse assessment. All areas specified in the 1990 contract are assessed. The trial, which is being conducted in 106 General Practices (45,000 patients aged 75 years and above) across the UK, will determine the cost effectiveness of these different strategies of screening and management with effectiveness measured by mortality, hospital and institutional admissions and quality of life.

There are strong arguments for assessment of elderly people on the basis of their special needs. It is likely that, unless specifically sought, these will not be identified. However, the results from the trials to date have been disappointing in that they have not provided a consistent or conclusive picture. This, in part, is due to methodological problems but also to the difficulties inherent in evaluating the effect of a package of assessments on wide, though important, outcomes, such as mortality, health service use and quality of life. Advocates for assessment of elderly people have tended to overemphasize the few positive findings from the trials and ignore results which are not supportive. More rigorous evidence is required on a variety of questions pertaining to regular assessment. Some of these are being addressed by current research, but additional studies are needed to address other important questions, such as the optimum frequency and the lower and upper age limits of assessment and the value of individual components of the assessment.

References

1   Williamson J, Stokoe IH, Gray S *et al*. Old people at home: their unreported needs. *Lancet* 1964; *i*: 1117–20
2   Thomas P. Experiences of two preventive clinics for the elderly. *BMJ* 1968; ii: 357–60
3   Williams EI, Bennett FM, Nixon JV *et al*. Sociomedical study of patients over 75 in general practice. *BMJ* 1972; ii: 445–8
4   Kane RA, Kane RL. *Assessing the Elderly*. Lexington, MA: Lexington Books, 1981
5   Barber JH, Wallis JB. The effects of a system of geriatric screening and assessment on general practice workload. *Health Bull* 1982; 40: 125–32

6   Taylor R, Ford G, Barber JH. The elderly at risk. A critical review of problems and progress in screening and case-finding. *Age Concern Research Perspective Monograph, No 6.* Mitcham, Surrey: Age Concern; 1983

7   Barber JH, Wallis J, McKeating E. A postal screening questionnaire in preventive geriatric care. *J R Coll Gen Pract* 1985; **35**: 288–90

8   Bowns I, Challis D, Tong MS. Case finding in elderly people: validation of postal questionnaire. *Br J Gen Pract* 1991; **41**: 100–4

9   Tulloch AJ, Moore V. A randomised controlled trial of geriatric screening and surveillance in general practice. *J R Coll Gen Pract* 1979; **29**: 733–42

10 Vetter NJ, Jones DA, Victor CR. Effect of health visitors working with elderly patients in general practice: a randomised controlled trial. *BMJ* 1984; **288**: 369–72

11 Hendriksen C, Lund E, Stromgard E. Consequences of assessment and intervention among elderly people: a three-year randomised controlled trial. *BMJ* 1984; **289**: 1522–4

12 Hendriksen C, Lund E, Stromgard E. Hospitalization of elderly people. A 3-year controlled trial. *J Am Geriatr Soc* 1989; **37**: 117–22

13 Department of Health. *Terms of Service for Doctors in General Practice.* London: DOH, 1989

14 McEwan RT, Davison N, Forster DP, Pearson P, Stirling E. Screening elderly people in primary care: a randomized controlled trial. *Br J Gen Pract* 1990; **40**: 94–7

15 Carpenter GI, Demopoulos GR. Screening the elderly in the community: controlled trial of dependency surveillance using a questionnaire administered by volunteers. *BMJ* 1990; **300**: 1253–6

16 Pathy MSJ, Bayer A, Harding K, Dibble A. Randomised trial of case finding and surveillance of elderly people at home. *Lancet* 1992; **340**: 890–3

17 van Rossum E, Fredericks CMA, Philipsen H, Portengen K, Wiskerke J, Knipschild P. Effects of preventive home visits to elderly people. *BMJ* 1993; **307**: 27–32

18 Fabacher D, Josephson K, Pietruszka F, Linderborn K, Morley JE, Rubenstein LZ. An in-home preventive assessment program for independent older adults: a randomized controlled trial. *J Am Geriatr Soc* 1994; **42**: 630–8

19 Stuck AE, Aronow HU, Steiner A *et al.* 3 year RCT of annual in home comprehensive geriatric assessment and follow-up of 414 people aged 75 years or older. *N Engl J Med* 1995; **333**: 1184–9

20 Wagner EH, LaCroix AZ, Grothaus L *et al.* Preventing disability and falls in older adults: a population-based randomized trial. *Am J Public Health* 1994; **84**: 1800–6

21 Rubenstein LZ, Robbins AS, Josephson KR, Schulman BL, Osterweil D. The value of assessing falls in an elderly population. A randomized clinical trial. *Ann Intern Med* 1990; **113**: 308–16

22 Vetter NJ, Lewis PA, Ford D. Can health visitors prevent fractures in elderly people? *BMJ* 1992; **304**: 888–90

23 Tinetti ME, Baker DI, McAvay G, Claus EB *et al.* A multifactorial intervention to reduce the risk of falling among elderly people living in the community. *N Engl J Med* 1994; **331**: 821–7

24 Rizzo JA, Baker DI, McAvay G, Tinetti ME. The cost-effectiveness of a multifactorial targeted intervention program for falls among community elderly persons. *Med Care* 1996; **34**: 954–69

25 Gillespie LD, Gillespie WJ, Cumming R, Lamb SE, Rowe BH. Interventions to reduce the incidence of falling in the elderly. In: Gillespie WJ, Madhok R, Murray GD, Robinson CM, Swiontkowski MF. (eds.) *Musculoskeletal Injuries Module of The Cochrane Database of Systematic Reviews* [updated 01 December 1997]. Available in The Cochrane Library [database on disk and CDROM]. The Cochrane Collaboration; Issue 1. Oxford: Update Software; 1998. Updated quarterly

26 Clarke M, Clarke SJ, Jagger C. Social intervention and the elderly: a randomised controlled trial. *Am J Epidemiol* 1992; **136**: 1517–23

27 Smeeth L, Illiffe S. Effectiveness of screening older people for impaired vision in the community setting: systematic review of evidence from randomised controlled trials. *BMJ* 1998; **316**: 660–3

28 Stuck AE, Siu AL, Wieland GD, Adams J, Rubensteiun LZ. Comprehensive geriatric assessment: a meta-analysis of controlled trials. *Lancet* 1993; **342**: 1032–6

29 Tremellen J. Assessment of patients aged over 75 in general practice. *BMJ* 1992; **305**: 621–4

30 Chew CA, Wilkin D, Glendenning C. Annual assessment of patients aged 75 years and over; general practitioners and practice nurses views and experiences. *Br J Gen Pract* 1994; **44**: 263–7

31 McIntosh IB, Power KG. Elderly people's views of an annual screening assessment. *Br J Gen Pract* 1993; **43**: 189–92
32 Brown K, Williams EI, Groom L. Health checks on patients 75 years and over in Nottinghamshire after the new GP contract. *BMJ* 1992; **305**: 618–21
33 Wilkieson CA, Campbell AM, McWhirter MN, McIntosh I, McAlpine CH. Standardization of health assessments for patients aged 75 years and over: 3 years experience in the Forth Valley Health Board Area. *Br J Gen Pract* 1996; **46**: 307–8
34 Illiffe S, Gould MM, Wallace P. *Evaluation of the 75 and over Health Checks*. Report to the NHS Executive. London. Department of Primary Care and Population Sciences, University College London Medical School and Royal Free Hospital School of Medicine, 1997

Screening in general practice and primary care

John Robson

Department of General Practice and Primary Care, St Bartholomew's and the Royal London School of Medicine and Dentistry, Queen Mary and Westfield College, London, UK

General practice and its associated primary care services are the final common pathway for the delivery of most screening programmes. The absence of nationally agreed priorities, guidelines and identifiable resources has meant that screening in primary care remains somewhat arbitrary, practice varies widely and programmes remain largely unevaluated. Discussion of screening has focused largely on test characteristics and performance with less attention being given to issues of policy formation, priority setting, implementation and quality assurance. Without these elements, quality and test performance deteriorate, recruitment and follow-up are incomplete and a poorly discriminating test of doubtful utility is applied inequitably and inefficiently.

For general practice there are two major concerns. The first is to improve delivery of programmes of proven efficacy, such as breast or cervical screening, that already have a national framework. The second is to develop and provide a national structure for preventive programmes for cardiovascular and smoking-related disease. For cardiovascular disease, the issue is no longer whether to screen and advise whole populations for multiple risk factors, but how best to implement this programme. In this chapter, the case for screening for cardiovascular disease is reviewed and potential strategies for improving delivery of screening in general practice and primary care discussed.

Correspondence to:
Dr John Robson,
Department of General
Practice and Primary
Care, St Bartholomew's
and the Royal London
School of Medicine and
Dentistry, Medical
Sciences Block, Queen
Mary and Westfield
College, Mile End Road,
London E1 4NS, UK

The last 20 years have witnessed increasing demands on general practitioners to carry out screening[1]. The absence of nationally agreed priorities, guidelines and identifiable resources has meant that screening in primary care remains somewhat arbitrary, practice varies widely and programmes remain largely unevaluated. The demand led, episodic health check has proved to be a lucrative procedure of doubtful efficacy[2,3]. In contrast, continuing systematic screening of whole populations with interventions of proven efficacy have been more successful. In the 1970s, preventive care became a major component of British general practice after Hart demonstrated that screening for raised blood pressure in general practice was feasible[4] and the Royal College of General Practitioners acknowledged that anticipatory care was a key component of clinical practice[5,6].

For general practice there are two major concerns. The first is to improve delivery of programmes of proven efficacy, such as breast or

Table 1 Proposed screening programmes in general practice and primary care by strength of evidence and consensus

High	Moderate	Low
Cervical cancer	Muliple risk factors for	Congenital dislocation of the hip
Breast cancer	ischaemic heart disease	Deafness (child distraction tests)
Phenylketonuria	Aortic aneurysm	Childhood squint
Congenital hypothyroidism	Haemoglobinopathies	Childhood development
Rhesus incompatibility	Rubella immunity in pregnancy	Vaginal chlamydia
Raised blood pressure	Diabetic retinopathy	Diabetes
Down syndrome	Pre-eclampsia	Gestational diabetes
Spina bifida	TB (school based Heaf test)	Iron deficiency anaemia
Smoking	Syphilis in pregnancy	(pregnancy and childhood)
	HIV in pregnancy in selected areas	Antenatal ultrasound for
	ABO incompatibility	congenital abnormality
	Family history of cardiovascular	Glaucoma
	disease under 55 years	Asymptomatic bacteriuria (childhood)
	Deafness (neonatal evoked	Domestic violence
	responses)	Depression
	Colorectal cancer	Falls in the elderly
		Alcohol dependence
		Testicular cancer
		Prostate cancer

cervical screening, that already have a national framework. The second is to develop and provide a national structure for preventive programmes for cardiovascular and smoking-related disease.

For cardiovascular disease, the issue is no longer whether to screen and advise whole populations for multiple risk factors, but how best to implement this programme. There is good evidence for effective intervention for smoking and raised blood pressure. In addition, there is a consensus on the treatment of those with established coronary heart disease and new evidence on treatment with aspirin and statins for those at increased risk of developing coronary heart disease.

In this chapter, the case for screening for cardiovascular disease is reviewed and potential strategies for improving delivery of screening in general practice and primary care discussed.

Conditions for which screening in general practice has been advocated are shown in Table 1, grouped into three categories based on strength of evidence and consensus. These include: (i) conditions for which there is good evidence of screening effectiveness and a high degree of consensus that implementation is desirable; (ii) conditions where the evidence or consensus is moderate or contested; and (iii) conditions in which the evidence or consensus is poor or even detrimental, as may be the case with screening for gestational diabetes[7,8]. While the allocation of specific conditions to these three groups is controversial, they serve to illustrate the number and diversity of conditions for which claims have been made and the difficulties facing GPs who have to decide which to support, which to prioritise and which to leave alone.

In the absence of comprehensive and authoritative review – including evidence of benefit, hazard, and costs – it is often difficult to know whether the advocates of these screening programmes are leading the pack or bringing up the rear. The situation is further confused when different conclusions are reached by different major reviews. National agreement on potential screening programmes, indicating priorities for support, is urgently needed. It is not clear whose responsibility is it to formulate such a list and respond to policy issues.

In the US, the Agency for Health Care Policy and Research provides a national focus for assessing the evidence and by ranking, affords some degree of prioritisation and Canada has a similar organisation[9]. In the UK, this role is undertaken by a number of bodies including the Population Screening Panel of the Standing Group on Health Technology, the NHS Centre for Reviews and Dissemination, the Cochrane Collaboration and the National Screening Committee. However, while assessment of the evidence is a necessary step, it is still a long way from policy formulation and strategies for implementation. The major implications of a screening policy for primary care services must not be underestimated. The assessment and prioritisation of competing claims on workload and resources is a complex task and policy formulation often has as much to do with the political process as it does with science[10].

Systematic and policy reviews in different countries have drawn very different conclusions from the same evidence, which indicates that the **process** and **context** of policy formation is at least as important as the final conclusion. The process remains even when the questions and their answers have long since altered. Attention to the way in which decisions are made influences implementation as much as the vagaries of shifting evidence. The failure to give general practice smoking cessation and blood pressure screening the degree of priority they deserve reflects, in part, a failure of policy formation. While yielding less community benefit[11], the cervical screening programme is better organised and supported.

Even after a policy has been formulated, the task of implementing a programme needs to be articulated with primary care teams. Preventive programmes for cardiovascular and smoking related disease such as those prioritised in *The Health of the Nation* initiative, could not be fully realised because of the lack of an effective infrastructure at practice level. There was no organisation which connected national strategy with local practice nor was there any mechanism for co-ordinating action within and between practices. The shift towards a primary care led NHS signals a change in perspective, but whether the new National Institute for Clinical Excellence and primary care led commissioning will provide these connections remains to be seen[12]. Recent Government and Medical Research Council reports on research and development in primary care suggest that some of these infrastructural issues are beginning to be debated[13,14]. There is no simple route from evidence to implementation and the absence of structures capable of bridging the gaps in this process remains a major obstacle to delivery of screening services within primary care. It is to be hoped that these organisational changes will provide new opportunities for more transparent priority setting and coherently organised implementation.

Risk factors and cardiovascular disease

Coronary heart disease remains the leading cause of premature death in Britain for both men and women, accounting for a quarter of all deaths. Among middle-aged men, 20% are at high risk with a 1 in 5 chance of death or a major cardiovascular event within the succeeding 10 years. Stroke makes a substantial contribution to the burden of cardiovascular death and morbidity accounting for 12% of all deaths in this age group.

Britain has one of the highest rates of coronary heart disease in the Western world. The UK epidemic peaked in the 1970s and has been slower to decline than in Finland, USA or Australia where changes in public consciousness in response to public health programmes have been more pronounced. In the UK, coronary heart disease deaths were halved between 1972 and 1992 and continue to show a decline of 4% per annum. This overall decline conceals major disparity between social groups. There has been a failure to generalise the benefits of the public health message. In the 1970s, there was a 50% difference in mortality rates between unskilled and professional workers which, by 1990, had increased to a 3-fold difference, as rates among the latter fell rapidly, whilst those of the unskilled declined little, if at all.

The decline in coronary heart disease is largely due to changes in smoking, blood pressure, diet and exercise. The absence of national legislation and initiatives on these issues has been notable. Increasing income inequality is also likely to have been an important underlying cause of increasing inequity in mortality from this cause[15].

Overall, smoking has declined and in 1995 was 39% among unskilled men and 32% among unskilled women compared to 18% and 13%, respectively, amongst professional workers. Diastolic blood pressure fell by 3 mmHg between 1991–5, while consumption of saturated fat declined by a quarter since 1975. However, total fat consumption remained constant with little change in serum cholesterol. Inadequate physical exercise remains the most ubiquitous risk factor affecting two-thirds of men and three-quarters of women, who are either sedentary or irregularly active. Though reliable data on trends of physical activity are not available, improvement, if any, has been small. In contrast, obesity shows a steady and massive increase, most pronounced in lower income groups but apparent across all sections of society, with trends in children indicating that things are likely to get worse[16].

Age is the most important risk factor for cardiovascular disease, followed by sex, smoking, blood pressure, obesity and physical exercise. A family history of coronary heart disease in first degree relatives under the age of 55 years predicts high risk; South Asian ethnic group or low income are also associated with higher risks.

With the possible exception of age, no single risk factor has a high level of predictive discrimination separating those who will have a heart attack from those who will not. By itself, serum cholesterol is a poor predictor of risk and is best combined as the ratio of total cholesterol/high density lipoprotein cholesterol in a multiple risk factor score which includes age, sex, smoking status, blood pressure and the presence or absence of diabetes or left ventricular hypertrophy[17].

While the task of reducing coronary heart disease is primarily an issue for government, organised medical intervention offers important benefits for people at increased risk as a result of either established cardiovascular disease or multiple risk factors. For the first time, there is almost universal consensus on interventions for established coronary heart disease. However, screening and intervention for those at high risk but without established disease lacks national consensus and is poorly applied.

Screening for high blood pressure is an accepted part of general practice. It is based on the level of blood pressure, rather than upon multiple risk factors. Guidelines offer a variety of levels of blood pressure as the treatment threshold, and interventions and population coverage and control remain less than optimal. Recording of smoking status and advice to stop smoking is also in widespread usage and again lacks single national guidelines. Early guidelines promoted screening for hyperlipidaemia and a treatment threshold based on serum cholesterol alone and relative, rather than absolute, risk. These have failed to gain widespread acceptance and have been superseded by risk ascertainment based upon absolute risk and multiple risk factors. There are a number of risk scores available[18] and the Framingham score (based on a cohort of people followed up in the American town of that name) has proved to be the most popular tool for this purpose. Factors include level of blood pressure, serum total and HDL cholesterol, smoking, and presence or absence of diabetes or left ventricular hypertrophy. The 5 or 10 year probability of a coronary event or stroke may be computed[19]. This has been adapted in both hospital outpatients[20] and on one of the larger GP computer systems[21], so that absolute risk is easily accessible in the clinical setting.

The big issue: screening for cardiovascular disease

Screening and management of cardiovascular disease is the single most important issue for primary care. For people who do not already have established cardiovascular disease, there is already general agreement that screening for individual risk factors for cardiovascular disease, such as blood pressure and smoking, is feasible and cost-effective. As GPs are already screening their populations for two major risk factors, the outstanding issue is not whether to screen whole populations for multiple risk factors, but **how** best to screen, and **at what level of risk** and **how intensely** to intervene.

The Oxcheck and Family Heart Studies tested the efficacy of screening and management of multiple coronary heart disease risk factors by general practice based teams in adult populations. In the intervention group, there were important improvements in diet, blood pressure and serum cholesterol, which were most pronounced for those at higher risk. However, the significance of these findings has been disputed, some considering that they demonstrate reasonable return on effort and cost[22-24], particularly as changes appeared to be sustained and might also have impacted on stroke[25]. Others considered that the improvements, if they were real at all, were not worth the effort or money[26,27].

In 1997, a review and meta-analysis of 14 relevant trials of multiple risk factor intervention was undertaken, 9 of which included deaths or coronary events as an outcome[28]. Systolic blood pressure decreased by 4.2 mmHg (SE 0.19 mmHg), smoking prevalence by 4.2% (SE 0.3%) and blood cholesterol by 0.14 mmol/l (SE 0.01 mmol/l). All were significant and important reductions.

However, trial methodology is likely to have exaggerated these reductions in risk factors and they were not reflected in reductions in mortality. Total mortality was reduced by 3% (odds ratio 0.97; 95% CI 0.92–1.02) and mortality from coronary heart disease was reduced by 4% (odds ratio 0.96; 95% CI 0.88–1.04). However, the sample was only large enough to confidently exclude a reduction in mortality of 8%. In order to have confidently excluded a reduction of 3%, 600,000 people would be required in each group, whereas group size averaged only 7000. The trials were, on average, of 5 years duration and the annual reduction in coronary mortality was about 0.8% per annum. This is not negligible when compared to annual reductions in coronary heart disease in men over the decade 1982–1992 of around 2% per annum for manual social classes and 4% per annum for non-manual classes[29]. No information was presented on cost-effectiveness.

This meta-analysis showed evidence of heterogeneity. The reduction in risk factors and mortality was greatest in those at highest risk, particularly those receiving drug treatment for high blood pressure. For these groups, reductions in mortality achieved significance. However, even amongst higher risk groups, the gains were only 1.1% per annum, around half that anticipated.

From these studies, it can be concluded that multiple risk factor screening, combined with systematic advice and treatment of raised blood pressure, results in a small improvement in risk factors and a small reduction in coronary mortality. The magnitude of change that is being debated is at best 1% per annum and national trends of decline are of a similar order of magnitude. Would a medical programme which improved the rate of decline by 50% or even 10% be worthwhile and at what cost? The question is whether the improvement is justified by the effort and the interpretation of current evidence on cost-effectiveness is contested. These studies were undertaken before the widespread introduction of statins and have failed to take account of the additional costs of a more comprehensive programme over existing programmes.

Cost-effectiveness

The threshold for intervention and the cost effectiveness of programmes continue to be contentious. While the utility of **intensive** advice rather than usual advice in addition to drug treatment is in doubt[30], prudent advice to whole populations is a necessary consequence of any screening programme and is associated with a small but demonstrable reduction in mortality.

Were the intensity of advice and results of the Oxcheck and Family Heart studies to be sustained for 5 years, these would be cost-effective interventions. Further cost-effectiveness analysis based on the Oxcheck trial reached similar conclusions[31]. This study examined a number of different options, ranging from simply recording blood pressure and asking about personal history of cardiovascular disease, to more extensive risk factor recording. The cost differences between the various options were relatively small and, for men, relatively cost-effective. Once

Table 2 Cost per year of life gained from six screening programmes[31]

	Screening programme	Cost (£ per discounted life year gained)	
		Men	Women
1	Blood pressure + personal history of cardiovascular disease	1240	4730
2	1+ Smoking	1640	5150
3	2+ Height and weight	2040	6270
4	3+ Dietary assessment	2090	6480
5	4+ Family history	2080	6700
6	5+ Blood cholesterol	2180	6850

smoking, height and weight had been included in the programme, there was little additional cost per year of life gained. The difference between maximum and minimum programmes was only £940 per discounted life year gained (Table 2). Compared to the cost of many medical interventions these are relatively small sums. Once again, those at highest risk gained added years at least cost.

Those at highest risk as a result of raised blood pressure or multiple risk factors can **only** be identified by screening and it is questionable whether screening for coronary heart disease should be assessed economically as a stand alone programme. Given that the cost-effectiveness of screening for raised blood pressure and smoking is already established, economic analyses in primary care need to consider the **additional** or marginal costs of multiple risk factor screening[31,32] to reduce both stroke and heart disease. For men, a more comprehensive programme of cardiovascular prevention can be established at an additional cost of £540 per discounted year of life gained and, for women, £1700[33]. This study confirmed that intervention for multiple risks in whole populations is cost effective, more so at older ages and at higher risks. If treatment with statins based on absolute risk derived from multiple risk factors were now included in these programmes, together with stroke as well as coronary heart disease as an outcome, cost-effectiveness would be further improved.

The way forward

The outstanding question is not whether, but how best to screen whole populations for multiple risk factors and what is the threshold for treatment. How many people should be treated with statins, aspirin and hypotensives and what intensity of advice should be given? For every person with established heart disease there are at least another two with multiple risk factors who are at a similar level of risk and who would benefit from treatment[18]. At what lower threshold do the benefits of treatment and advice outweigh the workload, costs and hazards?

Reviews of individual interventions on diet[34], smoking[35] and blood pressure[36] have all shown that benefit is greatest among those at highest risk, and that interventions to reduce blood pressure and smoking are cost effective. It has been proposed that management of raised blood pressure should also be based on absolute risk and should take account of other cardiovascular risk factors rather than simply depending upon the level of blood pressure[37].

In addition to the evidence on multiple risk factor intervention already cited, new evidence on the efficacy of statins[38,39] and aspirin[40,41] for those at higher risk of coronary heart disease provides further evidence of worthwhile benefit at reasonable cost. For the top 20% of the risk distribution, which for men is equivalent to an absolute risk of a coronary event of 2–3% per annum, treatment with statins reduces mortality by 20–30%, though whether the effects of statins and thrombolysis are additive remains uncertain.

In 1997, the Standing Medical Advisory Committee to the Department of Health proposed the biggest change in clinical practice for the past 20 years[42]. It recommended that people who had pre-existing ischaemic heart disease and those with multiple factors, generating an absolute risk of heart attack above 3% per annum, should be treated with statins[26]. This absolute risk is the treatment threshold and small changes in this threshold result in big changes in the numbers of people receiving treatment. As individuals with risks of 3% or more per annum constitute 8% of the older adult population under 70 years, the cost, resource and workload implications are enormous. The recommendation was criticised for ignoring cost effectiveness, policy issues and strategy for implementation[43]. However, although grey areas remain, there is more consensus on this issue than at any other time and the similarities between proposals are much more striking than the differences. What is at issue now is the threshold for intervention which determines numbers treated and total programme costs[44].

Unfortunately, the differences in view have obscured the areas of agreement. There is almost universal agreement that smoking and blood pressure programmes are the top health promotion priorities for implementation[45]. A national framework for their implementation, with well defined aims and standards comparable to those adopted by the breast and cervical screening programmes is lacking. For blood pressure, such a programme would need to rely on practice or shared hospital based recall[46] and there should be agreed specifications for ascertainment and intervention with a national system for collating agreed outcomes, processes and reporting of results[47].

However, screening and management of cardiovascular disease does not simply comprise a set of stand-alone programmes. Risk factors for stroke are almost identical to those for coronary heart disease and there is mounting evidence that treatment of both raised blood pressure and lipids should be based on absolute risk derived from multiple risk factors rather than on blood pressure or cholesterol alone[48,49]. In general practice, these programmes have a common organisation, common risk factors and common subjects. Screening using multiple risk factors for cardiovascular disease followed by drug treatment is now an effective option when absolute risk remains above agreed thresholds[37]. In the context of screening, the general population can be given prudent advice on smoking, diet and exercise – not because advice is likely to have a large effect, but because silence is not an option and advice is of some benefit.

The workload and cost implications of cardiovascular screening are considerable. The absolute risk threshold, which determines whether or not to treat, is a key consideration. Were the absolute risk threshold to be lowered to a coronary event rate of 2% per annum, 20% of men in the 35–69 year age group would require treatment with statins. Conversely, if the threshold were raised to 4% per annum, around 5% of this population would require treatment.

Primary and secondary care teams have so far been struggling to deal adequately with individuals with diabetes who constitute only 2% of the population. Implementing a programme such as that proposed by the Standing Medical Advisory Committee would amount to a major change in clinical practice, costing over £600 million per annum for statin treatment alone[50]. Without a national and local infrastructure and additional support and resources, programmes would only scratch the surface, missing many of those who have most to gain. The optimal risk threshold for intervention and the nature of the intervention remain controversial[44].

The impact of national policy on diet, smoking, exercise and transport outweighs the contribution of the medical sector. But as Susser has pointed out, the pace of change is glacial and will come too late for the current generation. Deaths from cardiovascular disease should no longer be regarded as a regrettable, but necessary, part of a consumer society. The growing inequalities in death from cardiovascular disease are a stark reminder of the cost of inaction[15]. The better off have been able to afford and effect changes in diet, smoking behaviour and exercise which have not been accessible to the majority of the population. Treatment and advice to people at high risk show unequivocal evidence of substantial benefit at reasonable cost and this has to involve whole populations in screening and advice. The outstanding issue is how best to implement and resource this programme. There is a greater consensus now than ever before on what is and what is not worth doing. If the NHS is to be primary care led, the prevention and amelioration of cardiovascular disease should be its first priority.

The need for developing and implementing screening for cardiovascular disease in primary care is compelling. Implementation has to fit in to the overall context of general practice and there are organisational issues that are shared with other screening and clinical programmes. These include disease registers, population coverage, equity of delivery, quality assurance and review.

How well are screening services delivered?

The implementation of new and existing screening programmes requires a common organisational framework within general practice. This includes accurate patient registers, computerised facilities for recall, follow-up and audit, and programmes to assist development and quality assurance. Potential obstacles to delivery of screening include the acceptability and accessibility of the intervention, inaccuracy of the patient register and poor quality screening and intervention. The concentration of risk factors in some inner city, industrial and other disadvantaged areas ensures that when national coverage is below 80%, the unscreened are inequitably distributed. National figures conceal the fact that many local communities are inadequately served by current services.

Equity

Although a key issue for screening services, equity has been given little priority over the past two decades. Where health services aim to provide maximum health gain for the nation at minimum cost, equity is likely to receive low priority as this strategy gives priority to those best able to make use of services, namely the young, white and better off. However, where the aim is to maximise the **potential** for good health in all individuals at minimum cost, then equity becomes a major consideration[32,51].

Geographical inequity in general practice and community services funding has been pronounced and has been exacerbated by fundholding. Deprivation payments to GPs, additional payment *per capita* for patients living in particularly deprived areas, were introduced to ameliorate some of the worst discrepancies. In such areas, workload is 50% above the national average and resources are often 50% below leaving little opportunity for anticipatory care. Although there has been substantial improvement in GP services, a minority continue to fall below adequate levels[52,53]. Such discrepancies have prompted review of basic funding formulae. Twenty years after such inequity in the hospital sector was reduced by the Resource Allocation Working Party, geographical financial inequity is finally, though slowly, being addressed for primary care through new allocation formulae.

Inequity by age, social class and ethnic group is as much a feature of screening services as other aspects of primary care[54,55]. The results of a survey among selected practices in an inner London Borough are summarised in Table 3. Differences in the coverage of selected preventive activities between white and minority ethnic groups and different socio-economic groups were most pronounced for centralised recall systems for breast and cervical cancer screening and less pronounced for activities such as blood pressure screening which are practice based and can utilise the opportunities presented by routine practice visits[56].

There is now substantial evidence from selected practices that, given organisation and resources, inequity of delivery of screening services can be largely eradicated and levels of coverage in excess of 85% or 90% achieved. In 1994, in one of London's most disadvantaged inner London

Table 3 Preventive activity by ethnic group. Sampled from records of 43 GPs in one inner London borough[56]

	White $n = 187$ (%)	Odds ratio standardised to age and sex of white population	All non-white $n = 294$ (%)	Odds ratio standardised to age and sex of white population	(95% CI)
Blood pressure	163 (87)	**1.0**	244 (83)	**0.9**	**(0.5, 1.5)**
Smoking	143 (76)	**1.0**	213 (72)	**0.9**	**(0.6, 1.4)**
Dietary advice	45 (24)	**1.0**	64 (22)	**1.0**	**(0.6, 1.6)**
Weight	141 (75)	**1.0**	209 (71)	**0.9**	**(0.6,1.4)**
Height	129 (69)	**1.0**	190 (65)	**0.9**	**(0.6, 1.4)**
Cervical smear	92/104 (88)	**1.0**	228/264(86)	**0.6**	**(0.3, 1.3)**
Mammography	17/37 (46)	**1.0**	4/20 (20)	**0.2***	**(0.1, 0.8)**

Number (percentage).   *P = 0.03.

Boroughs, 34% of practices achieved 80% cervical smear coverage and 16% failed to reach 50%. For the latter group, the major obstacles to change remain largely infrastructural: adequate premises, employment of a nurse and a practice computer are necessary prerequisites[57,58].

Registers

All screening programmes rely on population registers for selection of subjects, follow-up and audit. These registers are based on general practice populations registered with the Family Health Services Authority. The importance of a national and comprehensive system of registration should not be underestimated. Privately funded systems, characterised at one extreme by the American system, have major problems because there is no such thing as a whole population register. The uninsured in such systems are often effectively disenfranchised and national data are hard to come by because of fragmentation of services. In Britain, a national system of registration provides a unique opportunity to identify people at risk, audit population coverage and improve the quality of screening programmes. But although 98% of the population are registered, some outstanding problems remain.

Up until 1995, new patient registration, or change of details, depended on manual notification by the local practice. As people often fail to record their **previous** GP there is considerable potential for delay or failure to remove people from the register once they have left the area and little incentive for GPs to identify those who have left the practice. Conversely people moving into a new area may delay registration with a local GP, or fail to notify change of address within the same area.

In areas with high turnover there is substantial register inaccuracy[59]. In such areas, registers may be inflated by 25%[60] with up to 50% of addresses incorrect[61-63]. However, these are exceptional rates and nationally inflation is around 10–15%. Recent administrative change has improved the situation. From 1995, the notification of registration became computerised as GP-LINKS was introduced, which allowed connection between the central Family Health Services Authority computer and the local general practice computer. This shared register, on which details may be easily changed by either party, has substantially improved notification of change and matching of patients. The implementation of a new unique NHS number is likely to further enhance matching of details and register accuracy.

Opportunistic contact

A register is only one mechanism for patient contact. Each member of the population visits their GP on average four times per year, 70% of the population consults in any one year and 90% within five years. These contacts are an opportunity for personal invitations to participate in screening programmes. As registration data lag behind the patient's current residence, routine surgery visits enable opportunistic contact to be maintained. In many practices, additional systems are employed to identify those overdue for screening procedures or follow-up.

However, by itself, opportunistic contact is an inefficient method of contact. It needs to be an adjunct to a systematic programme and an organised framework. Combining opportunistic methods with systematic mailing or telephone contact to non-respondents is the most effective vehicle for improving coverage[56,64]. Failure to capitalise on opportunistic contact wastes a valuable and important resource and was the most remedial deficit in screening services for women found to have invasive carcinoma of the cervix[65].

Quality

Specification of quality standards for measurement, recording and intervention are as important for smoking cessation or raised blood pressure screening as they are for cervical or breast cancer. Although a number of authoritative guidelines exist in the UK, there are no nationally agreed specifications for smoking and blood pressure programmes between GPs and contracting authorities. For example, should mandatory components of ascertainment include the numbers of cigarettes smoked per day, age started and date stopped, or is it sufficient to simply record whether a smoker or non-smoker? Cuff size has an appreciable influence on measurement of blood pressure. Although the standard cuff is too small for the majority of arms, it persists in routine use in most NHS institutions including general practice. The proliferation of terminal zeros in many records indicate that measurement is often to the nearest 5 or even 10 mmHg rather than to 2 mmHg with which sphygmomanometers are calibrated[66]. The increasing use of electronic blood pressure measuring devices provides an opportunity to improve practice and requires clear national guidance and support[67]. A national specification based on evidence of best practice for measurement, ascertainment and intervention is needed to inform local practice.

The same considerations apply to other aspects of delivery. What information should be provided on smoking or diet for people with raised blood pressure? Although there is good evidence that written material significantly enhances verbal advice, its routine provision is not widespread. How often should individuals with raised blood pressure be reviewed and what should take place? Drug treatment of raised blood pressure is similarly variable. Existing guidelines vary and a national consensus is lacking to inform treatment thresholds and preferred drug regimes[48,68].

The quality and comparability of electronic data recording are also important. Agreement on code definitions may have pronounced effects on the apparent prevalence of hypertension. Data entry templates containing pre-agreed codes act as both check-lists and improve accuracy. For the majority of practitioners who currently maintain both paper and computerised records, the completeness of the latter requires verification by practice staff if it is to be relied upon.

Improving screening services

The expansion and improvement of screening in general practice has depended upon the employment and training of practice nurses[69]. In the decade up to 1995, the numbers of practice employed nurses more than doubled: 90% of general practices now employ at least one nurse[52]. Practice nurses have extended their role from a restricted list of activities to include a broad range of skills for screening and health promotion, including blood pressure measurement, venepuncture, cervical cytology, behavioural counselling, contraceptive services, pre-test counselling for inherited disorders, vision screening, spirometry, audiometry and many other techniques[70,71]. When records were paper based, nurses maintained manual call and recall systems for both screening and chronic disease management[72] and they now actively participate in the maintenance and recall of patients using computerised systems. The participation of nurses in these organised programmes significantly enhances uptake of screening[73].

During the 1980s, facilitation schemes were adopted in which administrative authorities employed nurse facilitators to help practice nurses and primary health care teams develop local health promotion and screening programmes. A National Association of Facilitators was formed and, in 1992, 200 were employed nationally[74,75]. Changes in the 1990s made it more difficult for health authorities to employ such staff using General Medical Services' money reserved for general practice activities. Although American experience confirms that it is as easy to facilitate procedures of doubtful effectiveness as those of proven value[76], the contribution of facilitators have played an important role in developing preventive care in general practice.

GPs employ a number of methods to improve uptake for screening programmes. These include opportunistic face-to-face advice during surgery visits for other reasons, flagging manual or computer records, identifying non-respondents systematically and sending them letters, using health advocates or interpreters from minority ethnic groups, providing home visits and the option of a test performed by female staff. With training, GP reception staff have been effective in improving uptake among non-respondents for breast screening, particularly for women in minority ethnic groups[56].

By 1995, local guidelines were being developed in many areas, comprised of local interpretation of national recommendations, research evidence and best practice[77]. Their importance lay in establishing collective objectives and co-operation between practices, providing criteria for local audit and review and a basis for continuing education and improvement. It is difficult to estimate the extent to which local screening services for raised blood pressure or cervical cytology are influenced, but guidelines have proved a useful focus for change and year on year improvement of patient coverage in most areas[78–80].

Information flow

For centrally organised screening programmes, there is a need to have a two-way flow of information. Not only does the central organisation require information regarding registration and tests from the practices up-the-pipe, but practices need information about individual results, lists of non-respondents and population coverage back down-the pipe. Computerisation of these functions is both feasible and necessary. The involvement of general practice and primary care as active participants in the recruitment and management of people involved in screening programmes is necessary for all but the most laboratory centred of programmes.

General practice computing has been transformed over the last 15 years and over 90% of practices are now computerised. Many GPs are actively maintaining call and recall systems for screening and disease registers for coronary heart disease, asthma/chronic lung disease, diabetes and raised blood pressure[81]. Around half are actively maintaining a Read (or similar) coded clinical record at each surgery consultation[82]. Paperless surgeries are not uncommon and the sophistication of software and hardware capabilities has transformed possibilities for decision support, audit and review, communications and linkage.

While linkage between central recall systems for breast and cervical screening and the Family Health Services Authority register is now routine, linkage of practice computers to the screening services is not generally available. However, in some programmes printed lists of non-respondents are sent to each GP and coverage by practice may also be available. As practice computers are often routinely linked with hospital pathology laboratories for blood and other results, it will hopefully be a short time before practice linkage with screening programmes is established. This will make redundant the tedious business of manually uploading central recall systems, and manually downloading screening results onto the practice computer. Conformance standards and accreditation of GP computing systems could ensure that a standard interface between the many different brands of local computers and central computer systems is facilitated.

Financial incentives

The investment and continuing costs of nursing and clerical time for preventive programmes in general practice are substantial, despite the fact that, in the UK, employing authorities reimburse 70% of practice nurse salaries and 50% of the capital cost of the practice computer. The introduction of target payments in 1990, to promote immunisation and cervical screening, provided financial resources pegged to performance. GPs currently receive a payment of £870 on reaching a 50% target for cervical cytology and £2160 for the 80% target. No such scheme exists for mammography and it is notable that many practices report rates of mammography substantially below their rate for cytology for women of the same age[83]. For cervical cytology, the combination of well-organised local recall registers and financial resourcing of general practices have transformed population coverage. In 1970, coverage was below 50% in many areas, but is now around 80%, although problems remain in disadvantaged areas and among some minority ethnic groups.

In 1990, the UK Government introduced payments for health promotion[84]. These initially took the form of payment for an extremely diverse range of health promotion activities, payment being generated by a clinic attended by 10 individuals. The doubtful benefit of this activity soon became clear and, in 1993, the government introduced a new patient registration check, together with an over 75 years check and chronic disease management payments for coronary heart disease, raised blood pressure, asthma and diabetes. Payment was dependent upon extensive recording of data and year on year rises in population coverage[85].

This approach was criticised as being too prescriptive, generating large amounts of centrally held data of variable quality with no obvious purpose. In addition, the requirement to routinely check urine glucose[86] and aspects of the over 75s check lacked an evidence base. In a climate which had already divided general practice into fundholders and non-fundholders, top down initiatives were viewed with some distrust[87]. The requirement to produce data on health promotion activities was discontinued in 1997 and practices were asked merely to submit outlines of their health promotion strategies, though payments for new patient, elderly checks and chronic disease management were continued.

Resourcing change through performance rather than facilitation failed to develop programmes. The ensuing controversy did nothing to enhance the progress of cardiovascular health or screening and the inclusion of screening unsupported by evidence further undermined credibility of health promotion in general. An important opportunity to develop the recording and organisation of preventive activities was missed during this turbulent decade and there were many who felt both baby and bathwater were jettisoned in the attempt to appease critics[88].

The alternative approach of supporting existing initiatives from the bottom-up has proved more productive. Organised local input from practices, combined with central co-ordination, has tended to be more successful than either component alone. The question is whether this model can be successfully applied not only to single-shot programmes such as cervical screening, where relatively small numbers of people are subsequently managed by secondary care, but also to conditions such as smoking or raised blood pressure, requiring continuing primary care management and behavioural change for large numbers of people. The emergence of locality diabetic registers suggest that it can. Whether the current initiative to promote clinical effectiveness can develop practice-based community registers, promote implementation and improve quality and audit remains to be seen[89].

Reviewing progress and quality

Routine review and audit of results, comparing individual practices with anonymised peers is a realistic proposition now that clinical computer systems are in day-to-day use in many general practices. Despite the additional payments designed to encourage recording of smoking, blood pressure and other cardiovascular risk factors, no systematic attempt was made to aggregate the large amounts of data generated by the chronic disease management and health promotion initiatives. Unlocking clinical data in a fashion which allows comparison of results remains an outstanding task for general practice.

While national programmes often generated more heat than light, sporadic initiatives in East London[60], Wales[90], Somerset[91], Wakefield[92], Buckinghamshire[93] and Northumberland[94] established locally valued programmes with published aggregated results from large groups of practices. Agencies involved include health authorities, Medical Audit Advisory Groups, University Departments and individual GPs. A pilot project by the National Health Service Executive (NHSE), *Collecting Data in General Practice*, aims to establish a national core dataset with agreed Read coded definitions and data collection from a range of general practice computer systems using a data extraction programme called MIQUEST. This includes training in establishing and maintaining datasets[95].

Unlike the *National Morbidity Survey of General Practice* which contains cross-sectional data, the NHSE Collecting Health Data in General Practice initiative will permit the linking of morbidity codes to process. For example, it will be possible to quantify the number of individuals with hypertension with a systolic blood pressure above 160 mmHg, or the number of hypertensive patients who have not had their blood pressure measured within the preceding year. As well as examining coverage and activities in whole populations, this in effect establishes disease registers for specific conditions which can then be examined in terms of their process. Not only will this allow coverage to be documented but it can also begin to address the quality of interventions.

Smoking and blood pressure ascertainment within the preceding 5 years in better organised practices averages around 80%, though hypertension definition is variable. These figures are derived from volunteer practices and the national or regional picture is likely to include a more diverse range[47]. Comparisons between practices or areas are difficult as treatment and control of raised blood pressure vary according to treatment thresholds and practice age structure. Age standardisation and an agreed range of target thresholds could address these problems. However, training of practice teams around agreed definitions and quality of data entry are essential if the value of such information is to be realised. The aim is to improve clinical practice: the production of information is only a means to that end.

Conclusion

There is now compelling evidence that general practice based screening and intervention are a valuable and cost-effective way of reducing cardiovascular mortality through the identification of smokers, raised blood pressure and other multiple risk factors for cardiovascular disease. However, the cost and resource implications are formidable and need to be considered within a national framework with explicit aims, as well as support for disease registers, quality assurance, implementation, audit and review. All screening programmes in general practice share common organisational elements which require support if delivery of screening services is to be equitably improved. A national framework to support evidence-based practice on screening and treatment is required which articulates with local development and clinical effectiveness groups. This would improve the coherence and implementation of current and new initiatives to prevent death from cardiovascular disease.

References

1   Li PL, Logan S. The current state of screening in general practice. *J Public Health Med* 1996; **18**: 350–6
2   Dales LG, Friedman GD, Collen MF. Evaluating periodic multiphasic health checkups: a controlled trial. *J Chronic Dis* 1979; **32**: 385–404
3   The South-East London Screening Study Group. A controlled trial of multiphasic screening in middle-age: results of the South-East London Screening Study. *Int J Epidemiol* 1977; **6**: 357–63
4   Hart JT. Semi-continuous screening of a whole community for hypertension. *Lancet* 1970; **ii**: 223–6
5   Report of a working party of the Royal College of General Practitioners. *Health and prevention in primary care. Report from general practice 18*. London: Royal College of General Practitioners, 1981
6   Van den Dool CWA. From multiple screening to anticipatory medicine. *Allgemeinmedizin Int* 1973; **3**: 100–1
7   Jarrett RJ. Should we screen for gestational diabetes? *BMJ* 1997; **315**: 736–7
8   Kerbel D, Glazier R, Holzapfel S, Young M, Lofsky S. Adverse effects of screening for gestational diabetes: A prospective cohort study in Toronto, Canada. *J Med Screen* 1997; **4**: 128–32
9   Logan AG. Lowering blood cholesterol level to prevent coronary heart disease. In: The Canadian Task Force on the Periodic Health Examination (ed) *The Canadian Guide to Clinical Preventive Health Care*. Canada: Minister of Supply and Services, 1994
10 Florin D. Barriers to evidence based policy. *BMJ* 1996; **313**: 894–5
11 Raffle AE. Deaths from cervical cancer began falling before screening programmes were established. *BMJ* 1997; **315**: 953–4
12 Secretary of State for Health. *The New NHS White Paper*. London: HMSO, 1997
13 Mant D. R&D in primary care – an NHS priority. *Br J Gen Pract* 1998; **48**: 871
14 Radda G. Primary care research: the MRC's proposals. *Br J Gen Pract* 1998; **48**: 872
15 Marmot M, Christie I, Dilnot A, Field A, Wilkinson M, Wilkinson R. The implications of social,political and economic trends in the prevention of coronary heart disease. In: National Heart Forum. (ed) *Coronary Heart Disease Prevention. Looking to the Future*. London: National Heart Forum, 1997; 119–36

16 National Heart Forum. *Coronary Heart Prevention. Looking to the Future.* London: National Heart Forum, 1997

17 Kannel WB. Framingham study insights into hypertensive risk of cardiovascular disease. *Hypertens Res* 1995; **18**: 181–96

18 Robson J. Information needed to decide about cardiovascular treatment in primary care. *BMJ* 1997; **314**: 277–80

19 Kannel WB. Office assessment of coronary candidates and risk factor insights from the Framingham study. *J Hypertens Suppl* 1991; **9**: S13–9

20 Vallance P, Martin J. Statins and hypercholesterolaemia. *Lancet* 1997; **350**: 1854

21 Robson J. *Framingham Risk Score on EMIS Computers.* Leeds: Egton Medical Services, 1997

22 Langham S, Thorogood M, Normand C, Muir J, Jones L, Fowler G. Costs and cost effectiveness of health checks conducted by nurses in primary care: the Oxcheck study. *BMJ* 1996; **312**: 1265–8

23 Wonderling D, Langham S, Buxton M, Normand C, McDermott, C. What can be concluded from the Oxcheck and British family heart studies: commentary on cost effectiveness analyses? *BMJ* 1996; **312**: 1274–8

24 Cruickshank JK. Health promotion in general practice. Refine the approach – don't abandon the principle. *BMJ* 1994; **308**: 852

25 Muir J, Jones L, Fowler G. Cost effectiveness of health checks. Effect of intervention was sustained. *BMJ* 1996; **313**: 624

26 Haq IU, Jackson PR, Yeo WW, Ramsay LE. Interventions in OXCHECK study waste resources. *BMJ* 1995; **311**: 260

27 Stott N. Screening for cardiovascular risk in general practice. *BMJ* 1994; **308**: 285–6

28 Ebrahim S, Smith GD. Systematic review of randomised controlled trials of multiple risk factor interventions for preventing coronary heart disease. *BMJ* 1997; **314**: 1666–74

29 Drever F, Whitehead M, Roden M. Current patterns and trends in male mortality by social class. *Popul Trends* 1996; **86**: 15–20

30 Lindholm LH, Ekbom T, Dash C, Isacsson A, Schersten B. Changes in cardiovascular risk factors by combined pharmacological and non-pharmacological strategies: the main results of the CELL Study. *J Intern Med* 1996; **240**: 13–22

31 Field K, Thorogood M, Silagy C, Normand C, O'Neill C, Muir J. Strategies for reducing coronary risk factors in primary care: which is most cost effective? *BMJ* 1995; **310**: 1109–12

32 Torgerson DJ, Spencer A. Marginal costs and benefits. *BMJ* 1998; **312**: 35–6

33 Winocour P. Cost effective strategies for reducing coronary risk in primary care. *BMJ* 1995; **311**: 573

34 Brunner E, White I, Thorogood M, Bristow A, Curle D, Marmot M. Can dietary interventions change diet and cardiovascular risk factors? A meta-analysis of randomized controlled trials. *Am J Public Health* 1997; **87**: 1415–22

35 Law M, Tang JL. An analysis of the effectiveness of interventions intended to help people stop smoking. *Arch Intern Med* 1995; **155**: 1933–41

36 Wood VA, Hewer RL. The prevention and management of stroke. *J Public Health Med* 1996; **18**: 423–31

37 Foss FA, Dickinson E, Hills M, Thomson A, Wilson V, Ebrahim S. Missed opportunities for the prevention of cardiovascular disease among British hypertensives in primary care. *Br J Gen Pract* 1996; **46**: 571–5

38 Scandinavian Simvastatin Survival Study Group. Randomised trial of cholesterol lowering in 4444 patients with coronary heart disease: the Scandinavian Simvastatin Survival Study (4S). *Lancet* 1994; **344**: 1383–9

39 Shepherd J, Cobbe MS, Ford I *et al.* Prevention of coronary heart disease with pravastatin in men with hypercholesterolaemia. *N Engl J Med* 1995; **333**: 1301–7

40 The Medical Research Council's General Practice Research Framework. Thrombosis prevention trial: randomised trial of low intensity oral anticoagulation with warfarin and low dose aspirin in the primary prevention of ischaemic heart disease in men at increased risk. *Lancet* 1998; **315**: 233–41

41 Verheught FWA. Aspirin, the poor man's statin? *Lancet* 1998; **315**: 227–8

42 Standing Medical Advisory Committee. *The use of Statins.* London: Department of Health, 1997

43 Freemantle N, Barbour R, Johnson R, Marchment M, Kennedy A. The use of statins: a case of misleading priorities? National guidance that does not link costs and benefits is worthless. *BMJ* 1997; **315**: 826–8

44 NHS Centre for Reviews and Dissemination. Cholesterol and coronary heart disease: screening and treatment. *Bulletin on Effectiveness of Health Service Interventions for Decision Makers* 1998; **4**: 1–16

45 Charlton BG, Calvert N, White M *et al.* Health promotion priorities for general practice: constructing and using `indicative prevalences'. *BMJ* 1994; **308**: 1019–22

46 McInnes GT, McGhee SM. Delivery of care for hypertension. *J Hum Hypertens* 1995; **9**: 429–33

47 Allan K, Murphy P, Singleton S, Edwards R. Audit of diagnosis and management of hypertension in primary care. Interpractice variation in prevalence of hypertension is due to inadequate detection. *BMJ* 1997; **315**: 314

48 Jackson R, Barham P, Bills J *et al.* Management of raised blood pressure in New Zealand: a discussion document. *BMJ* 1993; **307**: 107–10

49 Fahey TP, Peters TJ. A general practice-based study examining the absolute risk of cardiovascular disease in treated hypertensive patients. *Br J Gen Pract* 1996; **46**: 655–70

50 Pharoah PDP, Hollingsworth W. Cost effectiveness of lowering cholesterol concentration with statins in patients with and without pre-existing coronary heart disease: life table method applied to health authority population. *BMJ* 1996; **312**: 1443–7

51 Grimley Evans J. Rationing health care by age. The case against. *BMJ* 1997; **314**: 822–5

52 Leese B, Bosanquet N. Family doctors and change in practice strategy since 1986. *BMJ* 1995; **310**: 705–8

53 Leese B, Bosanquet N. Change in general practice and its effects on service provision in areas with different socioeconomic characteristics. *BMJ* 1995; **311**: 546–50

54 Coulter A, Baldwin A. Survey of population coverage in cervical cancer screening in the Oxford region. *J R Coll Gen Pract* 1987; **37**: 441–3

55 Dickerson JE, Brown MJ. Influence of age on general practitioners' definition and treatment of hypertension. *BMJ* 1995; **310**: 574

56 Atri J, Falshaw M, Pereira F, Robson J. Ethnic and socioeconomic influences on recording of preventive care in selected inner London practices. *BMJ* 1996; **312**: 614–7.

57 Majeed FA, Cook DG, Given-Wilson R, Vecchi P, Poloniecki J. Do general practitioners influence the uptake of breast cancer screening? *J Med Screen* 1995; **2**: 119–24

58 Moser K. *Cervical Screening Uptake in East London Practices.* Department of General Practice, Queen Mary and Westfield College, London. City and East London General Practice Database, 1995

59 Bowling A, Jacobson B. Screening: the inadequacy of population registers. *BMJ* 1989; **298**: 545–6

60 Robson J, Falshaw M. Audit of preventive activities in 16 inner London practices using a validated measure of patient population, the `active patient' denominator. Healthy Eastenders Project. *Br J Gen Pract* 1995; **45**: 463–6

61 Roe L, Mant D, Coulter A. Screening: the inadequacy of population registers. *BMJ* 1989; **298**: 1100

62 Shroff KJ, Corrigan AM, Bosher M, Edmonds MP, Sacks D, Coleman DV. Cervical screening in an inner city area: response to a call system in general practice. *BMJ* 1988; **297**: 1317–8

63 Boomla K, Moser K, Naish J. Uptake of breast screening. Accurate addresses will improve uptake rates. *BMJ* 1995; **310**: 1004

64 Pierce M, Lundy S, Palanisamy A, Winning S, King J. Prospective randomised controlled trial of methods of call and recall for cervical cytology screening. *BMJ* 1989; **299**: 160–2

65 Ellman R, Chamberlain J. Improving the effectiveness of cervical cancer screening. *J R Coll Gen Pract* 1984; **34**: 537–42

66 Petrie JC, O'Brien ET, Littler WA, de Swiet M. Recommendations on blood pressure measurement. *BMJ* 1986; **293**: 611–5

67 O'Brien E. Will mercury manometers soon be obsolete? *J Hum Hypertens* 1995; **9**: 933–4

68 Fahey TP, Peters TJ. What constitutes controlled hypertension? Patient based comparison of hypertension guidelines. *BMJ* 1996; **313**: 93–6

69 Carson I, Martin E, Shepherd P. Health screening by a nurse in general practice. *BMJ* 1985; **290**: 1792

70 Hibble A. Practice nurse workload before and after the introduction of the 1990 contract for general practitioners. *Br J Gen Pract* 1995; **45**: 35–7

71 Stilwell B. The rise of the practice nurse. *Nurs Times* 1991; **87**: 26–8

72 Kenkre J, Drury VW, Lancashire RJ. Nurse management of hypertension clinics in general practice assisted by a computer. *Fam Pract* 1985; **2**: 17–22

73 Robson J, Boomla K, Fitzpatrick S *et al*. Using nurses for preventive activities with computer assisted follow up: a randomised controlled trial. *BMJ* 1989; **298**: 433–6

74 Mant D. Facilitating prevention in primary care. *BMJ* 1992; **304**: 652–3

75 Fullard E, Fowler G, Gray M. Promoting prevention in primary care: controlled trial of low technology, low cost approach. *BMJ* 1987; **294**: 1080–2

76 Dietrich AJ, O'Connor GT, Keller A, Carney PA, Levy D, Whaley FS. Cancer: improving early detection and prevention. A community practice randomised trial. *BMJ* 1992; **304**: 687–91

77 Eccles M, Clapp Z, Grimshaw J *et al*. North of England evidence based guidelines development project: methods of guideline development. *BMJ* 1996; **312**: 760–2

78 Benech I, Wilson AE, Dowell AC. Evidence-based practice in primary care: past, present and future. *J Eval Clin Pract* 1996; **2**: 249–63

79 Burr AJ. Comparing hypertension guidelines. Audit in Mid-Glamorgan also shows major problems with management of hypertension. *BMJ* 1996; **313**: 1203

80 Hay S, Oakeshott P. Clinical guidelines in primary care: a survey of general practitioners' attitudes and behaviour. *Br J Gen Pract* 1996; **46**: 626

81 Pringle M, Ward P, Chilvers C. Assessment of the completeness and accuracy of computer medical records in four practices committed to recording data on computer. *Br J Gen Pract* 1995; **45**: 537–41

82 Hayes GM. Computers in the consultation. The UK experience. *Proceedings of the Annual Symposium on Computer Applications in Medical Care* 1993; 103–106

83 Rudiman R, Gilbert FJ, Ritchie LD. Comparison of uptake of breast screening, cervical screening, and childhood immunisation. *BMJ* 1995; **310**: 229

84 Lewis J. Primary care – opportunities and threats. The changing meaning of the GP contract. *BMJ* 1997; **314**: 895–8

85 Langham S, Gillam S, Thorogood M. The carrot, the stick and the general practitioner: how have changes in financial incentives affected health promotion activity in general practice? *Br J Gen Pract* 1995; **45**: 665–8

86 Mant D, Fowler G. Urine analysis for glucose and protein: are the requirements of the new contract sensible? *BMJ* 1990; **300**: 1053–5

87 Iliffe S, Munro J. General practitioners and incentives. *BMJ* 1993; **307**: 1156–7

88 Gillam S, McCartney P, Thorogood M. Health promotion in primary care. *BMJ* 1996; **312**: 324–5

89 Hayward J. Promoting clinical effectiveness. *BMJ* 1996; **312**: 1491–2

90 Anonymous. *General Practice Morbidity Database Project*. Cardiff: Welsh Health Common Services Agency, 1996

91 Anonymous. *Somerset Morbidity Review*. Taunton: Somerset Health Authority, 1996

92 Anonymous. *Final report of the Wakefield and Pontefract Primary Care Information Project*. Wakefield: Wakefield Health Care, 1995

93 Anonymous. *Buckinghamshire Primary Health Care Computing Progress Report*. High Wycombe: Oxford Health Authority, 1994

94 Anonymous. *Developing Information Systems for Purchasers. Use of primary care data in support of commissioning*. Morpeth: Northumberland Health, 1994.

95 Gearing D. *Collecting Health Data in General Practice*. London: National Health Service Executive, 1997.

Quality assurance in screening programmes

J A Muir Gray and June Austoker

Institute of Health Sciences, Oxford, UK

All screening programmes do harm; some also do good. The responsibility of the policy-maker is to decide which programmes do more good than harm at reasonable cost and then introduce them, once they are confident that the screening programme could and will reach the standard of quality required for success. The ratio of benefit to harm is not, however, constant and this relationship demonstrates a shifting balance.

This shifting balance was first elegantly described by the guru of quality assurance, Avedis Donabedian[1]. Donabedian pointed out that the relationship between the amount of resources invested and the benefit resulting from them demonstrated the law of diminishing returns – namely, that there was a rapid rise in benefit when resources were first invested but a point was reached at which the incremental benefit for each increment invested grew smaller and the cost benefit curve flattened off. For example, the increase in benefit between 3 yearly and 5 yearly cervical screening is much less than the benefit between no screening and 5 yearly screening on the one hand, and much more than the added benefit from moving from 3 yearly to 1 yearly cervical screening on the other hand (Fig. 1).

However, Donabedian also pointed out that the relationship between the adverse effects of care and the beneficial effects was usually linear,

*Correspondence to:
Dr J A Muir Gray,
Director of Research and
Development, Institute of
Health Sciences,
Oxford OX3 7LF, UK*

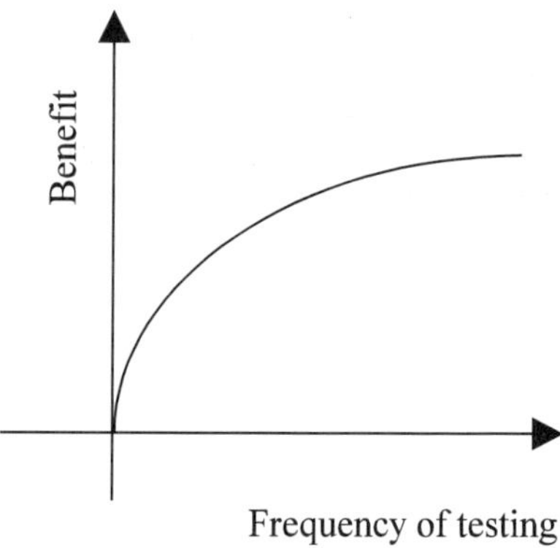

Fig. 1 Benefit as a function of frequency of testing.

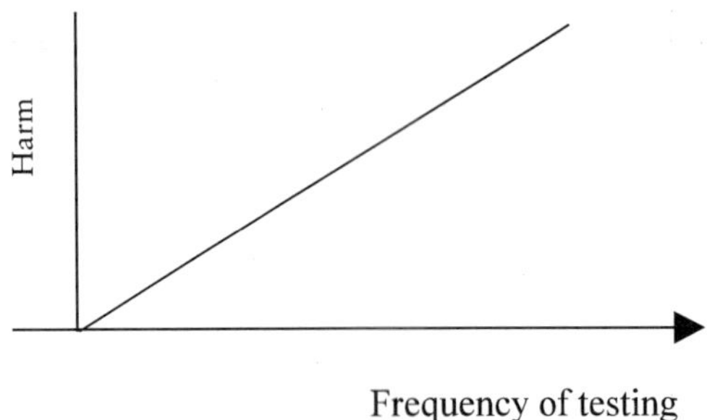

Fig. 2 The relationship between the adverse effects of care and the beneficial effects is usually linear.

namely the more people who receive a treatment, the more will have side effects (Fig. 2).

Thus any screening policy will have a balance of benefits to harms that varies depending upon the policy that is adopted. In cervical screening, the benefit to harm ratio for 5 yearly cervical screening is, all other things constants, more favourable than the benefit to harm ratio for 3 yearly screening, and that in turn is more favourable than the benefit to harm ratio for annual screening.

When other things are not equal

The relationship set out in Figures 1 and 2 is influenced by many factors, some of which, for example the incidence of the disease in the population, are outwith the control of the programme manager. However, the quality of the screening programme and, therefore, the size of the beneficial and adverse effects, is of central importance in determining the shape of both the cost benefit curve and the gradient of the straight line relationship between resources invested and adverse effects. The curve that is usually drawn by those advocating a screening programme is like that in Figure 1, but it is important to remember that those who are advocating a screening programme based on research results, are often basing this on the results obtained in research performed by dedicated and specialised teams working in a highly systematic and structured way.

Donabedian also pointed out the distinction between efficacy, namely the impact of a programme in ideal circumstances, and effectiveness, namely its impact in ordinary service settings. In the latter circumstance the benefits may be less and the harmful effects greater than in the research setting. In cervical cancer screening, for example, a lower quality programme has a higher rate of recall and, therefore, a higher

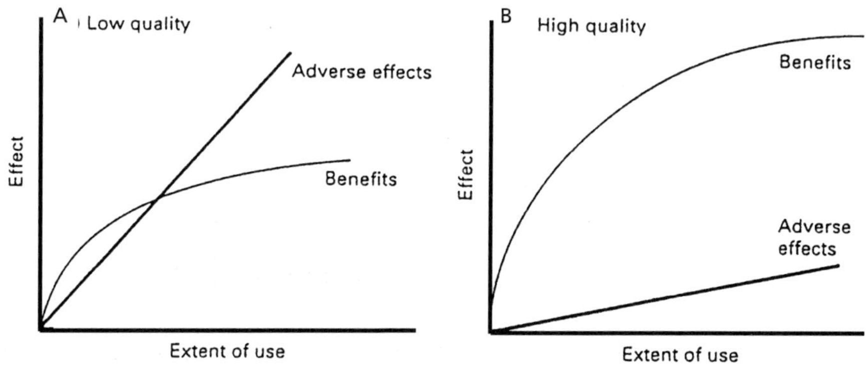

Fig. 3 Adverse effects can be greater than beneficial effects if the quality of screening is poor.

proportion of women are made anxious. Furthermore, the quality and, therefore, the balance of benefit to harm, may change with time. After some quality problems that may occur during the setting up of a programme have been overcome, quality may reach adequate levels but a new challenge may arise in years 6, 7 and 8 of a programme when the excitement of the programme launch is over and the steady grind and boredom of screening can take its toll.

When quality is low, the relationship between benefit and harm, at any level of screening intensity, changes, as shown in Figure 3, and it is possible for the harmful effects to be greater than the beneficial effects of screening. It is obviously essential, therefore, not only to choose the right screening policy but also to be assured that the screening actually offered is of high quality.

Quality jargon

Quality assurance has become an industry, for some people indeed a way of life, and like other such activities, has developed a language of its own. As with any language, differences in defining terms can lead to confusion and conflict, and it is appropriate at this stage to define how we use the jargon of quality.

'Quality control' was an early term and was, in its simplest form, the detection of quality failures, for example the identification and removal from an electric light bulb production line all the dud bulbs. Recognising that this had severe limitations, a more positive approach was developed which came to be called 'quality assurance' and which may be defined as all those activities designed not only to reduce the probability of quality failure but also to improve performance continuously. These two activities are distinct and different, albeit related. On the one hand, there is a need to ensure that quality failures do not occur. This in itself goes much further than the old concept of quality control which merely removed dud light bulbs from the production line, and includes, to extend the same example, the training of staff in the manufacture of light bulbs, the selection and use of the best materials for light bulb manufacture, and the adaptation and improvement of the conveyor belt itself to minimise failures arising during the process of production.

However, even this approach is not by itself sufficient, for it seems that it is the continuous and ceaseless drive to set higher and higher quality standards not only leads to high quality production but is the best insurance that quality failures will not occur. As the Japanese put it, unless quality standards and regulations are reviewed annually it is proof that they are not being used[2].

Different jargon is used by different people. One approach is to use the phrase 'quality assurance' for this whole range of activities; another is to talk of continuous quality improvement or total quality management. What is essential is the recognition that minimising the probability of failure is by itself insufficient and has to be complemented by measures which will lead to a continuous improvement in performance and a steady improvement in the standards by which quality is judged.

Lessons from industry

The history of industrial quality assurance is interwoven, like warp and woof, with the post-war history of Japan. Immediately after the Second World War, Japan was a byword for low quality and shoddy goods. Desperate for status and wealth, they listened and learned, in particular to the message of one man – Edward Demings. Demings was a classical prophet without honour in his own country, promoting his approach to quality assurance to US industry that was complacent and introverted in the balmy days of the 1950s. Rejected by his compatriots, Demings went to Japan and the managers there listened and learned. They adopted Demings' principles and the rest, as they say, is history[3].

Demings was not alone, and of course many companies and countries other than Japan adopted the principles of quality assurance and followed other gurus, for example Albert Juran. It was, however, Japan which took the quality revolution to its heart and some of the writings from Japan make fascinating and compelling reading, for example *Quality Control the Japanese Way* by Kaoru Ishigawa. Perhaps the most famous Japanese concept is Kaizen or continuous quality improvement[4]. The reasons why Japan became so successful are numerous and complicated. It is obvious that it is not necessary to be Japanese to be able to produce and sustain total quality management, for others have achieved it, but there is no country in which the approach has been adopted so fast by so many industries with such devastating results in industries and countries that did not get the message. Whatever happened to the Norton motorcycle, once the pride of British engineering?

Principles of quality assurance

It is possible to identify a number of principles that are common to quality assurance in any healthcare setting; a short list of principles is set out in Table 1. The terms 'quality' and 'effectiveness' are sometimes used interchangeably but, in this article, we are using the terms as distinct terms with different meanings. The **effectiveness** of an intervention or procedure or service is the degree to which it achieves desired objectives, while the **quality** of a service is the degree to which it conforms to pre-set standards of care.

Table 1 Principles of quality assurance

The primary responsibility for quality rests with the production worker, in health care the clinician.

Quality assurance systems aid, support and buttress production systems but are not simply a form of inspection.

Workers want to improve quality but need extra energy and skills to do so.

Vague exhortations, threats and blame are not effective quality improvement interventions.

Statistical methods should be used to measure performance and compare it with standards.

Quality assurance is a growth and not a control activity.

Quality assurance systems should cover all aspects of an organisation, including the process of management itself.

Quality assurance without consumer involvement is inadequate and incomplete.

Quality assurance focuses on systems and system failure, not on individuals and individual failure.

Developing systems and setting standards

Quality assessment by measuring the process of care

A standard is developed as part of a system of care, that system comprising a set of activities which have common objectives. The objectives for any service should be expressed in terms of the population

Table 2 Objectives on which the NHS Breast Screening Programme was planned

The aim of the programme is to reduce mortality from breast cancer in the population screened.

To identify and invite eligible women for mammographic screening.

To carry out mammography in a high proportion of those invited.

To provide services that are acceptable to those who receive them.

To follow up all women referred for further investigations.

To minimise the adverse effects of screening – anxiety, radiation and unnecessary investigations.

To diagnose cancers accurately.

To support and carry out research.

To make effective and efficient use of resources for the benefit of the whole population.

To enable those working in the programme to develop their skills and find fulfilment in their work.

To encourage the provision of effective acceptable treatment which has minimal psychological or functional side-effects.

To evaluate the service regularly and provide feedback to the population served.

served whenever possible, as demonstrated by the original objectives for the NHS Breast Screening Programme (Table 2). In a cervical screening programme, mortality rates from cervical cancer are the only measures required by those responsible for national policy but this outcome measure is not a good indicator of service quality for those responsible for 'local' services for two reasons. Firstly, changes in mortality rates are influenced by factors other than service quality, for example, changes in the incidence of cervical cancer. Secondly, changes in mortality rate reflect the quality of the service pertaining several years ago, whereas the manager or purchaser needs information about the current state of quality.

Outcomes are rarely of use in measuring quality. For any service, relevant healthcare activities need to be identified for each objective and the rate of delivery of these activities may be used to measure progress towards the objective. The healthcare activities chosen to indicate the rate of progress towards an objective were called process measures by Donabedian[1].

The processes measured should be those for which there is good evidence of effectiveness. For example, for an assessment of the quality of a maternity service, the proportion of women going into labour prematurely who were given antenatal steroids is an evidence-based process measure[5]. In assessing the quality of care received by those with acute myocardial infarction, the proportion of patients who receive streptokinase treatment within an hour of arriving at hospital is also an evidence-based process measure.

By using these evidence-based process measures, the performance of an individual or service can be defined; this is an objective assessment of what **is** being achieved. A standard is a subjective judgement of a level of performance that **could** be achieved. Different types of standard can be set.

Table 3 Setting achievable standards

Objectives	To cover the population who would benefit from cervical screening
Criteria	Percentage of women who have **not** had a hysterectomy who have had a readable smear in the last 5 years
Minimal standards	50%
Achievable standards	80%
Present position	1 out of 70 general practices less than 50%; 17 practices more than 80%
Year-end targets	70 general practices over 50%; 35 general practices over 80%

- The **minimum acceptable standard** is that below which no service should fall without urgent remedial action being taken.

- The **optimal standard** is the best level of service that can be achieved. Although this is a worthy standard, it is often achieved only by exceptional people and/or people working in exceptional circumstances. The optimal standard may be regarded by colleagues in other services as atypical and, therefore, of little use for motivating the majority of service providers.

- The **achievable standard** is that level of performance achieved by the top quartile of services. If one quartile of services can achieve a certain performance level, almost all services have the potential to do so.

A comparison of actual performance with the standard enables a target for quality improvement to be set. Targets are chosen arbitrarily, based on the target-setters' judgement of what constitutes a challenging but achievable goal. In selecting these targets, various factors are taken into account including: the past rate of improvement; the performance of other similar services, as well as any relevant changes, for example, the arrival of a new keen manager or the retirement of an older weary manager. Targets are best set by service providers with the advice of people responsible for quality assurance who may push the provider to set more challenging targets or, surprisingly often, rein in the provider's ambition and help them identify more modest but achievable targets. These elements can be combined into a system of care (Table 3).

Managing quality assurance

Quality assurance has to be managed with the same vigour and sensitivity as healthcare itself. For quality assurance to work, five preconditions are necessary (Table 4). Within the UK, the work of the National Screening Committee has revealed that, of the programmes

Table 4 Five preconditions for successful quality assurance

The right culture.

The existence of explicit standards of good performance.

An information system that allows each professional and programme to compare their performance with that of others and with the explicit standards.

Authority to take action if a quality problem is identified.

Clear lines of responsibility in managing the process of quality assurance itself.

currently on offer, only four have both a strong evidence base and satisfy these criteria, namely screening programmes for breast and cervical cancer, and the new-born screening programmes for congenital hypothyroidism and phenylketonuria.

It has been remarked that it appears paradoxical that the screening programmes with well developed quality assurance are the ones which receive most adverse publicity for quality failures, but the resolution of this paradox is obvious; without a quality assurance system, quality problems are not detected. Furthermore, it can be argued that unless quality problems were being detected regularly, it could be concluded either that the quality standards were too low and insufficiently exacting, or that the quality assurance system was not detecting quality failure. This is not the message that the media portray or the public perceives, illustrating the delicate relationship between quality assurance and the system whose quality is being assured on the one hand, and the professionals providing that service and the public on the other. Quality assurance systems are not thumbscrews that can be tightened and tightened; they are delicate systems which can have adverse as well as beneficial effects.

Benefits and harms of quality assurance

At first sight it might seem that quality assurance is only beneficial, but quality assurance can have adverse effects when applied to screening, particularly that type of screening in which the distinction between positive and negative rests solely on the perception of the observer.

When the distinction between a positive screening test and a negative screening test is based solely on a numerical value, quality assurance is relatively straight forward and free from individual bias. Where, however, the distinction between positive and negative rests solely on the perception of the individual in, for example, mammography, the reading of cervical smears, or the interpretation of the Ortolani-Barlow test for hips, a quality assurance system can shift the threshold of the screener usually to increase sensitivity while at the same time increasing the false positive rate.

Imagine working in a cervical screening laboratory when a press story about cases that are 'missed' breaks; imagine that the press are interested in your laboratory. The emphasis is always on 'missed' cases, and the pressure is always to identify the individual who has not identified the positive smear. Three things can happen, sometimes simultaneously. One is that the laboratory staff may increase the proportion of smears deemed unreadable, unwilling to commit themselves on a doubtful smear and preferring to ask for a repeat smear rather than make a decision that the smear is negative. Secondly, where there is any doubt at all, the screener may find it more reassuring to classify the smear as positive rather than negative. Thirdly, the screener may request a more rapid recall, for example one year recall instead of a customary three year recall.

Pressure from media interest or the quality assurance system itself can lead to increases in the rate of inadequate smears, the false positive rate and the proportion of women deemed 'at risk' and recalled at shorter intervals. All of these trends have adverse effects on both the women in the population screened and on the laboratory staff. The experience of the women screened has been clearly documented. The experience of the laboratory staff has not yet been adequately documented but the problems of recruitment and retention of staff can be increased by these types of pressure.

Returning to the first principles

Screening programmes present a daunting challenge to managers. Members of the public, perhaps remembering what now seems an old-fashioned concept of zero defect manufacturing as a principle in quality control, assume that the well-managed screening programme will have neither false positives nor false negatives (Fig. 4). Because there is no screening test that is 100% sensitive and 100% specific, this is impossible and the screening programme manager must, like Blondin inching his way across Niagara Falls, lean neither to one side nor the other.

As a consequence, it is all too easy to develop increasingly complicated and prescriptive quality assurance programmes. There may come a point, however, at which increased investment in quality assurance will be counter-productive if it results in those who actually have to deliver the screening service becoming anxious or defensive or demoralised. Screeners who become defensive or anxious can all too easily change screening criteria, albeit unconsciously, leading usually to an increase in the false positive rate and, therefore, the proportion of people who are screened who are made anxious. It is important to remember that

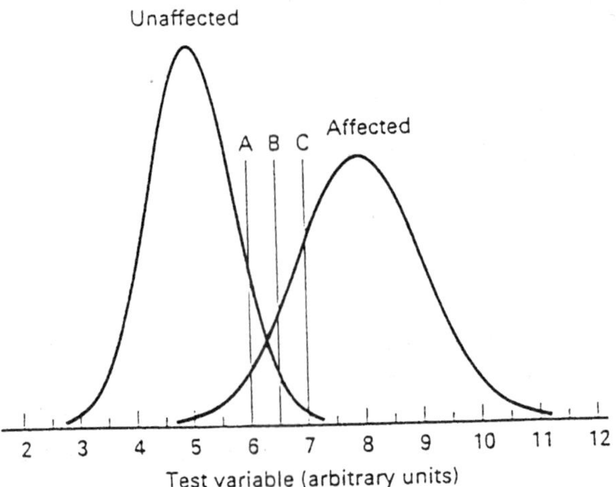

Fig. 4 Hypothetical example of the detection rate and false positive rate of a screening test at three different cut off levels, A, B and C.

screening programmes are lifetime experiences for those who are screened, with a cumulative chance of having a false positive test result increasing with each screening round.

Furthermore, it is important to appreciate that when quality assurance is introduced, quality problems are revealed. This is an inevitable consequence of quality assurance and the screening programme with quality assurance in place receives more adverse publicity than the screening programme with no quality assurance in place in which no-one can be below standard. As a result of this, those involved in screening may find themselves criticised by either national media or, just as distressing, by the newspapers provided to the population they are serving. The lesson the Japanese have taught us above all others is that the responsibility for quality rests not with an inspector or a quality manager but with the person responsible for producing the product or delivering the service, and all quality assurance should be developmental and not inspectorial if it, like screening, is to do more good than harm.

References

1   Donabedian A. The definition of quality: a conceptual exploration. In: Explorations in Quality Assessment and Monitoring. Vo I: The definition of quality and approaches to its assessment. Ann Arbor: Health Administration Press, 1980
2   Ishikawa K. What is Total Quality Control? Englewood Cliffs, NJ: Prentice Hall, 1985
3   Walton M. The Deming Management Method. London: Mercury Books, 1989
4   Imai M. Kaizen: the Key to Japan's Competitive success. New York: McGraw-Hill, 1986
5   Crowley PA. Corticosteroids prior to Preterm Delivery. The Cochrane Library (database on disk and CDROM). The Cochrane Collaboration, Oxford: Update Software, 1998 (updated quarterly)

The economic perspective

Jackie Brown and **Martin Buxton**

Health Economics Research Group, Brunel University, Middlesex, UK

The rationale for the economic perspective on screening is presented and the particular relevance of economic evaluation highlighted. The principles of economic evaluation are described in terms of measuring and valuing the costs and outcomes associated with screening. The different types of economic evaluation are described with discussion of data sources. The problematic issues associated with time preferences and discounting and with the measurement and valuation of outcomes other than true positives are discussed. Issues associated with antenatal screening, in particular the inclusion of averted costs due to the termination of an affected pregnancy and the inclusion and valuation of the unborn child's utility, are also raised.

Rationale for the economic perspective

The principles of screening formulated by Wilson and Junger[1] three decades ago are still used as a basis for reviewing the evidence for screening programmes[2,3]. These criteria, and other modifications of these original criteria[4,5], encompass the need for economic evaluation of screening programmes in that they recognise the economic costs of the programme have to be considered in relation to the benefits of early detection. They do not, however, provide any formal structure for undertaking an assessment of the benefits and costs of introducing a screening programme. Economic principles are being increasingly applied as part of the formal evaluation of health care interventions, and methods for such assessments have been developed and refined.

Today there is widespread acceptance of the need to address the economic question, specifically whether the benefits of a proposed or existing intervention are sufficient to justify that particular use of scarce health care resources. The use of any scarce resources, be they manpower, buildings or equipment, has an opportunity cost in terms of the benefits foregone by denying those resources to other competing claims. Choices, sometimes harsh choices, have to be made in all health

*Correspondence to:
Dr Jackie Brown, Health
Economics Research
Group, Brunel
University, Uxbridge,
Middlesex UB8 3PH, UK*

care systems: none can offer patients and public all technically feasible, or even all potentially beneficial interventions[6].

Economics is concerned principally with allocating resources efficiently. Efficiency is not about cost cutting, but about making choices which derive the maximum total benefit from the finite resource available. In the same way as evidence-based medicine stresses the need to use the best available formal evidence on effectiveness, rather than relying simply on educated guesses or 'gut feelings' to make individual treatment decisions, health economics emphasises the need to assess formally the implications of choices over the deployment of resources. A number of economic evaluation techniques have been developed to aid this formal assessment and to help identify the most efficient allocation of resources.

Economic evaluation is particularly relevant to screening for a number of reasons. Firstly, screening is discretionary: the case for intervention can be made relatively dispassionately in the light of the probabilistic expectation of benefit to a proportion of those screened. Screening is not normally subject to the pressures from the social 'rule of rescue'. Most individuals offered screening are well and it is not possible to distinguish at the outset those individuals who have the potential to benefit from treatment. In contrast, treatment of symptomatic patients offers the potential of immediate benefit to those who are identifiably 'ill'. Secondly, within any one screening programme a number of different strategies for screening exist. Each of these can be informed by economic evaluation. For example, choices have to be made as to the tests or screening technologies to use, the thresholds to use, and hence the specificity and sensitivity of the test, the frequency of screening, age at screening, and whether the screening test should be used universally or selectively in a group identified on the basis of known risk factors.

Thirdly, formal screening programmes require substantial investment and infrastructures. Decisions about screening programmes tend to be made, in the UK at least, at national, or regional level, rather than at the level of the individual practitioner. As a result, a number of examples of economic evaluation being undertaken to support policy decisions relate to screening. For example, decisions about whether to introduce breast screening in a number of European countries have been informed and influenced by analyses of its likely cost-effectiveness[7,8]. In the UK National Health Service Breast Screening Programme, the number of mammography views taken at a woman's prevalent screen have been influenced by the findings of economic analyses[9,10]. Indeed, one of the earliest examples in the UK was the decision to abandon the routine use of mass-miniature radiography screening for tuberculosis, a decision supported by an economic analysis showing that screening was no longer cost-effective with changes in prevalence and improved therapy[11].

Economic evaluation can contribute to decisions about whether a new screening programme for a particular disease or disorder should be introduced, and can also aid decisions about changes to existing programmes. It should be recognised, however, that economic evaluation is a way of structuring, measuring and valuing the expected consequences of alternative courses of action. It is an aid to decision making, but criteria other than efficiency will also be relevant when making value judgements as to whether or not to provide a particular screening programme. In particular, issues of equity, which are not formally addressed in most economic analyses, may have an important impact on decisions.

Principles underlying the economic evaluation of screening programmes

Economic analysis is concerned with systematically comparing both the resource use consequences (or costs) and non-resource use consequences (or outcomes) of alternative courses of action. These may be alternative screening strategies, a comparison of formal screening with the current policy, or, where no current screening policy exists, with the *status quo* or 'no screening' scenario. The precise methods used to identify, measure and value costs and outcomes will depend on the specific screening context, the particular economic question being posed, and the form of analysis adopted to answer that question. A number of broad principles exist that govern the way costs and outcomes are usually handled, and these are set out in detail in a number of texts and guidance manuals[12–16]. The following sections highlight some key issues in the measurement and valuation of costs and health outcomes which are important in understanding the application of economic evaluation to screening.

Measuring and valuing the costs

The resource costs relevant to an economic evaluation are those incurred and those avoided as a result of undertaking a particular programme. The perspective adopted in a particular study will determine how widely the net of costs is cast. Typically economic evaluation studies adopt a broad societal perspective, and aim to estimate all important costs no matter on which bodies or individuals they fall. This is particularly important when examining the resource consequences of a screening programme, since the burden of resource provision and the benefit of resource savings may fall on sectors of society other than the health service, such as social, educational or voluntary services.

Whatever the perspective adopted, direct costs associated with organising and operating a screening programme, such as the labour involved and the equipment and facilities, need to be estimated. While the cost per individual screened may be relatively small, the total cost of the programme may be substantial. In the case of a cervical screening programme, for example, this would include the costs associated with recruiting women to the programme; taking, transporting and reading the smears; the costs associated with informing women of the results and, for the suspected cases detected (the screen positives) the costs of further confirmatory diagnosis and treatment. In part these costs may be offset by the savings in health service costs associated with a reduced number of patients requiring diagnosis and radical treatment at a later date.

One argument often given in favour of screening is the expectation of cost savings associated with reducing the amount of treatment of advanced diseases. In the case of breast screening, for example, it was estimated in a Dutch study that 47% of the costs of screening would be offset by cost savings in the treatment of advanced disease[17]. Others have been much more conservative in their estimate[18], the differences being due to different treatment patterns. The potential savings to the health service due to the reduction in advanced disease and mortality, as a result of a mass cervical screening programme was found to be relatively small compared to the total cost of the screening programme, offsetting 10% of the costs of screening plus the incremental cost of diagnosis and treatment of primary disease[19].

Screening also imposes resource costs directly on the individuals concerned. Individuals are likely, for example, to incur out-of-pocket expenses on travel and other costs (for example, child care) when they, or a member of their family, attend for screening. Individuals will also incur indirect costs in terms of the value of their time devoted to attending for screening: they may forgo productive time at work or forgo time pursuing leisure activities or doing household tasks[20–23]. A recent study showed that the costs incurred by the individuals' attending for breast screening or for further assessment following screening were of similar magnitude to those incurred by the health service[23,24]. Costs incurred by individuals are likely to have an important effects on behaviour, particularly attendance rates need to be considered carefully, if only to begin to understand and to be able to influence take-up of screening services[25].

If a broad societal perspective is adopted these private costs should be included in the costs of screening. Direct valuation of these costs using earnings as a measure of the opportunity cost of the time spent being screened is controversial and raises important distributional issues[12]. For example, with this approach the time lost by an active male in the work force would be valued more highly than time lost by the elderly. Less controversial in a societal costing are the differences in 'care' costs falling on services other than health, for example social services or education, as a result of the reduction in disability brought about by screening.

In measuring costs, it is important to focus on the difference in costs between the options under consideration. Thus, if the policy question is whether or not to increase the frequency of screening, the costs identified should be the net additional cost of the greater frequency compared with the lesser frequency. The principle underlying costing for economic studies is to identify and measure resource use, by estimating the quantities of the resource inputs that are used in the intervention, such as the hours of particular types of manpower, use of specific equipment, types and quantities of drugs, other consumables, and applying appropriate unit costs to these units of resource. Resource use is usually valued using market prices, but adjustments may be necessary, for example, where resources are subsidised by a third party[12]. Some unit costs will be readily available from published sources and others will need to be estimated in the context of a specific study.

In some situations, this cost calculation will be complicated by the existence of spare capacity. For example, if a local mammography service was operating below capacity, the incremental cost of screening a small additional cohort is likely to be less than the existing average cost per screen, since the current average costs will already include the costs of some specialised equipment and staff which may not need to be increased to accommodate a small increase in the number screened. Estimated costs need to reflect a particular context and question, and may well differ significantly between screening centres[26].

Measuring and valuing outcomes

Economics is not simply about costs, but about the relationship between costs and outcomes. The identification and measurement of non-cost consequences is usually the conceptually most challenging issue. Screening programmes have a number of health and non-health related effects depending on whether the result of the screen is positive or negative and whether this result is true or false.

Typically, economic studies have focused on the outcomes associated with true positive findings. The major change in outcomes associated with screening will be experienced by this group. While the identification of a true positive case can be used as a measure of screening outcome, the value of this approach will depend upon the impact of early detection or diagnosis of the condition on future life expectancy and/or quality of life. For most screening situations, true positive results will bring forward the time of detection and allow earlier treatment. In the case of non life-threatening conditions, such as hearing loss in childhood, earlier treatment is associated with improved future quality of life. In the case of screening programmes for conditions which are life threatening, such as cancer, or abdominal aortic aneurysms, the main outcome would be reduced mortality, although quality of life may also be affected. In both situations, improvements in quality of life are experienced mainly by the individuals concerned, but may also have implications for the quality of life of immediate family and close friends. Economic evaluation requires evidence that screening is effective in identifying true positive cases, as well as evidence that earlier diagnosis and treatment results in better long-term outcome.

However, there are likely to be other health outcomes from a screening programme. False negative screening results may not simply fail to bring forward detection, but may provide false reassurance, thereby delaying subsequent clinical diagnosis. Thus, for some individuals, there may be a measurable reduction in survival and quality of life that needs to be set against the gains experienced by individuals who are true positives.

The most immediate and widespread impact of screening may be in terms of anxiety and or reassurance. A positive screening result will inevitably be received with negative feelings, whereas a negative result is usually reassuring[27]. However, anxiety may be experienced as a result of receiving an invitation for screening, attending the screen and the follow-up examination. This anxiety may be short-lived if the results are negative, but may remains for several months, or in some cases years, after a false positive result[28,29]. Anxiety may also be experienced by non-attenders[30]. In adults, most of these anxieties will be experienced by the individual being screened, although they may have implications for family and friends. In addition, there may be some pain or discomfort directly associated with the test or screen[31], and there may be small, but potentially important, risks associated with screening, for example from a radiation dose.

Information gained from a screening test may be valued even where it does not affect prognosis or subsequent treatment. For example, parents may value the information regarding the risk to their fetus of a specific disorder, even though they have no intention of terminating the pregnancy[32].

Thus, a number of health states are likely to be experienced by the target population of a screening programme and, in some cases, their families. Moreover, different individuals will not necessarily experience the same health state. How such outcomes of a health care programme are measured and valued in an economic evaluation will depend on the technique used.

Methods of economic evaluation

Economic evaluations are generally categorised into four main types: cost-minimisation; cost-effectiveness analysis; cost-benefit analysis; and cost-utility analysis. Each technique, or form of analysis handles costs in the same manner: resource use is identified, measured and then valued in monetary terms. The techniques differ, however, in how they measure and value the non-resource use consequences of alternative actions[12]. Equally important is the nature and source of the evidence available on which to base these analyses. There is often a tension between the clinical science pressures to use only evidence directly obtained from clinical trials and the economist's need to model a broader picture of the consequences of interventions than such trials typically provide.

Forms of economic analysis

Cost-minimisation analysis is the simplest form. It is relevant only when there is good evidence, usually from previously published studies, to indicate that the outcomes of the alternatives being evaluated are the same in all important respects. This might be the case in comparing two different tests with identical sensitivity and specificity or alternative logistic arrangements for running a screening service. In such restricted circumstances, it is only necessary to compare the resource use, and hence costs, of the alternatives. It then makes obvious economic sense to implement the least costly alternative. In most circumstances, however, the outcomes will differ in some way and then a technique that can consider differences in both costs and outcomes is required.

Cost-benefit analysis is, in principle, the most comprehensive technique available. The criterion of efficiency is based upon a comparison of the value placed on the outcome of implementing a new programme, or changes to an existing programme, with that placed on the resource use implications. Thus, an efficient programme is one whereby the value placed on the outcome exceeds the value of the resource consumed. Where there are multiple alternatives under comparison, the implication is that priority should be given to the one with the greatest net value. This technique requires that the outcomes of a programme (for example, improvements in quality of life and survival gains) are valued in the same unit of account as resources, *i.e.* in monetary units. Methods to obtain monetary outcome values exist, such as 'willingness to pay' and these have been used, for example in the context of antenatal screening for cystic fibrosis[33], but are generally considered experimental[12]. Thus, despite the common use of the term cost-benefit analysis, in practice true cost benefit studies are rarely undertaken to evaluate health care programmes because of the practical difficulty and the social dislike of putting monetary values on life and suffering.

Cost-effectiveness analysis attempts to avoid this problem by defining the outcome or 'effectiveness' of a health care programme in terms of natural units. Ideally the outcome measure should be all embracing, and must at least capture the main objective of the programme. No attempt is made to value this outcome. In assessing screening programmes, process measures such as the proportion of cases detected are often used as the measure of effectiveness[21,22,34]. In the case of antenatal screening, reproductive choice over the outcome of an affected pregnancy could be seen as an appropriate measure of effectiveness[35].

It obviously makes economic sense to implement the programme which costs less and is at least as effective as the alternative, or which costs the same but is more effective than the alternative. These so-called situations of dominance are, however, relatively rare. What is more usual is for one alternative to cost more but also to be somewhat more effective. The additional costs and effects of a programme are then presented in terms of an incremental cost-effectiveness ratio, such as the additional cost per additional case detected. This raises the question as to what is an acceptable incremental cost-effectiveness ratio. An indication of what has been acceptable historically is useful but a value judgement has to be made as to what a decision-maker or society as whole is willing to pay for an additional unit of effect.

Cost-effectiveness analysis can be useful for determining technical efficiency, *i.e.* the most efficient way of delivering a particular programme, such as which test to use in a screening programme. It may also be useful for comparing alternative programmes whose effects can be measured in the same units. However, it is more limited than cost-benefit analysis since comparison cannot be made across health care programmes where different outcome measures are used. Moreover it is unlikely that all the important outcomes are captured by a uni-dimensional measure of effectiveness.

Cost-utility analysis attempts to provide a broader comparability between different programmes than cost-effectiveness analysis by measuring the health effects of all programmes in a generic unit. Effectively, it is a special case of cost-effectiveness analysis whereby a programme's effects are measured in terms of utility. Utility reflects the preferences of individuals or society and, in the context of health care appraisal, refers to the relative value placed on a specific health status or an improvement in health status. The most common measure of utility used in such analyses is the quality adjusted life year or QALY. It incorporates both the programme's impact on survival as well as health related quality of life. The quality of life associated with a health state is measured on a scale of zero to one, where death is assigned a value of zero and full health is assigned a value of one. A number of techniques exist to elicit utility values for specific health states. These techniques include the time trade-off and standard gamble[12,36]. The duration of each health state is then weighted, or multiplied, by its utility value. Where options lead to a series of health states, the weighted durations are summed to give the number of quality adjusted life years.

Where outcomes are multi-dimensional, as in the case of screening, QALYs may be more useful than uni-dimensional natural units used in cost-effectiveness analysis. As with cost-effectiveness analysis, it obviously makes economic sense to implement the programme which costs less and is at least as effective as the alternative, or which costs the same but is more effective. Where this is not the case, the additional costs and effects of a programme are then presented in terms of an incremental cost-utility ratio, such as the additional cost per QALY gained. Again this raises the question as to what is an acceptable incremental cost-utility ratio.

Cost-utility analysis is useful for addressing the most efficient way of providing a particular programme, that is technical efficiency. More controversially, QALYs can also be used to help judge relative priorities across different health care programmes. Programmes can be ranked according to their incremental (additional) cost per QALY gained and, in the context of a fixed budget for health care, those programmes offering additional QALYs at lowest additional cost per QALY should be given priority. In the UK, for example, the additional cost per QALY for breast screening, as recommended by the Forrest report[7], was estimated to be £3309. This was compared with the cost per QALY gained for various other health care procedures and found to fall somewhere between the cost per QALY for kidney transplant and heart transplant. It was argued that the cost per QALY gained for breast screening was not dissimilar from other health service activities undertaken at the time.

One of the main implications of these so-called 'QALY league tables' is that as the only output of the health service is health, health outcomes are the only outcomes arising from the resource use considered in these tables. This means that resource use from outside the health budget and non health outcomes, such as the productivity gains referred to earlier, are difficult to incorporate into such tables. Reservations have also been expressed with regards to the quality of data used in such studies and the difficulties of comparing studies undertaken in different years. Analysts have also been criticised for not providing an adequate account of the incremental analysis undertaken. In addition, individual cost-utility studies are often locally specific as the appropriate comparator for the decision making context may differ between localities. It may also be inappropriate to transfer results to another area if, for example, the incidence and prevalence of the disease or level of service differs between two areas. Caution has to be exercised when using such tables[37-39]. It should, nonetheless, be recognised that resource allocation does take place and that QALYs can be used to aid such decisions, but they should be viewed as being indicative rather than determinate.

Furthermore, it is not possible to conduct a cost-utility analysis if data on the effectiveness of final outcomes are not available and it is unnecessary if the programmes under comparison are all equally effective, or quality of life can be captured in easily understood natural units, or the results cannot be altered by the use of utility values[36].

Sources of data: trials and modelling

Economic evaluation requires good evidence on outcomes, and is often limited by the lack of evidence on clinical outcomes. For example, it is not possible to conclude whether or not screening for prostate cancer is cost-effective because there is a lack of data on the effectiveness of available screening tests and treatment options for the early detected cancers[40]. The decision not to recommend prostate cancer screening at the present time in the UK is based on lack of proven effectiveness, rather than on cost considerations[29].

Ideally, the evidence on effectiveness of screening should come from population-based prospective randomised controlled trials. Such trials would ideally be long-term to trace the survival and quality of life effects of earlier detection. This implies that they need to be large, if differences in mortality are to be estimated with reasonable confidence. Ideally, economic and psychological evaluations are incorporated into the trial design, so allowing relevant data to be collected on the outcomes and resource use from individuals participating in the trial. This is the case in a UK randomised trial investigating the effectiveness of undertaking ultrasound screening of 65 year old men to identify asymptomatic abdominal aortic aneurysms. This trial, involving 66,000 men who are being followed for 5 years, will cost approximately £4.5 million.

Possibilities for setting up such trials are infrequent, not least because of the costs entailed. For some situations, the length of follow-up required may need to be even greater, and the sample size even larger, than that cited above. Where a clinical trial is not feasible, or it is not practical to incorporate an economic evaluation into a clinical trial, available data can be synthesised using modelling techniques. In such circumstances it is likely that estimates of costs and outcomes will be subject to greater uncertainty than where data comes directly from an appropriate trial in a relevant population. Sensitivity analysis can be used to establish whether the results are sensitive to uncertainty or variation in the values of key parameters, and to assess the potential significance of parameters for which no reliable estimates are available.

Even when economic evaluation has been incorporated in a clinical trial, some modelling is likely to be necessary to allow for differences between the trial participants and the target population, to extrapolate from short-term outcomes to long-term survival and quality of life, or to estimate QALYs using a combination of within trial classification of health states and externally generated utility values[41]. Modelling studies undertaken before a clinical trial is initiated can help identify the key parameters that need to be estimated within the planned trial[42]. They can also ensure that there is a reasonable prospect that the screening programme in question will prove cost-effective, and hence be of policy interest, and can help to show the likely value of undertaking the planned research study[43].

Problematic issues for the economic evaluation of screening

Dealing with time preferences and discounting

Economic evaluation takes into account the timing of costs and outcomes. This is because both as individuals and collectively as a society we are not indifferent to when costs or benefits arise. We exhibit a degree of 'positive time preference'. That is to say that individuals and society prefer resources now rather than later and would prefer to postpone costs. This time preference is evidenced by the existence of real interest rates (after allowing for inflation) paid on money saved. This is allowed for in economic evaluation by 'discounting' future costs to estimate their 'present value' to us now. The rate of discount will vary between societies and over time. Currently in the UK, the Treasury recommends a rate of 6% per annum for discounting cost of public sector projects[44], and internationally a rate of 5% is common[45].

What is less clear is the degree of time preference that relates to health benefits, measured for example as years of life or QALYs gained. Evidence suggests that both individuals and societies exhibit time preference for such benefits[46], preferring them sooner rather than later, but the degree of preference that should be reflected in economic evaluation is still controversial[47]. Traditionally the argument has been to discount benefits at the same rate as costs, but in the light of recent debate the Department of Health now recommends that life years and QALYs should be discounted at 1.5–2%[48,49].

The discount rate for costs and benefits is of great significance for screening, where invariably the costs will occur before the outcomes, and where sometimes the benefits may only arise after several decades. For example, in a Dutch study, the total number of life years gained from cervical screening was estimated to be 68,300 without discounting. After discounting at a rate of 7%, the number of life years gained was reduced to 7,900, 12% of the undiscounted life years gained. On the other hand, the total additional costs amounted to 510 million Dutch Florins (DFL) before discounting and were reduced 277 million DFL after discounting at a rate of 7%, amounting to 54% of the undiscounted costs[50]. The higher the rate of discount applied to benefits the less attractive screening will appear, particularly when compared with those treatment interventions that give immediate benefits. This means that when evaluating screening, analysts should use sensitivity analysis to examine the impact of different and differential discount rates. Similarly, those considering economic evidence should check carefully the discount rates applied in individual studies.

Valuing outcomes other than true positives

While there may be health outcomes and other non-cost consequences associated with the offer of screening, economic evaluations, in common with most clinical studies, have tended to focus on the main health effects for true positives. Many cost-effectiveness studies simply measure cost per case detected[21,22,34,51,52], while those that estimate mortality and quality of life often do so only for the detected cases[7,53,54].

This may be an adequate approximation if other effects are very small. While anxieties and other effects associated with the invitation and screening test may be short lived, they may affect a large number of individuals and this could have significant implications for the cost-effectiveness of a screening programme[27,29]. Potentially economic evaluation in terms of QALYs provides a metric in which the balance of these various effects can be judged.

The problem is that in practice our measurement instruments for utility are generally not sufficiently refined to be sure that we can reliably measure the small but real degree of disutility associated with temporary increases in anxiety that may be associated with many programmes. Some research has been undertaken to explore the use of willingness to pay and conjoint analysis to measure the relative values respondents place on aspects of services other than health effects, such as the informational value[55-58], but these approaches are still essentially in development.

However, as there is increasing debate about the limitations of screening programmes and more reservations are expressed about their possible harmful effects[27,29], the omission of an estimate of these effects in most economic studies will become less acceptable. The issue should have a priority in any research agenda concerned with making economic evaluation more relevant to the policy questions relating to screening.

The particular case of antenatal screening

The cost implications of screening pregnant women for conditions which might affect their fetus are generally more complex than for programmes which screen individuals for conditions which might only affect those individuals. Antenatal screening raises the issue of saved resources, or averted costs, associated with the termination of affected pregnancies. Had the affected pregnancy not been detected through screening and terminated, costs would have been incurred throughout the affected child's lifetime to treat the condition for which it was screened. These are costs over and above the cost of a 'replacement' child without the condition[59]. If a health service perspective is adopted, the excess costs avoided can be considered equivalent to the health service costs of treating the condition which would otherwise have been detected clinically at a later stage. When comparing the costs of a universal antenatal screening programme with a selective antenatal programme, averted costs are only associated with those additional affected pregnancies identified and terminated as a consequence of the universal screening programme. These additional affected pregnancies, and the costs associated with them, would otherwise have been missed by a selective programme. When comparing a universal or selective antenatal screening programme with a policy of no screening, all terminated pregnancies are associated with an averted cost since the affected children would otherwise all have been detected at a later stage.

Analysts often feel morally uncomfortable about including the resource savings due to terminating a life. These averted cost are thus often excluded without explanation, or with an explanation which may be confused. For example, in a study looking at the cost-effectiveness of antenatal screening for Down syndrome, the savings associated with lifetime care were excluded on the basis that the objective of screening was not to save the costs of care, but to give couples the opportunity of choosing not to have a child with a severe abnormality[60]. The savings associated with lifetime care are, however, nothing to do with the outcome or non-resource use consequences of the programme, but part of the resource or cost implications.

Saved or averted costs can also be associated with those affected pregnancies which are detected early by antenatal screening but are not terminated. Here the saved or averted costs relate to cost reductions due to improved prognosis achieved as a result of the early detection of an affected newborn, *i.e.* the difference in cost between treating an early and late detected case.

Not all conditions, however, will be associated with averted costs due to the improved prognosis of an early detected affected case. The treatment for thalassaemia, for example, is not altered through early detection. In addition, for some conditions it might be that early detected cases actually cost more because the individual survives longer.

When the resource use implications for other sectors of society are considered the issue becomes more complicated: for example, the avoided excess costs associated with educational and institutional care, would need to be considered, as well as the costs of voluntary services and care incurred by the family. Furthermore, the implementation of antenatal screening may affect family size by dissuading couples from having further children, in which case, it could be argued that the cost of caring for these children is saved. Alternatively, it may actually encourage the conception and birth of unaffected children who would otherwise not have been born, as a result of the clearer indication of risk given to couples, as well as the opportunity to terminate an affected fetus[61].

Some analyses have considered outcome only in terms of the number of affected pregnancies and resource use only up to the detection of those affected pregnancies[51,62]. Whilst, arguably, this approach handles outcomes and resource use symmetrically, it provides neither an adequate measure of the true effect (what happens as a result of the identification of affected pregnancies) nor the full resource implications of instituting a programme of screening.

As discussed earlier, the use of the proportion of cases detected through screening as a measure of outcome is limited in as much as it does not capture all the important outcomes. This is particularly true in the case of antenatal screening, where a number of individuals are likely to be affected by screening. Antenatal screening has implications for the existing family, as well as for the future life of an affected fetus. Although this raises practical difficulties, particularly in whether and how to include the utilities of the unborn child, in theory these would be best captured in a cost-utility analysis where the QALYs associated with the different individuals are summed and the lifetime costs averted considered[59].

Thus, although economic evaluation is particularly relevant to screening, it raises several important and challenging issues which are mainly related to outcome measurement and valuation and where further research is needed. Even where such problems exist, explicit and well presented economic analysis can help to illuminate the difficult policy decisions that have to be made.

References

1 Wilson JMG, Junger G. *Principles and Practice of Screening for Disease.* Geneva: World Health Organization, 1968

2 Seymour CA, Thomason MJ, Lord J, Chalmers RA *et al.* Newborn screening for inborn errors of metabolism: a systematic review. *Health Technol Assess* 1977; **1**(11)

3 Snowden SK, Stewart-Brown S. *Preschool Vision Screening: results of a systematic review.* York: NHS Centre for Reviews and Dissemination, CRD Report 9, 1997

4 Cuckle HS, Wald NJ. Principles of screening. In: Wald NJ. (ed) *Antenatal and Neonatal Screening.* Oxford: Oxford University Press, 1984

5 Holland WW. Screening for disease. Taking stock. *Lancet* 1974; **ii**: 1494–7

6 Buxton M. Scarce resources and informed choices. In: Ashton D, (ed) *Future Trends in Medicine.* London: Royal Society of Medicine Press, 1993; 36–9

7 Forrest APM. *Breast Cancer Screening: report to the health ministers of England, Wales and Scotland.* London: HMSO, 1986

8 Health Committee. *Breast Cancer Services. Third report,* Vol 1. London: HMSO, 1994–

9 NHS Executive. *Quality in the National Health Service Breast Screening Programme.* Leeds: Quarry House, 1995

10 Wald NJ, Murphy P, Major P, Parkes C, Townsend J, Frost C. UKCCCR multicentre randomised controlled trial of one and two view mammography in breast cancer screening. *BMJ* 1995; **311**: 1189–93

11 Pole JD. Mass radiology: a cost/benefit approach. In: McLachlan G., (ed) *Problems and Progress in Medical Care.* London: Oxford University Press, 1971; 46–55

12 Drummond MF, O'Brien B, Stoddart GL, Torrance GW. *Methods for the Evaluation of Health Care Programmes.* Oxford: Oxford University Press, 1997

13 Russell LB, Gold MR, Siegel JE, Daniels N, Weinstein MC; for the Panel on Cost-Effectiveness in Health and Medicine. The role of cost-effectiveness analysis in health and medicine. *JAMA* 1996; **276**: 1172–7

14 Weinstein MC, Siegel JE, Gold MR, Kamlet MS, Russell LB; for the Panel on Cost-Effectiveness in Health and Medicine. Recommendation of the panel on cost-effectiveness in health and medicine. *JAMA* 1996; **276**: 1253–8

15 Siegel JE, Weinstein MC, Russell LB, Gold MR. Recommendations for reporting cost-effectiveness analysis. *JAMA* 1996; **276**: 1339–41

16 Canadian Coordinating Office for Health Technology Assessment. *Guidelines for Economic Evaluation of Pharmaceuticals: Canada.* 2nd edn. Ottawa: Canadian Coordinating Office for Health Technology Assessment, 1997

17 de Koning HJ, van Ineveld BM, de Haes JCJM, van Oortmarssen GJ, Klijn JGM, van der Maas PJ. Advanced breast cancer and its prevention by screening. *Br J Cancer* 1992; **65**: 950–5

18 Salkeld G, Gerard K. Will early detection of breast cancer reduce the costs of treatment? *Aust J Public Health* 1994; **18**: 388–93

19 van Ballegooijen M, Koopmanschap MA, Tjokrowardojo AJS, van Oortmarssen GJ. Care and costs for advanced cervical cancer. *Eur J Cancer* 1992; **28A**: 1703–8

20 Bryan S, Buxton M, McKenna M, Ashton H, Scott A. Private costs associated with abdominal aortic aneurysm: the importance of travel and time costs. *J Med Screen* 1995; **2**: 62-6.

21 Bryan S, Brown J, Warren R. Mammography screening: an incremental cost-effectiveness analysis of two view versus one view procedures in London. *J Epidemiol Community Health* 1995; **49**: 70–8

22 Brown J, Bryan S, Warren R. Mammography screening: an incremental cost effectiveness analysis of double versus single reading mammograms. *BMJ* 1996; **312**: 809–12

23 Brown J, Johnston K, Gerard K, Morton A. Attending breast screening and assessment: women's costs and opinions. *Radiography* 1998; **4**: 121–4

24 Johnston K, Gerard K, Brown J. *Generalising NHS Costs from the Breast Screening Frequency and Age Trials.* HERG Discussion Paper No. 19. Uxbridge: Brunel University, 1997

25 Torgerson DJ, Donaldson C, Reid DM. Private versus social opportunity cost of time: valuing time in the demand for health care. *Health Econ* 1994; **3**: 149–55

26 Johnston K, Gerard K, Morton A, Brown J. *NHS Costs for the Breast Screening Frequency and Age Trials*. HERG Discussion Paper No. 16. Uxbridge: Brunel University, 1996

27 Marteau TM. Psychological costs of screening. *BMJ* 1989; **299**: 527

28 Marteau TM. Reducing the psychological costs. Screening in practice. *BMJ* 1990; **301**: 26–8

29 Stewart-Brown S. Screening could seriously damage you health. *BMJ* 1997; **314**; 533–4

30 MacLean U, Sinfield D, Klein S, Harden B. Women who decline breast screening. *J Epidemiol Community Health* 1984; **38**: 278–85

31 Gram IT, Slenker SE. Cancer anxiety and attitudes towards mammography among screening attenders, nonattenders and women never invited. *Am J Public Health* 1992; **82**: 249–51

32 Cains J, Shackley P. Sometime sensitive, seldom specific: a review of the economics of screening. *Health Econom* 1993; **2**: 43–53

33 Miedzybrodzka Z, Shackley P, Donaldson C, Abdalla M. Counting the benefits of screening: a pilot study of willingness to pay for cystic fibrosis screening. *J Med Screen* 1994; **1**: 82–3

34 Davis A, Bamford J, Wilson I, Ramkalawan T, Forshaw M, Wright S. A critical review of the role of neonatal hearing screening in the detection of congenital hearing impairment. *Health Technol Assess* 1997; **1**(10)

35 Zeuner D, Ades AE, Karnon J, Brown J, Dezateux C, Anionwu EN. *Antenatal and neonatal haemoglobinopathy screening in the UK: review and economic analysis*. Report prepared for the Health Technology Assessment Panel of the NHS Executive. London: NHS Executive, 1997.

36 Torrance GW. Measurement of health-state utilities for economic appraisal: a review. *J Health Econom* 1986; **5**: 1–30

37 Gerard K, Mooney G. QALY league tables: handle with care. *Health Econom* 1993; **2**: 59–64

38 Drummond MF, Torrance G, Mason J. Cost-effectiveness league tables: more harm than good? *Soc Sci Med* 1993; **37**: 33–40

39 Mason J, Drummond M, Torrance G. Some guidelines of the use of cost effective ness league tables. *BMJ* 1993; **306**: 570–2

40 Chamberlain J, Melia J, Moss S, Brown J. *Report prepared for the health technology assessment panel of the NHS executive on diagnosis, management, treatment and costs of prostate cancer in England and Wales. Br J Urol* 1997; **79** (**Suppl** 3): 1–32

41 Buxton MJ, Drummond MF, van Hout BA *et al*. Modelling in economic evaluation: an unavoidable fact of life. *Health Econom* 1997; **6**: 217–27

42 Sculpher M, Drummond M, Buxton M. The iterative use of economic evaluation as part of the process of health technology assessment. *Health Serv Res* 1997; **2**: 26–30

43 Townsend J, Buxton M. Cost effectiveness scenario analysis for a proposed trial of hormone replacement therapy. *Health Policy* 1997; **39**: 181–94

44 HM Treasury. Appraisal and evaluation in central government. Treasury guidance. London: HMSO, 1997

45 Lipscomb J, Weinstein MC, Torrance GW. Time preference. In: Gold MR, Siegel JE, Russell LB, Weinstein MC. (eds) *Cost-effectiveness in Health and Medicine*. Oxford: Oxford University Press, 1996: 214–35

46 Parsonage M, Neuberger H. Discounting health benefits. *Health Econom* 1992; **1**: 71–6

47 Cairns J. Discounting and health benefits: another perspective. *Health Econom* 1992; **1**: 76–9

48 HM Trsury. *Economic appraisal in central government: a technical guide for government departments*. London: HM Treasury, 1991

49 Department of Health. *Policy appraisal and health. A guide from the Department of Health*. London: Department of Health, 1995.

50 Koopmanschap MA, Lubbe KTN, van Oortmarssen GJ, van Agt HMA, van Ballegooijen M, Habbema JDF. Economic aspects of cervical cancer screening. *Soc Sci Med* 1990; **30**: 1081–7

51 Cuckle HS, Richardson GA, Sheldon TA, Quirke P. Cost effectiveness of antenatal screening for cystic fibrosis. *BMJ* 1995; **311**: 1460–4

52 Sprinkle RH, Hynes DM, Konrad TR. Is universal neonatal hemoglobinopathy screening cost-effective? *Arch Pediatr Adolesc Med* 1994; **118** ; 546–54

53 Hall J, Gerard K, Salkeld G, Richardson J. A cost-utility of mammography screening in Australia. *Soc Sci Med* 1992; **34**: 993–1004

54 Whynes DK, Neilson AR, Walker AR, Hardcastle JD. Faecal occult blood screening for colorectal cancer: Is it cost-effective? *Health Econom* 1998; 7: 21–9
55 Berwick DM, Weinstein MC. What do patients value? Willingness to pay for ultrasound in pregnancy. *Med Care* 1985; **23**: 881–92
56 Grimes DS. Value of a negative smear. *BMJ* 1988; **296**: 1133
57 Donaldson C, Shackley P, Abdalla M, Meidzybrodzka Z. Willingness to pay for antenatal carrier screening for cystic fibrosis. *Health Econom* 1995; **4**: 439–52
58 Vick S, Scott A. Agency in health care. Examining patients' preferences for attributes of the doctor-patient relationship. *J Health Econom* 1998; **17**: 587–605
59 Karnon J, Brown J, Zeuner D, Briggs A. *Issues in the economic evaluation of antenatal screening programmes for genetic disorders*. Uxbridge: Health Economics Research Group, Discussion Paper No. 18, 1997
60 Wald NJ, Kennard A, Hackshaw A, McGuire A. Antenatal screening for Down's syndrome. *J Med Screen* 1997; **4**: 181–246
61 Marteau TM. Psychological implications of genetic screening. *Birth Defects* 1992; **28**: 185–90
62 Fletcher J, Hicks NR, Kay JS, Boyd PA. Using decision analysis to compare policies for antenatal screening for Down's syndrome. *BMJ* 1995; **311**: 351–6

Ethical and legal issues

Ian S Markham

Department of Theology and Religious Studies, Liverpool Hope University College, Liverpool, UK

This article considers the general issues surrounding screening, in particular the problems involved in the collection and use of information derived from screening. Different forms of screening entail particular problems, which have their own ethical complexities. The legal and ethical issues arising from screening are likely to assume greater significance. The screening opportunities afforded by the Human Genome Project will provide humanity with choices that would have been inconceivable to any previous generation.

The purpose of screening is to accumulate information for the benefit of the individual tested and the population at large. Armed with this information, we should be able to prevent certain diseases or at least mitigate their effects. This at least is the theory. The ethical and legal issues mainly revolve around the collection, use, value, and cost of the information.

Both ethically and legally, the principle of the autonomy of the individual is central to medical ethics. Autonomy is the right to 'self-determination'; for adults to decide for themselves what they want to do; that I am not entitled to interfere with you unless you give me permission. It has its roots in John Stuart Mill's famous 'Harm-to-others' Principle. Mill wrote[1]: *The only purpose for which power can be rightfully exercised over any member of a civilised community against his will is to prevent harm to others. His own good, either physical or moral, is not sufficient warrant.* Even Mill conceded that this principle cannot be an absolute. Parents make decisions for their child in the belief that this is for the child's good without the child's permission. Parents are permitted to be paternalistic. However, doctors are not parents and adults are not children. Although it is tempting for the doctor to use their expertise to decide what is best, respect for an individual's autonomy should forbid this.

Information obtained in the course of screening should not be collected or recorded without the full knowledge and consent of the individual being screened. Furthermore, the information should be directly relevant to that individual, and should not be collected to benefit others, without their express permission. The expectation is that the interests of the individual should be central. The principle of autonomy means that informed consent and confidentiality are important.

Correspondence to:
Prof Ian S Markham,
Liverpool Chair of
Theology and Public Life,
Liverpool Hope University
College, Hope Park,
Liverpool L16 9JD, UK

Different types of screening programmes raise different issues which adds to their complexity. With pre-implantation screening, whose interests are central: the embryo's or those of the future parents? With prenatal screening, is the mother really in a position to give informed consent to a fairly technical procedure that provides an indication of 'risk'? These two cases concentrate on parental rights. However, as with other screening programmes, society clearly has an interest. In a world of limited resources and unlimited needs, we (collectively) have to arrive at priorities. Screening for certain medical conditions can be extremely expensive, and may not obviously represent the best use of resources, even if it does detect certain difficulties at an earlier, and potentially more treatable, stage. Consider the following dilemma: we may have a very effective treatment for a very rare condition which can be identified through screening. We also have a less effective treatment for a relatively common condition that can be identified through screening. Which screening programme ought to get priority? Policy makers have tended to determine priorities by taking the utilitarian principle of 'the greatest good for the greatest number'. This means that programmes that benefit more people tend to be preferred over programmes that benefit smaller numbers. This is linked to the principle of equity: limited resources should be distributed in ways that are fair and benefit the majority, not small minorities.

At the heart of the screening debate lies the ethics of information. It is tempting to imagine that all information is helpful and, therefore, 'ethically' neutral; it is, one might imagine, the action taken on the basis of the information that involves ethical reflection. In fact information is much more ambiguous. First, descriptions of the information generated by screening are difficult to describe accurately. For chronic conditions or ones that have very different levels of severity between different affected individuals (such as cystic fibrosis and sickle cell disease), it can be very difficult to present a single 'truth' about a condition for which screening is offered. At present, we do not understand what contributes to variability and so, at an individual level, we cannot predict the likely level of severity. So parents have to be given an average picture with some concept of the worse and best scenarios. In a screening programme, it is important that information is given consistently by different personnel by arriving at a consistent 'truth': it can be difficult for the clinicians as they will vary in the emphasis they give to some aspects of day to day life for families of affected children. Second, many of us may not want to know that there is a high probability of developing an incurable disease in 20 years' time. Not only would we have to become highly skilled in understanding the 'probability theory' involved, but it may, almost certainly, affect our quality of life now. We might find ourselves pre-occupied and miserable, even though welcoming the chance to plan in accordance with our probable plight.

So, in the screening debate, we are examining the ethics of information. The ethical and legal contours of this debate can be grouped under four headings: (i) provision of information; (ii) the value of the information; (iii) handling the information; and (iv) the costs of screening. Each of these will be discussed in turn.

Provision of information

The instincts of the law in most western countries are to require that individuals should provide information, where possible, on a voluntary basis. Although a government may encourage screening (for example, for cervical cancer), it is unlikely to make it compulsory. The autonomy of the individual gives her the right to decline such tests.

As has been already stressed, both ethically and legally, individual autonomy is considered important. Responsible health authorities make informed consent central. Legally, informed consent, explains Ian Kennedy[2], has 'three discrete and equally important aspects: first, consent is only valid if the person giving it is competent to do so; second, the person giving consent must be properly informed; and third, the consent must be given voluntarily'. This is not simply a matter of signing a form, but an individual must be aware of the complexity of the decision. Good practice, however, is time consuming. For example, when amniocentesis is recommended following a positive serological screening test for Down syndrome, parents should be provided with a clear statement of the risks involved. For a woman aged 35 years, the 1 in 300 risk of pregnancy loss due to miscarriage needs to be interpreted in the context of her risk of 1 in 192 of carrying a fetus with Down syndrome.

However, there is some evidence that social pressure can undermine the principle of informed and voluntary consent. Callahan writes[3]: *When prenatal diagnosis was being introduced in the late 1960s, every assurance was given that no woman would be forced to have such a diagnosis, much less be forced into an abortion if the diagnosis turned up a terrible genetic defect. The great anxiety focused on government coercion of those who would be judged unfit mothers. The worry about direct coercion was misplaced, but that did not mean influence was absent. Not at all. Social pressure and developing mores on prenatal diagnosis soon turned into a routine 'medically indicated' procedure, as common and standard for women over the age of 35 as taking blood pressure. It takes a tough and determined woman these days to exercise the 'free choice' of not choosing prenatal diagnosis, and a still tougher and more determined woman not to have an abortion if a serious defect is discovered in her fetus after that diagnosis. Here, as elsewhere, social pressure can accomplish quite nicely and smoothly what could never be legislated directly.* It is clearly inappropriate for a woman to be compelled to undergo an abortion and the need to ensure that good practice triumphs is important.

In some cases the subject of the test is not capable of giving consent. This is seen most clearly in the debate over pre-implantation screening. In this situation, the law regulates the screening closely. In the UK, alteration of the embryo's genes is illegal and clinics are forbidden by the government-appointed authority to screen for the sex of the child. For some this is insufficient. Roman Catholics, for example, believe that human life begins at conception and, therefore, all such screening is wholly illegitimate. Of course, the Roman Catholic view of human life also prohibits many of the infertility treatments that require this screening; for example, they are opposed to *in vitro* fertilisation.

In other areas there are pressures for mandatory screening. One area, which has attracted a lot of interest, is the call by some for mandatory HIV antibody testing[4]. The current position is that one can only test for HIV after counselling and consent. Some have been attracted to the idea that hospital patients and prisoners should be routinely tested. However, the dangers are considerable. Along with the temptations to deny certain forms of treatment (in hospital) or to segregate in an inhumane way (in prison), it is not obvious in these situations that the information gleaned would significantly assist care. Therefore, for most legislators, the drawbacks of such screening are sufficient to outweigh any potential benefit.

One compromise between completely voluntary screening and mandatory screening is to opt for mandatory offering. The recent report from the Royal College of Paediatrics and Child Health[5], which tackled the problem of maternal-to-child transmission of HIV infection, was that, for mothers considered high risk, it should be 'obligatory on those providing care to offer and recommend HIV testing'. As some 300 infants are born to HIV infected mothers each year in the UK, and the chances of transmission are significantly reduced by certain treatments and the avoidance of breastfeeding, the advantages of screening are almost overwhelming. One potential danger of mandatory offering is that the offering appears to the mother to be compulsion. Yet, given the human tragedy of transmission from mother to child, 'mandatory offering' seems a sensible way of recognising the principle of 'consent' yet maximising the chances of identifying HIV infected women.

An additional complication of screening is that in many cases the process leads to diagnostic procedures that carry certain risks. For amniocentesis, major centres have a loss rate of 1 in 300, although this is improving all the time as techniques improve[6]. Although this is a small risk, it is a factor that needs to be taken into account in relation to the benefits to the individual derived from the programme.

Finally, under this heading, there is a gender and race dimension to consider. Given their greater role in the childrearing process, women are often the ones who are expected to make the decisions about antenatal screening. Given that often this involves the careful evaluation of 'risk', this is not easy. As Murray and Botkin observe[7]: *In carrier screening programmes especially, though potentially also in presymptomatic screening, women typically bear a disproportionate burden. They often are tested first, with men tested later if at all; when decisions are made whether to continue a pregnancy, women must bear the direct consequences, whatever choice is made.*

The race dimension emerges particularly when screening for certain conditions is targeted at particular ethnic groups at high risk of these disorders. With carrier screening, especially, race is central. Cystic fibrosis is found mainly among Northern European whites, sickle-cell anaemia occurs among Africans and some Asians, while Tay-Sachs disease is found almost exclusively among Ashkenazic Jewish people. Stigmatisation and, as a result, discrimination have been significant problems. Carriers of sickle cell disorders in the US have been[8] 'refused health and medical insurance, and difficulties in securing or retaining employment and in interactions with adoption agencies have been reported'. The US has made such discrimination illegal. Successful screening programmes today work hard to carry the support of the communities most affected.

The value of the information

Our information-orientated age tends to work on the assumption that all information is useful. However, when it comes to screening, it is not always the case. It has already been noted how, if it were to be introduced, mandatory HIV antibody testing for hospital patients and prisoners might generate information which is of limited value. Generally, the important question is whether this screening is in the interests of the individuals being screened, for whom the outcome of screening varies. Screening for prostate cancer provides a good example. At first sight this seems a wholly legitimate area for screening: our ageing population has led to a significant increase in mortality from this cancer. We have a fairly reliable means of screening, namely the measurement of serum levels of prostate specific antigen. However, there is a significant ethical difficulty. The fact is that autopsy studies show that many men die **with** prostate cancer but not **from** prostate cancer. The danger is obvious. A screening programme might well identify slowly developing prostate cancer, which will not be responsible for the person's death. This, coupled with the fact that radical treatment can be highly invasive and have unpleasant side effects (*e.g.* incontinence and impotence) makes one question the value of the information because it may not be in the best interests of the individual who has been screened.

Handling the information

Undoubtedly this is the most contentious ethical and legal area. The first difficulty is that the information generated by screening is rarely 100% reliable. Indeed, Russell has argued that the entire debate is surrounded by 'pseudo-truths'. She writes[9]: *The straightforward recommendations about screening tests and the information that usually accompanies them are pseudo-truths. They convey rules of thumb developed by experts and leave out the complexities and trade-offs, the mixture of solid information and educated guesses, that have gone into their development.* Russell provides the example of the cervical cancer smear and argues that the health services propagate the illusion that screening can lead to a longer life through early detection and treatment. There is, however, a possibility of a wrong result. The cancer might be missed: abnormal cells might be present in the cervix, but may not be included in the scraping of the cervical tissue; or the abnormality may be missed by the technician responsible for examining the thousands of cells on the slide. To those who believe that these dangers can be mitigated by regular testing, another danger arises, that of borderline or false positive due to a non-cancerous inflammation or injury to the cervix. The odds of a such false positive result will increase with the number of tests the woman has over her lifetime. To reduce the proportion of false positives in a screening pro-gramme, all positive smears may be either repeated, or confirmed by procedures such as colposcopy, with attendant risks to the woman. Never-theless, with almost all forms of screening, there is a risk of misdiagnosis.

This leads to a second consideration. Legally and ethically, education and information giving are essential components of most screening programmes. Those being screened need to be made aware of the limitations of a screening test and, in addition, need to understand the expressions used to convey risk. For example, if a husband and wife discover they both carry a gene for an autosomal recessive disorder, it would be important for them to realise that they have a one-in-four chance of giving birth to a child with that disorder **with each pregnancy**. Even following diagnostic amniocentesis, there remains a small chance that a normal pregnancy may be terminated or that parents will proceed with an apparently normal pregnancy, only to deliver an affected child.

Counselling is important because the information that is provided as a consequence of screening can be very distressing. As the genetic basis for many conditions becomes increasingly understood, it is now possible to screen for diseases that are incurable. Consider for example a fetus that is found to carry the gene for Huntington's disease, a progressive neurological condition manifesting in early adult life. This is a disease that cannot be prevented, treated, or cured; the potential for distress is considerable. In addition, the status of the fetus is now, after the test, ambiguous. Prior to screening, the fetus was considered healthy, but now it has a potentially fatal illness. It is inevitable that our perception of health will change as greater screening possibilities become available. We shall have to come to grips with the concept of a 'genetically ill person'.

Coupled with education, the next major issue is confidentiality. Legally this is considered essential, although in the UK a number of exceptions are recognised. These are[10]: *where the law requires disclosure, to assist in the investigation or prosecution of a serious crime, to prevent a continuing and serious threat to health of either specific identifiable persons or the public at large, where disclosure is necessary in the performance of a public or statutory duty and where it is necessary in the public interest.* However, these are viewed as exceptions, and this is for very good reasons. For, along with the person screened, there are numerous other parties who would like access to the information derived from screening. Partners might want to know about the genetic potential for reproductive purposes; employers are interested in the health of their employees; insurance companies would love to be able to levy premiums on the basis of reliable health information. The current position in the UK is that Insurers should regard genetic testing in the same way as any other medical testing, that is a test that has been carried out should be declared on proposal forms. Legally, the *Access to Medical Reports Act 1988* states that disclosure of test results should be entirely at the discretion of the individual[11].

For most screening procedures, confidentiality is guaranteed. However, ensuring confidentiality in practice is very tricky. If a person makes certain genetic discoveries about him or herself, this has implications for their immediate family. While they are at liberty to share this information with their family, doctors and others concerned with screening would need the explicit consent of the individual to release this information to family members.

Costs of screening

Thus far our discussion has concentrated on the interests of the patient. Now it is necessary to consider the legitimate interests of society as a whole. Much of the recent debate about screening in this area has evolved around the costs involved. One might expect screening to be much cheaper; after all, the advantage of prevention is that one detects the potential problem early on (perhaps even prior to its onset). Given that the task of 'curing' a person can be very expensive, then surely it is better to prevent the illness arising.

However, the truth is that screening can be very expensive. Screening by its very nature will require the medical examination of large numbers of people who do not have and never will get the disease. Russell, writing in 1994, suggests that screening all American adult women for cervical cancer would cost $6 billion a year. This means, Russell explains, that it costs $1 million for each additional year of life for each woman detected[9]. Mant and Fowler cite a UK 1985 study which reported that 40,000 smears and 200 excision biopsies were required to prevent one death from cervical cancer in Britain. Thus the cost involved per life could have been as high as £300,000[13]. Russell goes on to argue that, given the limited resources available for healthcare, it is not obvious that this is the best use of such resources.

In summary, key ethical concepts in the discussion of screening include the individual's interests and autonomy. From this, two further principles are important: informed consent (through education and counselling) and confidentiality. Strictly this means that at every stage (collection, value, use of information), the individual should be in control. Screening programmes ought to operate with the co-operation of individuals. The legal and ethical consensus strongly discourages medical paternalism. It is a fundamental right of all adults that they have control over their body's integrity. The law recognizes that, in principle, screening, examination, and diagnostic procedures are potential battery (*i.e.* the application of force) unless clear consent has been given. (In the absence of consent, then one would have to show either necessity or statutory sanction.) Building on this foundation, a social policy should emerge which is based on decisions about the balance of benefit and harm relating to any specific screening programme. Generally, the criteria for a screening programme are as follows: it must be in the interests of all individuals screened; it should be targeted at a particular problem; it should yield an accurate result, preferably a clear pass/fail one; an effective treatment should be available; and it should be cost-effective.

Screening and the future

The science of screening is moving on rapidly. An important task is to identify the priority conditions and the rationale for screening. Governments remain committed to the principle that prevention is better than cure. Given this, the research and medical industry now revolving around screening is considerable.

Anticipating future trends and analysing them from an ethical and legal perspective is always tricky. Yet I shall conclude this article by reflecting on two contradictory trends: one, driven by resources, which is leading to a more focussed approach to screening (*i.e.* the discriminating and strict use of certain criteria by policy agencies/government committees as a basis for deciding whether to introduce, continue or discontinue screening programmes); and the other, driven by technology, which could lead to less discriminating use of screening tests with its inherent problems.

Screening and resources

There is a clear trend toward a more focussed approach in determining screening priorities, based on scientific evidence. With pressure on resources, there is a much greater sensitivity to the issue of opportunity cost. Every decision to spend limited resources on one need must involve deciding not to spend on other needs. We have already noted how our social priorities tend to be determined by the utilitarian principle of the 'greatest good for the greatest number'. This is considered fairer. Social policy will deny the minority who need a reliable screening programme that can identify a treatable disease. The cost is just too great.

Screening and the new genetics

The Human Genome Project started in 1990 and is a continuing project to map and sequence the entire human genome. Progress has been dramatic. We are already in a position to diagnose, with much greater accuracy, those who are affected by the fragile-X syndrome. Progress has been made in the battle against cancer, the Human Genome Project having enabled us to identify the genes involved in certain of its forms. Clinical trials of gene therapy are underway (*i.e.* the augmentation of the bad gene with a normal gene). In addition, it is now possible to identify those who have a susceptibility to developing diabetes, arthritis, hypertension, and heart disease. In short, over 3000 genetic disorders have been identified.

We already have a potentially lucrative source of genetic information about newborn babies. The blood specimen taken from each newborn infant to test for conditions such as phenylketonuria is an obvious source of DNA[14]. We are already in a position to screen comprehensively every newborn baby for a large number of genetic disorders. These advances in genetics have the potential to generate much wider screening programmes and the ensuing ethical and legal problems are considerable. First, the need to identify the precise meaning of the knowledge we are acquiring. As there is a complex relationship between genetic and environmental factors, our forecasts about potential illnesses can only be statistical judgements. While this is also true when screening for non-genetic conditions or for medical or surgical treatments, the factors involved in genetic analysis makes the judgement even harder. We shall be taking life and death decisions based on predictions about a future that cannot be certain.

Second, we have the issue of extent of screening in the light of the new knowledge. Should we screen *in utero* for incurable diseases that are not realised for at least 40 years? And if we do, should we disclose that information to the patient or other interested parties?

Third, there is a whole host of potential liabilities[15]. Would physicians be liable for not disclosing the availability of genetic tests to a patient? With non-genetic diagnostic tools, there is an obligation on the physician to make them available. It is almost certain that the public would be interested in taking advantage of genetic testing. However, some physicians will hesitate to permit widespread testing of this kind, while others will encourage such testing. Would physicians be liable if they declined to reveal a genetic risk to a patient? Would physicians be liable if they declined to reveal a genetic risk to the patient's family or siblings? These decisions need to be made at a societal level.

An additional problem in screening for genetic conditions is that testing may reveal that the putative father of the child is not the biological father, that is, that there is false paternity. Wertz and Fletcher[16] discuss a case of false paternity, discovered inadvertently when evaluating a child with an autosomal recessive disorder for which carrier testing is possible and accurate. When testing the relatives for genetic counselling, the doctor discovers that the mother and half the siblings are carriers, whereas the husband, who believes he is the father, is not. The consequences of disclosure could be traumatic. The husband's relationship with the child and mother could be changed dramatically for the worse; yet surely he has a 'right' to know? It is clearly very difficult to know how this information should be handled.

Fourth, there are implications for employment and education. The temptation to screen potential employees for genetic diseases to avoid the risk of employing someone susceptible to certain exposures in the workplace might be overwhelming. In addition, given that certain aptitudes, such as mathematical skills, may have a genetic base, the value of supplementing IQ tests with a genetic one may be attractive to some educationalists.

Acknowledgements

I am grateful for the assistance of Dr Mike Speed, Dr Helen O'Sullivan, Rose-Marie Newport and Fr Michael O'Dowd.

References

1 Mill JS. Three essays: On liberty, representative government, the subjection of women (original 1859, reprinted 1975). London: Oxford University Press, 1985

2 Kennedy I. Treating me right. Essays in medical law and ethics. Oxford: Clarendon Press, 1988

3 Callahan D. 'The genetic revolution'. In: Birth and Death: Science and Bioethics. Thomasma D, Kushner T. (eds) Cambridge: Cambridge University Press, 1996: 13–20

4 O'Brien M. Mandatory HIV testing policies: an ethical analysis. Bioethics 1989; **34**: 273–300

5 Intercollegiate Working Party. Reducing mother to child transmission of HIV infection in the United Kingdom. London: Royal College of Paediatrics and Child Health, 1998

6 Evans MI, Hallak M, Johnson MP. Genetic testing and screening: prenatal diagnosis. In: Reich WT. (ed) Encyclopaedia of Bioethics, 2nd edn. New York: Macmillan, 1995; 986–90

7 Murray TH, Botkin JR. Genetic testing and screening: ethical issues. In: Reich WT. (ed) Encyclopaedia of Bioethics, 2nd edn. New York: Macmillan, 1995; 1005–10

8 Laird L, Dezateux C, Anionwu EN. Neonatal screening for sickle cell disorders: what about the carrier infants? BMJ 1996; **313**: 407–11

9 Russell L. Educated guesses. Making policy about medical screening tests. California: University of California Press, 1994

10 Haigh R, Harris D. AIDS: a Guide to the Law, 2nd edn. London: Routledge, 1995

11 Mason JK, McCall Smith RAA. Law and Medical Ethics. London: Butterworth, 1994

12 Mant D, Fowler G. Mass screening: theory and ethics. BMJ 1990; **300**: 916–8

13 Seashore MR, Walsh-Vockley C. Introduction: new technologies for genetic and newborn screening. Yale J Biol Med 1991; **64**: 3–7

14 Schwartz R. Genetic knowledge: some legal and ethical questions. In: Birth and Death: Science and Bioethics. Thomasma D, Kushner T (eds) Cambridge: Cambridge University Press, 1966; 21–33

15 Wertz DC, Fletcher JC. Privacy and disclosure in medical genetics examined in an ethics of care. Bioethics 1991; **5**: 212–32

Index

NEXT ISSUE   BRITISH MEDICAL BULLETIN   Volume 55 Number 1 1999

Impact of genomics on healthcare

Scientific Editors

George Poste, John Bell, Kay Davies, Peter Goodfellow, Nick Hastie